Global Mental Health Trials

Global Mental Health Trials

Edited by

Graham Thornicroft

Vikram Patel

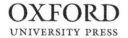

OXFORD
UNIVERSITY PRESS

OXFORD
UNIVERSITY PRESS

Great Clarendon Street, Oxford, OX2 6DP,
United Kingdom

Oxford University Press is a department of the University of Oxford.
It furthers the University's objective of excellence in research, scholarship,
and education by publishing worldwide. Oxford is a registered trade mark of
Oxford University Press in the UK and in certain other countries

Published in the United States of America by Oxford University Press
198 Madison Avenue, New York, NY 10016, United States of America

British Library Cataloguing in Publication Data
Data available

Library of Congress Control Number: 2014930060

ISBN 978–0–19–968046–7

Printed in Great Britain by
Clays Ltd, St Ives plc

Contents

Contributors

Daisy Acosta
Department of Internal Medicine,
Universidad Nacional Pedro
Henríquez Ureña,
Santo Domingo, Dominican Republic;
Former Chairperson,
Alzheimer's Disease International,
Santo Domingo, Dominican Republic

Nancy Amador
Ramón de la Fuente National Institute
of Psychiatry,
Mexico City, Mexico;
François-Xavier Bagnoud Center
for Health and Human Rights,
Harvard University,
Boston, MA, USA

Judith Bass
Applied Mental Health Research Group,
Department of Mental Health,
Johns Hopkins University Bloomberg
School of Public Health,
Baltimore, MD, USA

William Beardslee
Harvard Medical School and Boston
Children's Hospital,
Boston, MA, USA

Theresa S. Betancourt
Department of Global Health
and Population,
Harvard School of Public Health,
Boston, MA, USA

Justin I. Bizimana
Rwinkwavu District Hospital,
Ministry of Health,
Rwinkwavu, Rwanda

Paul Bolton
Applied Mental Health Research Group,
Department of International Health,
Johns Hopkins University Bloomberg
School of Public Health,
Baltimore, MD, USA

Sudipto Chatterjee
Sangath,
Goa, India

Cheryl Cherpitel
Alcohol Research Group,
Emeryville, CA, USA

Neerja Chowdhary
Consultant Psychiatrist,
Mumbai, India
(prior affiliation: Sangath,
Goa, India, and London School
of Hygiene and Tropical
Medicine,
London, UK)

Alex Cohen
Centre for Global Mental Health,
London School of Hygiene
and Tropical Medicine,
London, UK

Hamid Dabholkar
Parivartan,
Satara, India

Mary J. De Silva
Centre for Global Mental Health,
London School of Hygiene
and Tropical Medicine,
London, UK

Amit Dias
Assistant Professor,
Department of Preventive Medicine,
Goa Medical College;
Chairperson, Sangath, Secretary,
Dementia Society of Goa;
Coordinator, 10/66 Dementia
Research Group,
Goa, India

Lara Fairall
Knowledge Translation Unit,
University of Cape Town,
Cape Town, South Africa

Buddhika Fernando
Institute for Research
and Development,
Colombo, Sri Lanka

Katrina Hann
François-Xavier Bagnoud Center
for Health and Human Rights,
Harvard University,
Boston, MA, USA

Viviana E. Horigian
Department of Public Health Sciences,
Miller School of Medicine,
University of Miami,
Miami, FL, USA

Sujit John
Schizophrenia Research Foundation
(SCARF),
Chennai, India

Joop T.V.M. de Jong
Amsterdam Institute for Social Science
Research,
University of Amsterdam,
Amsterdam, The Netherlands;
Boston University School
of Medicine,
Boston, MA, USA;
Rhodes University,
Grahamstown, South Africa

Mark J.D. Jordans
Research & Development,
HealthNet TPO,
Amsterdam, The Netherlands;
Centre for Global Mental Health,
King's College London,
London, UK

A.T. Jotheeswaran
Assistant Professor,
Indian Institute of Public Health,
Public Health Foundation of India,
India

Fredrick Kanyanganzi
Partners In Health/Inshuti Mu Buzima,
Rwinkwavu, Rwanda

Catherine Kirk
François-Xavier Bagnoud Center
for Health and Human Rights,
Harvard University,
Boston, MA, USA

Mirja Koschorke
Center for Health and Human Rights,
Institute of Psychiatry,
King's College London,
London, UK

Shuba Kumar
Social Scientist, Samarth, Chennai,
Tamil Nadu State, India

Ralph N. Martins
Foundation Professor,
Ageing and Alzheimer's Disease,
Centre of Excellence for Alzheimer's
Disease Research and Care,
Edith Cowan University,
Perth, Australia

Paul McCrone
Centre for the Economics of Mental
and Physical Health,
Institute of Psychiatry,
King's College London,
London, UK

David McDaid
London School of Economics
and Political Science,
London, UK

María Elena Medina-Mora
Ramón de la Fuente National
Institute of Psychiatry,
Mexico City, Mexico

Iris Mosweu
Centre for the Economics of Mental
and Physical Health,
Institute of Psychiatry,
King's College London,
London, UK

Dilip Motghare
Professor and Head,
Department of Preventive Medicine,
Goa Medical College,
Goa, India

Morris Munyana
Partners In Health/Inshuti Mu Buzima,
Rwinkwavu, Rwanda

Christine Mushashi
Partners In Health/Inshuti Mu Buzima,
Rwinkwavu, Rwanda

Abhijit Nadkarni
Centre for Global Mental Health,
London School of Hygiene
and Tropical Medicine,
London, UK
Sangath,
Goa, India

Smita Naik
Sangath,
Goa, India

Rodrigo Marín Navarrete
Clinical Trial Unit on Addiction
and Mental Health,
Ramón de la Fuente National Institute
of Psychiatry,
Mexico City, Mexico

Sairat Noknoy
Department of Social Medicine,
Chonburi Hospital and Medical
Education Center,
Chonburi, Thailand

R. Padmavati
Schizophrenia Research Foundation
(SCARF),
Chennai, India

Vikram Patel
Centre for Global Mental Health,
London School of Hygiene
and Tropical Medicine,
London, UK;
Public Health Foundation of India,
Sangath, India

Melissa Pearson
Research Project Manager,
University of Edinburgh and South
Asian Clinical Toxicology Research
Collaboration,
Edinburgh, UK

Atif Rahman
University of Liverpool,
Liverpool, UK

Tania Real
Ramón de la Fuente National Institute
of Psychiatry,
Mexico City, Mexico

Jacob Roy
Chairperson,
Alzheimer's Disease International,
London, UK

Athula Sumathipala
Professor of Psychiatry,
Research Institute for Primary Care
and Health Services,
School for Primary Care Research,
Faculty of Health,
Keele University,
Staffordshire, UK

Dessy Susanty
HealthNet TPO South Sudan,
Wau, South Sudan;
previously Church World Service
Indonesia,
Jakarta, Indonesia

Rangaswamy Thara
Schizophrenia Research Foundation
(SCARF),
Chennai, India

Graham Thornicroft
Professor of Community Psychiatry,
Centre for Global Mental Health,
Institute of Psychiatry,
King's College London,
London, UK

Wietse A. Tol
Department of Mental Health,
Johns Hopkins Bloomberg School
of Public Health,
Baltimore, MD, USA;
Research & Development,
HealthNet TPO,
Amsterdam, The Netherlands;
Peter C. Alderman Foundation,
Bedford, NY, USA

Román Pérez Velasco
Health Intervention and Technology
Assessment Program,
Department of Health,
Ministry of Public Health,
Muang, Nonthaburi, Thailand

Helena Verdeli
Teachers College, Columbia University,
New York, USA

Lakshmi Vijayakumar
Founder Trustee,
SNEHA,
Head of Department of Psychiatry,
Voluntary Health Services,
Adyar, Chennai, India;
Honorary Associate Professor,
University of Melbourne,
Melbourne, Australia;
Adjunct Professor,
Griffith University,
Brisbane, Australia

Helen Weiss
London School of Hygiene
and Tropical Medicine,
London, UK

Moses Zombo
Green Africa,
Kenema, Sierra Leone

Merrick Zwarenstein
Centre for Studies in Family
Medicine Department of Family
Medicine,
Schulich School of Medicine
and Dentistry,
Western University,
London, Ontario,
Canada

Part 1

Principles of global mental health trials

Chapter 1

The importance of trials for global mental health

Graham Thornicroft and Vikram Patel

Introduction

Global health has been defined recently as 'an area for study, research and practice that places a priority on improving health and achieving equity in health for all people worldwide' (1) or, more succinctly, as 'public health for the world' (2). Global mental health is the application of these broad principles to the specific domain of mental health (3). The mission of global mental health is to reduce suffering caused by mental disorders, guided by the twin foundations of scientific evidence of effective interventions and respect for human rights, in all countries of the world. Iniquity lies at the heart of global health, both between and within populations. The greatest iniquities, however, are those between countries. Despite the fact that over 80% of the global population live in low- and middle-income countries (LAMIC), virtually every indicator of mental health resources shows the reverse distribution: more than 80% are concentrated in high-income countries (HIC). Naturally, then, the focus of the emerging discipline of global mental health is on addressing the burden of mental disorders in the less-resourced countries of the world. This task requires an interdisciplinary approach to developing and evaluating interventions which seek to promote mental health, prevent mental disorders, and enable recovery when mental disorders occur.

A key question in designing mental health programmes is selecting interventions, and randomized controlled trials (RCTs) are the study design of choice to guide us in making the appropriate decision. RCTs have been described as the 'most scientifically rigorous method of hypothesis testing available in epidemiology' (4). Although, as discussed below, RCTs have their limitations and cannot be applied to all evaluation questions, they occupy the pole position in the hierarchy of evidence due to their unique experimental design which offers the highest degree of confidence with which one can infer the causal relationship between an intervention and a health outcome (see Table 1.1). However, as with other mental health resources, there is a great iniquity in the global distribution of RCTs of mental health interventions. As part of the 2007 Lancet series on Global Mental Health, a systematic review of all RCTs for the treatment or prevention of four priority mental disorders (depression, alcohol dependency, mental retardation, and schizophrenia) was carried out (5). Of the 11,039 trials identified, only 14% were conducted in LAMIC and only 1% (104/1521) were conducted in low-income countries (LIC) (Fig. 1.1). Two-thirds (954/1521) of all LAMIC trials were conducted in China (Fig. 1.2). Over half of all trials in LAMIC (841/1521) evaluated interventions for schizophrenia in China.

Table 1.1 Advantages of RCTs

- Controls for confounding variables
- Eliminates effects of spontaneous remission
- Eliminates regression to mean
- Eliminates placebo effect
- Independent of rater bias if blinded
- Basis for systematic reviews (see Cochrane Library, <http://www.thecochranelibrary.com/view/0/index.html>)

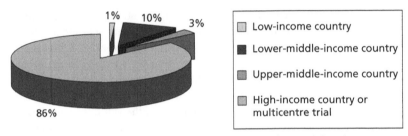

Fig. 1.1 Setting of all trials for the treatment or prevention of mental disorders.

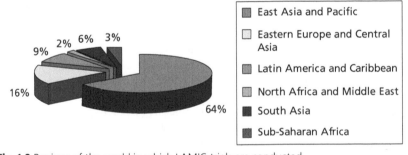

Fig. 1.2 Regions of the world in which LAMIC trials are conducted.

Why should it be important for RCTs to be carried out in LAMIC? It should be because the vast differences in how mental health conditions are conceptualized and how mental health care is organized across countries may influence the generalizability of RCT evidence on mental health interventions (6). A major goal of global mental health is to generate evidence from a wider range of contexts and address a wider range of mental health conditions. Such research would not only generate knowledge that is of practical value to local health systems but also build a truly global evidence base as the foundation of the public mental health sciences.

When to use trial study designs

The main reason for using the RCT design is that public health is likely to suffer as a result of avoiding such high-quality evidence (7). The origin of the RCT is generally attributed to Sir Austin Bradford Hill, and Bull has provided an extensive account of their historical development (8). The first well-documented RCT of medical treatment was organized by the Medical Research Council (MRC) in the UK (9). Nevertheless, similar methodologies, called 'experiments', had been used outside medicine by psychologists before this, and have therefore a much longer tradition than the clinical trial (10). Following the earlier work of Sir Ronal Fisher in 1926 on agricultural research, the contribution of Sir Bradford Hill (the prime motivator behind these MRC trials) is considered pre-eminent in making systematic the methodology for conducting RCTs (11, 12).

RCTs have well-recognized advantages and disadvantages (13, 14) (see Table 1.1). In particular the key advantage is the minimization of both known and unknown confounders by the random allocation of individuals or groups of individuals (15, 16). At the same time, there are conditions under which trials may be impossible or inadvisable to use, as Black has indicated in Table 1.2 (17).

RCTs have been applied in relation to research on mental disorders over the last 50 years. It is likely that the first controlled clinical trial was published in 1955 (18). It reported a double-blind study of reserpine versus placebo, conducted at the Maudsley Hospital in London and involving 54 patients with symptoms of anxiety and depression. The first large-scale RCT appeared some years later, in 1965. This study was a multicentre MRC study on the treatment of depression and compared the effects of electroconvulsive therapy, a tricyclic antidepressant, a monoamine oxidase inhibitor antidepressant, and placebo in hospitalized psychiatric patients (19).

More generally, some important questions, for example the impact of clinical guidelines, may only be researchable in real-world settings, and will therefore bypass the efficacy study stage (20). In relation to mental health interventions within primary care, Wells has defined effectiveness trials as those that 'duplicate as closely as possible the conditions in the target practice venues to which study results will be applied' (21).

Table 1.2 Conditions in which trials are inadvisable or impossible (19)

◆ *Trials are unnecessary*, for example when the effect is so dramatic that unknown confounding factors could be ignored, such as the treatment of diabetic coma with insulin

◆ *Trials are inappropriate*, such as when outcome is rare, for example completed suicide, or when an excessively long follow-up period is required

◆ *Trials are impossible*: for example when practitioners do not agree to participate, or where the use of any of the intended intervention arms is unethical

◆ *Trials are inadequate*: for example in cases of trials that may have a high internal validity but low external validity

---

Overall it is fair to say that the evidence that stems from RCTs is usually seen as the strongest form of evidence available to support individual/treatment-level decision-making in health care (22, 23). At present the 'hierarchy' of evidence is usually understood to consist of (in descending order of strength) (24):

1a Systematic review of RCTs

1b Individual RCT

2a Systematic review of cohort studies

2b Individual cohort study, low-quality RCT

2c Ecological studies

3a Systematic review of case-control studies

3b Individual case-control study

4   Case series, poor-quality cohort, and case-control studies

It seems to us to be true that RCTs are both beautifully simple in concept and devilishly complex in practice! With great insight Bradford Hill wrote that 'the essence of a successful controlled clinical trial lies in its minutiae—in a painstaking and sometimes very dull attention to every detail' (11). The need for such attention to detail in clinical trials is equally applicable for trials in high-, medium-, and low-resource settings.

Trials within the translational medicine continuum

The wider context of the phases of research before and after RCTs is discussed in more detail in Chapters 2 and 3. In brief, it is important to understand that trials are just one possible part of a chain of evidence that can inform practice. This sequence of steps can be seen as a whole continuum of phases along a translational medical research continuum, and Fig. 1.3 displays these as flowing from the most basic/fundamental research, addressing fundamental mechanisms of action at the left, moving through to the most applied/clinical practice domain to the right. In this schema Phase 4 can be understood as the arena that is increasingly referred to, in understanding the fundamental mechanisms of knowledge transfer into clinical practice, as 'implementation science' (25–27).

Within this phased picture of how medical and health care research can follow particular lines of enquiry, this book particularly focuses upon those forms of evidence generated by research that can have practical utility, and in particular effectiveness trials. Since the

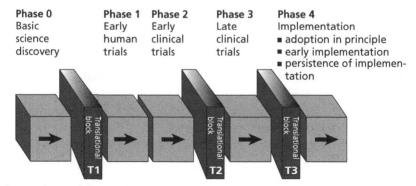

Fig. 1.3 Phases of the translational research continuum.

seminal paper by Schwartz and Lellouch, it is now common to distinguish between efficacy trials (which tend to be explanatory) at Phase 2 and effectiveness trials (sometimes otherwise called pragmatic, practical, or management trials) at Phase 3 (28, 29). This categorical distinction has its uses, although in reality we may rather see efficacy and effectiveness trials as falling along a continuum. Efficacy trials, which usually precede effectiveness studies, refer to those conducted under more ideal, experimental conditions, while effectiveness trials are RCTs carried out in more routine clinical conditions (15, 30, 31).

Criteria to use in assessing effectiveness trials

When either assessing a proposal for an effectiveness trial or evaluating the results of such a study, it may be useful to use a structured approach by considering the following criteria (see Table 1.3).

Study question/hypothesis

In planning an effectiveness trial, the first task is to ask a clear and important question, relevant to clinical practice (e.g. symptom severity) and/or to public health (e.g. burden of disability). The background to defining the study question will usually be clinical uncertainty about whether two or more interventions produce different or similar outcomes, for example in comparing pharmaceutical products. Indeed some ethicists have argued that all trials should be based upon some degree of equipoise (genuine uncertainty about which is the best treatment, or if there is no difference between treatments, i.e. non-inferiority). In this case the likely outcome is that one intervention will be shown to be better than the other.

The choice of the primary hypothesis for a trial is one of the most central decisions. This will lead to the selection of the primary outcomes measures, and to the necessary sample size, but will itself follow an a priori decision on the single most important question to investigate (32). The selection of primary and secondary outcomes can be seen along a spectrum from simple, easily collectable, and often dichotomous variables, on the one hand (such as medication change, relapsed/not relapsed, or admitted/non-admitted), to more complex outcomes (such as symptoms, quality of life, carer impact or disability) on the other. The former (larger, simpler, and more realistic trials) will allow smaller treatment effect sizes to be detected. The latter will be more costly and time-consuming and may yield a lower follow-up rate, but will produce a far greater richness of data to understand the interrelationships between key variables, and so the possible mechanisms of action of the intervention. In each trial a trade-off therefore needs to be struck between simplicity and depth in outcome selection.

Reference population

In contrast to efficacy RCTs, effectiveness trials by definition aim to establish the external validity of their results in terms of the relevance of the findings to a wider reference population of similarly affected individuals. Interestingly, effectiveness trials rarely specify, or even discuss, this wider reference group (to which the trial results are intended to be generalized) and so do not allow judgements to be made about how far the patient sample is in fact representative of the intended reference group (33).

Table 1.3 Criteria to use in assessing effectiveness trials

1 Study question

- Who defines the aim of the study?
- What process is used to identify the question addressed?
- Is the study question expressed in an answerable way (as a clear hypothesis)?
- Prior evidence of intervention effect size
- Is the answer to this question really unknown?
- Why is this question important now?
- Is there initial evidence from efficacy trials or effectiveness studies (observational or trials)?
- What is the public health importance of the policy or practice question addressed?
- What is the clinical necessity of the question?
- Sample size and statistical power for primary/secondary aims and related hypotheses

2 Reference population

- What is the reference group (or sub-group) to which the trial results should be generalized?
- What are their sociodemographic and clinical characteristics?
- What are the ethnic and cultural characteristics of the target group?
- What is the resource level in this population?
- What is the nature and standard and coverage of health and social care?
- At what time point is the population identified?

3 Patient sample

- What are their sociodemographic and clinical characteristics?
- What are the inclusion criteria?
- What is the not invited to participate rate?
- What is the non-participation rate?
- Patient preferences
- What are the exclusion criteria?
- How far does the sample reflect the target population?
- What level of heterogeneity is there?
- Selection of incident or prevalent cases (true incidence/prevalence or treated incidence/prevalence?)
- What are the rates of adherence and non-adherence to treatment as recommended?

4 Study settings

- Characteristics and representativeness of professional staff
- Levels of resources available
- Research-oriented culture
- Staff morale and sustainability of intervention
- Incentives for research collaboration
- Opportunities for data linkage
- Centre/professional non-participation

5 Study intervention

- Is intervention acceptable?
- Total time needed to deliver intervention
- Frequency of interventions
- Simplicity/complexity of the intervention
- Single/multicomponent intervention
- Is intervention manualized?
- Do usual professional staff deliver the intervention during the study?
- Can the treatment process be measured (fidelity)?
- Degree of fit/feasibility for current practice
- Exit strategy–who pays after the end of study?

6 Control condition

- Treatment as usual or specific control
- Acceptability to patients of control condition
- Cost and feasibility of control condition
- Variation between control condition within and between sites (fidelity)
- Are the key characteristics of the control condition well described?

7 Bias

- Does contamination take place?
- Degree of blinding
- Choice of primary and secondary outcomes
- Perspectives prioritized in outcome choice
- Time(s) at which outcomes measured
- Total length of follow-up and late effects
- Sources of outcome data
- Respondent burden
- Consent rate
- Recruitment rate
- Attrition/drop-out and follow-up rates

For a satisfactory understanding of the wider reference patient population, we would need, for example, to report the number of screened, randomized, and excluded patients, with reasons for exclusion, and to know (1) key clinical and sociodemographic characteristics, (2) features of the relevant health care-related services available to the reference population, (3) service coverage to population sub-groups, and (4) the wider context, such as the overall level of resources in those sites.

Patient sample

Having decided upon the wider reference patient population, effectiveness trials then need to recruit patients who reflect that target group, using relatively wide inclusion and few exclusion criteria. This will usually mean far higher heterogeneity between patients in effectiveness than in efficacy studies, and this may be determined by clinically meaningful eligibility criteria, for example by explicitly including cases with co-morbid disorders. High rates of participation are also necessary; otherwise the trial will move along the continuum towards the status of an efficacy study. In addition, patient motivation may vary. Typically, in effectiveness trials it is important that the eligibility criteria be as simple as possible, so that these should be as generalizable as the intervention. Study groups other than patients may be also important for some research questions, such as the identification of effective interventions to support family members of people with schizophrenia.

Study settings

Another important aspect of effectiveness trials is that their results should be relevant not only to other patients but also to other staff and health care settings. To establish if this is the case, it will be necessary to assess key staff characteristics, including training, clinical experience, available resources, and how far the context is research-oriented. It may also be important to measure staff morale and burnout, and if the particular intervention is sustainable over time, for example whether it places high demands upon clinicians. One implication of this is that effectiveness trials will often need to be set in real-world settings where the majority of mental health care takes place, such as primary care.

Study intervention

The choice of the intervention is of central importance in effectiveness studies (28). A critical question is: can the experimental intervention, if effective, be realistically generalized? For example, is the intervention ethically and practically acceptable to patients and to clinicians? Further, is the intervention sufficiently manualized (especially for more complex treatment packages) to be taught and practiced in a similar way by routine clinical staff? If effective, is the new intervention affordable in ordinary practice, in medium- and low-resource countries and regions? Who will pay for the continuation of a successful project after the trial ends? A related question better considered at the start than at the end of a study is whether there will be a market for the new technology, and who will own its intellectual property? This may not be a straightforward issue, as in some cases mental health trials evaluate complex interventions which combine multiple components, for example for depression (34–36), post-traumatic disorders (37), or psychotic disorders (38).

Control condition

Trial protocols and reports commonly do not pay sufficient attention to the control condition. Interestingly, the results of effectiveness trials are often discussed in terms of the impact of a new treatment or intervention, while in fact any differences between the experimental and the control conditions are as much due to the latter as the former.

The choice of the control condition is often difficult to make. For example, in a trial of supported work placement, is it preferable to choose usual local rehabilitation services or a manualized and specific control intervention as the comparison? A 'treatment as usual' control condition may also need to be viewed cautiously, as it may not be fully representative of the range of settings in the intended reference population. Further, the content of the 'treatment as usual' should be consistent with the range of practices current in routine clinical sites relevant to the larger reference population. One must also ask: is the control acceptable to patients, carers, and staff? Particular ethical issues arise, especially in low-resource settings, where no care is the usual provision for most people with mental disorders, and such situations are discussed in Chapter 8.

Bias

Bias can be defined as any factor or process that tends to deviate the results or conclusions of a trial systematically away from the truth, leading to an under- or overestimate of the effect of an intervention (13, 39). In fact the twin key strengths of the RCT design are random allocation (to reduce selection bias) and blinding (to reduce information bias) (30, 40). Bias is an ever-present threat at every stage of a trial, and some types of bias are more specific to effectiveness than to efficacy trials. Blinding (also known as masking), for example, may be compromised in an effectiveness trial. Blinding (not knowing patient status in a trial) can apply to treating staff, patients, or researchers, or to any combination of these, and may therefore be termed nil, single, double, or triple blinding. However, in a comparison of community or hospital treatment, for example, it is likely that blinding of staff and patients is not feasible, and that even single blinding of researchers is difficult or impossible. For this reason blinding may be less complete in complex interventions than in simple pharmacological trials. Every effort needs to be made to preserve at least the single blindness of researchers to patient status, for example by basing them away from the clinical site.

A further source of bias in effectiveness trials is a high attrition rate (between baseline and follow-up), which may relate to the nature of the assessments (invasive or non-invasive tests), the study burden (number and duration of the measures), or to the acceptability of the experimental and control treatments (primary care participants may be less likely to engage with mental health interventions). Bias may also be increased by contamination between conditions. This means that the distinction between the two treatment or intervention packages may be diminished or even lost by blurring what staff deliver in practice. Where this risk is substantial, then a cluster randomization design needs to be considered (41).

Implications of RCT data

If 'efficacy is the potential effectiveness of a treatment', then a clear direction of travel is established in moving from efficacy to effectiveness studies of mental health interventions, and then to the implementation of the new interventions that do work. Very often adding health economic analyses, to assess cost-effectiveness for example, will considerably enhance the relevance of the results for policy makers, especially where these produce information directly relevant to the concerns of health and finance ministry staff in LAMIC. Indeed it is increasingly clear that for research grants for RCTs to offer value and a return on investment, the implementability of their interventions needs to be considered from the very beginning of a line of investigation. This approach particularly needs to address how far an intervention used in an RCT in LAMIC settings could later be used in routine practice, if it is found to show patient benefit at the trial stage, such as is being currently adopted by two large-scale research programmes in LAMIC, PRIME (<http://www.prime.uct.ac.za>), and EMERALD (<http://www.emerald-project.eu>).

A key use of RCT evidence is to develop guidelines for health care workers. The Grading of Recommendations Assessment, Development and Evaluation (GRADE) framework (42, 43) is an approach for creating clinical practice guidelines based on an explicit assessment of the evidence base. This framework, developed by an international network of methodologists with an interest for grading quality of evidence and strength of recommendations (Box 1.1), is now used by WHO in its production of clinical guidelines (44). It has been developed to produce a standardized method to review and summarize evidence to improve the transparency and replicability of this process. An example of such use relevant to global mental health is the development of the World Health Organization (WHO) Mental Health Global Action Programme (mhGAP) Intervention Guide (45–47). This was based upon over 100 systematic reviews of the literature, synthesizing RCTs in particular, but most evidence was from

---

Box 1.1 Key features of the GRADE methodology

GRADE is an approach for creating clinical practice guidelines based on an explicit assessment of the evidence base.

GRADE is not a system for performing systematic reviews and meta-analyses (it is not a systematic review tool as, for example, the RevMan software of the Cochrane Collaboration (see <http://www.cc-ims.net/revman>)).

The GRADE approach is suitable for: (1) summarizing the evidence extracted from systematic reviews and meta-analyses into 'Summary of Findings (SoF) tables'; (2) grading the quality of evidence summarized in SoF tables; (3) grading the strength of treatment recommendations.

GRADE separates the judgement on quality of evidence from strength of recommendations.

An application called GRADE Profiler (GRADEpro) has been developed to summarize the evidence and grade its quality. GRADEpro can be freely downloaded at <http://www.gradeworkinggroup.org/toolbox/index.htm>.

Additional information on the GRADE methodology and on the GRADE working group can be found at <http://www.gradeworkinggroup.org/index.htm>.

(Adapted from Barbui et al. (51).)

HIC or high-income settings, and most designs were efficacy trials, so such evidence was subjected to a dual filter: which of the HIC study results were (1) feasible and (2) ethically acceptable and appropriate in LAMIC (48)?

Thus, a key challenge in generalizing this efficacy trial evidence to the global context is that much of the evidence is generated in HIC and from specialist settings. This is, of course, in contrast to the reality that the vast majority of people with mental disorders live in LAMIC and do not have access to mental health specialists. Thus, global mental health practitioners have needed to innovate on delivering efficacious treatments using non-specialist health workers (NSHWs) in routine health care platforms, such as primary or general health care and community platforms (a strategy referred to as task-shifting or task-sharing). The past decade has witnessed a rapid growth in the number of such trials from LAMIC, some of which have been profiled in this book. A recent Cochrane review of task-sharing controlled trials (both randomized and non-randomized) for any mental health condition from any LAMIC identified 38 studies from seven LIC and 15 middle-income countries (MIC). Most interventions were for common mental disorders (16) and post-traumatic stress disorder (PTSD) (12), were performed by lay health workers (LHWs) (22 studies), and had specialists as supervisors or educators. The authors concluded that NSHWs and teachers have 'some promising benefits in improving patients' outcomes for common mental disorders (depression and anxiety), perinatal depression, post-traumatic stress disorder and alcohol use disorders, and patients and carer outcomes for dementia'. A key element of task-sharing is that the non-specialist health workers typically deliver interventions in a collaborative care framework, with diverse health care providers playing complementary roles and delivering multiple treatments tailored to the needs of the individual patient. Such 'packages' of care can also be evaluated through RCTs, though some may be better evaluated through other types of study designs; the evidence underpinning such 'packages of care' and their integration into routine platforms of care have been published in two series of articles in *PLoS Medicine* (49, 50).

There is an ongoing revolution in global mental health research, fuelled by the recent publication of the Grand Challenges in Mental Health (50). This initiative sought to identify the key research investments to reduce the global burden of mental disorders. The priority-setting exercise was unique in several respects: its global scope with participation of over 400 stakeholders from diverse communities and countries; the use of a multistage Delphi process; the coverage of a full range of mental, neurological, and substance use disorders; and the explicit goal to build a community of global mental health research funders. The priority challenges were aimed at improving access to care, for example, by integrating the screening and packages of services in routine primary health care and providing effective and affordable community-based care and rehabilitation (both of which are the goals of trials profiled in this book). Several government and private donors have responded to these challenges, with commitments exceeding 50 million dollars in the past couple of years. These include the National Institute of Mental Health (NIMH) funding of four 'hubs' to promote international mental health, all of which are conducting RCTs, and five stand-alone RCTs (see Fig. 1.4). Grand Challenges Canada has invested to date CAN $28,006,876 committed in 49 grants and contracts in 28 LAMIC to develop and evaluate mental health

- Healthy Options: Group psychotherapy for HIV-positive depressed perinatal women (Smith Fawzi)
- Integrated care for co-morbid depression and diabetes in India (Ali)
- The depression hypertension COACH study (Yeates)
- Integrating depression care for acute coronary syndrome patients in low-resource hospitals in China (Wu)
- COBALT: Comorbid Affective Disorders, AIDS/HIV, and Long-Term Health (Thornicroft)

Fig. 1.4 Integrating mental health into chronic disease care. Projects in LAMIC funded by the NIMH.

interventions, a number of which involve RCTs. Another call for up to CAN $6 million has recently been announced.

This flourishing of RCTs will generate a rich resource of evidence in the coming years which will need effective knowledge synthesis and exchange to facilitate uptake by the many potential users, notably governments, researchers, and mental health practitioners. Indeed, the growing momentum for research evaluating mental health interventions is complemented by an equally vigorous policy response, both at the international and national levels, for scaling up services for people with mental disorders. The *Mental Health Innovation Network* funded by Grand Challenges Canada (<http://www.mhinnovation.net>) was recently launched to perform this task, and its key product is an open-access database which provides a description of each innovation and its impact, along with images, videos, and links to further information including websites, published papers, and reports. Global mental health trial investigators are encouraged to submit their innovations and findings to the database to enhance their visibility and uptake. In addition to the efforts of countries like India and Brazil to incorporate evidence-based practices in their national efforts to scale-up services, the landmark WHO Comprehensive Mental Health Global Action Plan (2013–2020) provides a robust platform for the generation and uptake of RCT evidence (51). The Plan has four objectives, three of which are directly relevant to the subject of global mental health trials: to provide comprehensive, integrated, and responsive *mental health and social care services* in community-based settings; to implement strategies for *promotion and prevention* in mental health; and to strengthen *information systems, evidence, and research* for mental health.

Conclusion and overture to the book

In the following chapters you will find a wealth of detailed discussions about global mental health trials. In the next chapter in Part 1, Lara Fairall and colleagues discuss the question of effectiveness trials in more detail and illustrate the application of a particular way to assess effectiveness trials, the pragmatic trials and the PRagmatic Explanatory Continuum Indicator Summary (PRECIS) tool. In Chapter 3 Abhijit Nadkarni and colleagues consider the key stages in developing mental health intervention studies, using the Wellcome Trust-funded PRogram for Mental health Interventions in Under-resourced health systeMs (PREMIUM) in India as a case study. Critical issues in the design of RCTs are then dealt with in detail from a statistical point of view by Helen Weiss in Chapter 4. Just as interventions need to be tailored to particular contexts, so too the outcomes chosen for trials may need to be customized to specific settings, and this is discussed with specific examples by Paul Bolton and Judith Bass in Chapter 5. Iris Mosweu then leads a chapter to address the issues associated with how to include a cost/health economic dimension to global mental health trials. Populations in LAMIC are often exposed to humanitarian crises and there is often a need to sensitively address the needs of vulnerable populations when conducting trials, and Theresa Betancourt and colleagues illustrate these issues with examples from their own research practice. The first part of the book is drawn together with a detailed account of the important ethical issues to be considered in global mental health trials, led by Athula Sumathipala.

Part 2 of the book deals with trials seeking to address the needs of people affected by six major categories of mental disorders: depression, alcohol use disorders, dementia, stress-related mental health conditions, schizophrenia, and suicidal behaviour. In each chapter, the authors have first briefly described the global burden of these conditions and the mhGAP guidelines for their treatment and care, followed by a review of the RCT evidence for these conditions from LAMIC. The main body of each chapter then describes a specific RCT as a case study, detailing the design, major findings, and, importantly, the challenges faced, the strategies used to address these, and the key methodological lessons arising from the trial. The latter are information that are rarely available through the primary publications of trials and are a key to the objectives of this book.

In drawing together the many strands of the book, in Part 3 David McDaid has written a chapter to detail how RCT data can be used to extrapolate the findings and the implications to other settings through the use of economic modelling techniques. Finally Mary de Silva and colleagues describe the methods that can be used to evaluate scaled-up mental health interventions which require a wider array of information and data sources, for example data on quality, access/coverage, and cost/expenditure.

The good news, as captured in this book, is that global mental health trials are a rapidly growing endeavour. This book is an attempt to synthesize the knowledge gained on the design, conduct, interpretation, and utilization of evidence generated from RCTs in the global context, with the goal of serving as a resource for future generations of investigators committed to strengthening the evidence base to address the global burden of mental disorders. We trust that you will find this book informative but, more importantly, that you will find it useful to address the challenge of finding out what works to improve global mental health.

References

1 Slade M, Leese M, Ruggeri M, Kuipers E, Tansella M, Thornicroft G (2004) Does meeting needs improve quality of life? Psychother Psychosom, **73**(3):183–9.

2 Ruggeri M, Lasalvia A, Bisoffi G, Thornicroft G, Vazquez-Barquero JL, Becker T, et al. (2003) Satisfaction with mental health services among people with schizophrenia in five European sites: results from the EPSILON study. Schizophr Bull, **29**(2):229–45.

3 Patel V, Prince M (2010) Global mental health: a new global health field comes of age. JAMA, **303**(19):1976–7.

4 Gaite L, Vazquez-Barquero JL, Arrizabalaga Arrizabalaga A, Schene AH, Welcher B, Thornicroft G, et al. (2000) Quality of life in schizophrenia: development, reliability and internal consistency of the Lancashire Quality of Life Profile—European Version. EPSILON Study 8. European Psychiatric Services: Inputs Linked to Outcome Domains and Needs. Br J Psychiatry Suppl, (39):s49–54.

5 Patel V, Araya R, Chatterjee S, Chisholm D, Cohen A, de Silva M, et al. (2007) Treatment and prevention of mental disorders in low-income and middle-income countries. Lancet, **370**(9591):991–1005.

6 McCrone P, Leese M, Thornicroft G, Schene AH, Knudsen HC, Vazquez-Barquero JL, et al. (2000) Reliability of the Camberwell Assessment of Need—European Version. EPSILON Study 6. European Psychiatric Services: Inputs Linked to Outcome Domains and Needs. Br J Psychiatry Suppl, (39):s34–40.

7 Edwards SJL, Lilford RJ, Braunholz DA, Jackson JC, Hewison JC, Thornton J (1998) Ethical issues in the design and conduct of randomised controlled trials. Health Technol Assess, **2**(15):i–vi, 1–132.

8 Bull JP (1959) The historical development of clinical therapeutic trials. J Chronic Dis, **10**:218–48.

9 Medical Research Council (1948) Streptomycin treatment of pulmonary tuberculosis. A Medical Research Council investigation. BMJ, **2**:769–82.

10 Tansella M (2002) The scientific evaluation of mental health treatments: an historical perspective. Evid Based Ment Health, **5**(1):4–5.

11 Hill AB (1963) Medical ethics and controlled trials. BMJ, **1**(5337):1043–9.

12 Hill AB (1966) Reflections on controlled trial. Ann Rheum Dis, **25**(2):107–13.

13 Jadad AR (1998) Randomised controlled trials. London: BMJ Books.

14 Everitt B, Wessely S (2004) Clinical trials in psychiatry. Oxford: Oxford University Press.

15 Cochrane AL (1999) Effectiveness and efficiency: random reflections on health services. CRC Press, Boca Raton.

16 Kleijnen L, Goetzsche P, Kunz RH, Oxman AD, Chalmers I (1997) So what's so special about randomisation? In: Maynard A, Chalmers I (eds) Non-random reflections on health services research. London: BMJ Publishing, pp. 93–106.

17 Black N (1996) Why we need observational studies to evaluate the effectiveness of health care. BMJ, **312**(7040):1215–18.

18 Davies DL, Shepherd M (1955) Reserpine in the treatment of anxious and depressed patients. Lancet, **ii**:117–20.

19 Medical Research Council (1965) Clinical trial of the treatment of depressive illness. BMJ, **1**:881–6.

20 Andrews G (1999) Randomised controlled trials in psychiatry: important but poorly accepted. BMJ, **319**(7209):562–4.

21 Wells KB(1999) Treatment research at the crossroads: the scientific interface of clinical trials and effectiveness research. Am J Psychiatry, **156**(1):5–10.

22 Thornicroft G, Tansella M, Becker T, Knapp M, Leese M, Schene A, et al. (2004) The personal impact of schizophrenia in Europe. Schizophr Res, **69**(2–3):125–32.

23 Thornicroft G, Tansella M (2004) Components of a modern mental health service: a pragmatic balance of community and hospital care: overview of systematic evidence. Br J Psychiatry, **185**:283–90.

24 Howard LM, Thornicroft G, Salmon M, Appleby L (2004) Predictors of parenting outcome in women with psychotic disorders discharged from mother and baby units. Acta Psychiatr Scand, **110**(5):347–55.

25 Thornicroft G, Lempp H, Tansella M (2011) The place of implementation science in the translational medicine continuum. Psychol Med, **41**(10):2015–21.

26 Thornicroft G, Alem A, Antunes Dos Santos R, Barley E, Drake RE, Gregorio G, et al. (2010) WPA guidance on steps, obstacles and mistakes to avoid in the implementation of community mental health care. World Psychiatry, **9**(2):67–77.

27 Tansella M, Thornicroft G (2009) Implementation science: understanding the translation of evidence into practice. Br J Psychiatry, **195**(4):283–5.

28 Schwartz D, Lellouch J (1967) Explanatory and pragmatic attitudes in therapeutic trials. J Chronic Dis, **20**(20):637–48.

29 Peto R, Collins R, Gray R (1993) Large scale randomised evidence. Annal NY Acad Sci, **703**:314–40.

30 Lilienfeld AM (1982) The Fielding H. Garrison Lecture: ceteris paribus: the evolution of the clinical trial. Bull Hist Med, **56**(1):1–18.

31 Haynes B (1999) Can it work? Does it work? Is it worth it? The testing of healthcare interventions is evolving. BMJ, **319**(7211):652–3.

32 Essock SM, Drake RE, Frank RG, McGuire TG (2003) Randomized controlled trials in evidence-based mental health care: getting the right answer to the right question. Schizophr Bull, **29**(1):115–23.

33 Bauer MS, Williford WO, Dawson EE, Akiskal HS, Altshuler L, Fye C, et al. (2001) Principles of effectiveness trials and their implementation in VA Cooperative Study #430: 'Reducing the efficacy–effectiveness gap in bipolar disorder'. J Affect Disord, **67**(1–3):61–78.

34 Patel V, Weiss HA, Chowdhary N, Naik S, Pednekar S, Chatterjee S, et al. (2011) Lay health worker led intervention for depressive and anxiety disorders in India: impact on clinical and disability outcomes over 12 months. Br J Psychiatry, **199**(6):459–66.

35 Bolton P, Bass J, Betancourt T, Speelman L, Onyango G, Clougherty KF, et al. (2007) Interventions for depression symptoms among adolescent survivors of war and displacement in northern Uganda: a randomized controlled trial. JAMA, **298**(5):519–27.

36 Araya R, Rojas G, Fritsch R, Gaete J, Rojas M, Simon G, et al. (2003) Treating depression in primary care in low-income women in Santiago, Chile: a randomised controlled trial. Lancet, **361**(9362):995–1000.

37 Thornicroft G, Rose D (2005) Health services research: is there anything to learn from mental health? J Health Serv Res Policy, **10**(1):1–2.

38 Chatterjee S, Leese M, Koschorke M, McCrone P, Naik S, John S, et al. (2011) Collaborative community based care for people and their families living with schizophrenia in India: protocol for a randomised controlled trial. Trials, **12**(1):12.

39 Sackett DL (1979) Bias in analytic research. J Chronic Dis, **32**:51–63.

40 Maynard A, Chalmers I (1997) Non-random reflections on health services research. London: BMJ Publishing.

41 Medical Research Council (2002) Cluster randomised trials: methodological and ethical considerations. London: Medical Research Council.

42 Oxman AD, Lavis JN, Fretheim A (2007) Use of evidence in WHO recommendations. World Hosp Health Serv, **43**(2):14–20.

43 Guyatt GH, Oxman AD, Vist GE, Kunz R, Falck-Ytter Y, Alonso-Coello P, et al. (2008) GRADE: an emerging consensus on rating quality of evidence and strength of recommendations. BMJ, **336**(7650):924–6.

44 Hill S, Pang T (2007) Leading by example: a culture change at WHO. Lancet, **369**(9576):1842–4.

45 World Health Organization (2008) mhGAP: Mental Health Gap Action Programme: scaling up care for mental, neurological and substance use disorders. Geneva: WHO.

46 World Health Organization (2010) mhGAP intervention guide for mental, neurological and substance use disorders in non-specialized health settings: mental health Gap Action Programme (mhGAP). Geneva: WHO.

47 Dua T, Barbui C, Clark N, Fleischmann A, Poznyak V, Van OM, et al. (2011) Evidence-based guidelines for mental, neurological, and substance use disorders in low- and middle-income countries: summary of WHO recommendations. PLoS Med, **8**(11):e1001122.

48 Barbui C, Dua T, Van OM, Yasamy MT, Fleischmann A, Clark N, et al. (2010) Challenges in developing evidence-based recommendations using the GRADE approach: the case of mental, neurological, and substance use disorders. PLoS Med, **7**(8):e1000322.

49 Patel V, Thornicroft G (2009) Packages of care for mental, neurological, and substance use disorders in low- and middle-income countries: PLoS Medicine Series. PLoSMed, **6**(10):e1000160.

50 Collins PY, Patel V, Joestl SS, March D, Insel TR, Daar AS, et al. (2011) Grand challenges in global mental health. Nature, **475**(7354):27–30.

51 World Health Organization (2013) Global Mental Health Action Plan 2013–20. Geneva: WHO.

Chapter 2

The applicability of trials of complex mental health interventions

Lara Fairall, Merrick Zwarenstein, and Graham Thornicroft

Introduction

The evidence on *what* interventions are currently known to be effective in mental health was recently summarized in the 2009 *PLoS Medicine* series on packages of care for mental, neurological, and substance-use disorders in LAMIC (1–3) and the WHO mhGAP guidelines published in 2010 (3, 4). But far less is known about *how* best to deliver and scale-up these interventions in real-life settings. How to translate this evidence into practice, in ways that are culturally appropriate and sensitive, has been identified as the key research priority in global mental health (1).

This chapter discusses the potential contribution of trials to the genesis of interventions that are both effective *and* highly applicable to real-world settings. It does so by considering two frameworks for understanding the place of trials in the development of such interventions: the development–evaluation–implementation process proposed by the MRC in Britain in its 2000 and 2008 guidance on developing and evaluating complex interventions (5–7), and the PRECIS tool developed by pragmatic trialists to help researchers understand where their trial fits on the explanatory–pragmatic spectrum (8). The role of evaluation designs other than trials in the evaluation of mental health interventions during implementation and scale-up in real-world settings is discussed in Chapter 15.

MRC guidance on developing and evaluating complex interventions

Overview of the guidance

At an individual clinical level, care for mental health conditions is by its nature complex, involving the combination of pharmacological and psychological treatments, targeting carers and family members as well as the person affected by the disorder, and requiring a fairly high level of tailoring. This is before the complexity of the health system is considered, with its complex interactions between a cast of providers, and variable access to, and in, quality of care.

The MRC in Britain has provided a framework for developing and evaluating complex interventions, first published in 2000 (5) and revised in 2008 (6, 7), which has become the go-to resource for researchers embarking on such a journey.

There are many recommendations in the 2008 guidance that resonate strongly with researchers from the global mental health community, including:

1 the attention paid to the documentation and role of *context* in facilitating or ameliorating the effectiveness of an intervention;

2 the involvement of *end-users* in the design of the intervention and evaluation;

3 the requirement to *carefully describe the intervention*, so that those reading the evaluation may understand exactly what was evaluated, and help those who wish to reproduce the intervention elsewhere; and

4 the importance of *process evaluation* to elucidate the mechanisms by which the intervention produced the observed effects and to contribute to the understanding of how an intervention works, or doesn't, and how it could be optimized in future.

The guidance urges researchers to carefully consider randomization in their evaluations, as 'the conditions under which non-randomized designs can provide reliable estimates of effect are very limited'. It provides a list of alternatives to the conventional individually randomized parallel group trial, including cluster trials and stepped-wedge designs. These designs are described in more detail in Chapter 4.

Two frameworks for understanding the translational continuum

The earlier version of the MRC guidance proposed a framework for understanding the sequence of evaluation activities during the process of developing a complex health intervention, drawing on the phases used during clinical drug development (Fig. 2.1).

This early framework suggested a sequential process of moving through phases from conception and initial design, through an exploratory trial, to long-term monitoring alongside implementation, and in so doing proposed what could be viewed as a 'translational continuum'. The 2000 framework was subsequently revised following criticism that it drew too heavily on the clinical drug development model, implied that the development process was linear, and did not adequately address the importance of context in the evaluation of complex interventions.

The replacement framework (Fig. 2.2) clearly highlights the iterative nature typical of processes to develop complex interventions. The accompanying guidance recommends that researchers adopt a systematic approach to developing interventions, committing substantial effort to preparatory work in the design and piloting of the intervention before launching a definitive evaluation.

Phase II in this schema can be helpfully disaggregated further. The 'exploratory trial' phase may in fact include a pilot sub-phase before the exploratory trial per se. The pilot may serve a series of important functions including:

1 testing whether the invention is in fact feasible to delivery in the exploratory trial;

2 assessing how far the intervention, if later shown to be effective, is practicable for future routine clinical use;

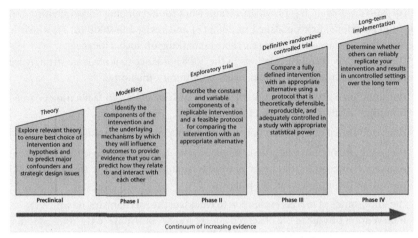

Fig. 2.1 Framework for design and evaluation of complex interventions to improve health (5). (Reproduced from *British Medical Journal*, Campbell M, Fitzpatrick R, Haines A, Kinmonth AL, Sandercock P, Spiegelhalter D, et al., 16;321(7262):694–6, 2000, with permission from BMJ Publishing Group Ltd).

3 assessing whether the intervention is acceptable to staff and to patients, for example in terms of local ethical and cultural norms, and also in terms of the time and effort needed to deliver the intervention;

4 evaluating the proposed outcome scales to see whether they perform adequately in the initial pilot study, if they are able to detect change, and also whether these outcome scales are acceptable to staff and patient participants;

5 making an initial estimate of effect size that can then be used in sample size/statistical power calculations for the exploratory trial.

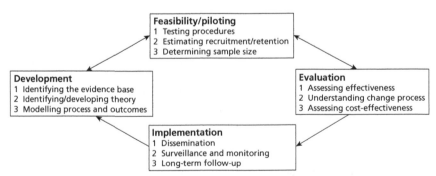

Fig. 2.2 Framework of the feasibility, development, evaluation, and implementation process (7). (Reproduced from *British Medical Journal*, Craig P, Dieppe P, Macintyre S, Michie S, Nazareth I, Petticrew M, 29;337(sep29 1):a1655–a1655, 2008, with permission from BMJ Publishing Group Ltd).

For grant applications it is common that funding is sought both for these pilot study activities and for the conduct of the subsequent exploratory trial, but it can also be clarifying to keep these two elements conceptually distinct.

Limitations of the MRC complex interventions framework

Both frameworks pose useful questions for researchers to consider in the design of their interventions and accompanying evaluations. But neither provide sufficient guidance on the trade-offs required between what is 'best practice', and most likely to yield a positive result within a trial setting, and what can be feasibly implemented in the real world. The temptation to load an intervention with everything that is known or thought to work in pursuit of a positive trial, widely cited publication, and policy change needs to be tempered by the numerous constraints encountered in the practice setting, if that intervention is to have some chance of being implemented at scale.

In reality, drug delivery is compromised by inappropriate prescribing, drug stock depletion, poor and varying ability to pay for medication, and limited patient compliance. The 'rule of halves', where only half of all people with an index condition are diagnosed, and only half of all dispensed medication is estimated to be consumed, may come from the area of hypertension research (9), but the implications for all health researchers are global. Psychological interventions typically depend on skilled practitioners and privacy for their delivery. In reality neither is readily available in real-world settings. At a systems level, insufficient provision for support of staff in peripheral facilities is usual, and referral services are often lacking. At a staff and community level, stigma may impair care-seeking or ability to comply with treatment plans.

Researchers need to carefully consider such constraints when designing their intervention, and aim to realize a trade-off between what is ideal and what is feasible, when implemented at scale. In the context of closing the treatment gap for mental health care, this likely means aiming to develop interventions of lesser quality that could be delivered to many people with mental health conditions (e.g. provision of counselling by lay health workers), rather than providing high-quality interventions to a select few (e.g. delivery of specific psychological interventions by skilled psychologists). The scale-up of antiretroviral treatment (ART) services within South Africa provides useful insights in this regard (see Box 2.1).

The 2008 framework places a great emphasis on the context of the intervention and on developing a theoretical understanding of the intervention, claiming that this is necessary to develop an intervention that is more likely to be effective compared with one with purely an empirical or pragmatic basis, and that it is helpful in determining relevant process outcomes for the evaluation. While both these claims are sensible, any theoretical framework for the intervention should be carefully interpreted within the context of existing evidence. Traditionally 'existing evidence' means knowing what has been shown to work. Equally important is being aware of what has been shown *not* to work. More so because the controlled conditions under which most trials are completed means that if an intervention doesn't work under ideal conditions it is likely not to work in real-world settings. Further effort in testing such an intervention is therefore unwarranted.

Box 2.1 Realizing trade-offs between best practice and what is feasible—the South African ART programme

South Africa is home to the largest number of people living with HIV (estimated 5.9 million) and has the world's largest ART programme (19). When the public-sector ART programme started in 2004, it was as a Rolls Royce version, strongly imitating the standard of care provided in HIC. Patients were thoroughly assessed and underwent intensive drug readiness training before starting treatment, treatment was always initiated by a doctor, and monitoring was intensive, with monthly clinical assessments and frequent (expensive) laboratory tests. Outcomes among patients who received treatment were excellent and similar to those achieved in high-income settings (20). However, the demand for treatment quickly exceeded the health system's capacity to supply it. Mortality among patients waiting to be assessed and initiated onto treatment by a doctor was unacceptably high (20, 21). Task-shifting prescribing from doctors to nurses (22, 23), relaxing adherence assessments before starting treatment, and doing away with the frequent laboratory monitoring have all followed, but so too has a gratifying reduction in mortality, especially among the country's young adults (19). Lessons learned from the scale-up of ART programmes provide a timely reminder to keep interventions simple, and to take system constraints, such as the absence of sufficient numbers of skilled health workers, into account at the design stage.

The 2008 MRC guidance provides a menu of randomized alternatives to a conventional individually randomized parallel-group trial, but little advice on what to do when randomization is either not necessary or not possible. Randomization can be viewed as unnecessary in determining treatment effects when these are dramatic, either because a high proportion of patients improve (e.g. insulin for diabetes) or because the treatment effect rapidly follows the intervention (e.g. pressure or suturing for arresting haemorrhage) (10). But examples of such dramatic treatment effects are rare generally and almost unheard of in mental health.

Randomization is frequently viewed as not possible because a decision regarding large-scale implementation has already been made, and it is considered unethical to limit access to an intervention that has some evidence of effectiveness from a trial performed under controlled conditions. In reality, large-scale implementation is rarely instantaneous, and randomization offers policy makers an equitable mechanism for determining who gets an intervention first as opposed to later, while providing further opportunity to undertake rigorous evaluation of its effects in real-world settings. But many policy makers come with firm views on who should receive the intervention first, so in practice examples of where this has been negotiated are in fact rare. Several alternatives to randomized trials for evaluating interventions in the context of large-scale implementation are described in Chapter 15.

Pragmatic trials and the PRECIS tool

Overview of pragmatic trials

A development not fully considered by the MRC framework has been the emergence of pragmatic RCTs as a methodology that sites the statistical tool of randomization in real-world settings. Pragmatic trials have arisen out of the realization that while many trialists have gone to great lengths to minimize bias and preserve internal validity, many such trials are of limited applicability (also known as generalizability or external validity) beyond the exact setting in which the intervention was tested.

Consider the case of most drug trials, which, in order to maximize the chance that the drug will be shown to be beneficial and to meet regulatory requirements, are conducted under tightly controlled and specialized conditions. Typically drug trials involve extra resources to implement the intervention 'properly'; more detailed follow-up of the recipients of the intervention to ensure full outcome information for the evaluation (which sometimes results in extra care being given to subjects in the trial as a result of this intensive follow-up that ordinary recipients of usual care would not receive); and lastly, the participants in the trial, both those who receive care and those who provide it, may be highly selected to ensure optimal delivery and uptake of the intervention: practitioners may be unusually well trained or highly skilled, patients may be selected to ensure that they are above-average in their adherence to treatment regimens, and health care facilities may be selected for the trial on the basis that they are particularly good at sticking to guidelines or extra-careful in their dealings with patients. This means that many of the standard attributes of randomized trial evaluations are distinctly non-standard and, indeed, unrealistic in the real world of usual care delivery, where the tested intervention might be later used, if it was shown to work in the trial. And this means that when applied in the real-world setting, an intervention that did well in its original trial might do much worse, as most of these differences between real world and trial settings favour a better outcome under idealized conditions—the results of widespread implementation may well be disappointing.

This question of applicability is central to those who have to choose between treatments and interventions for groups of patients (policy makers), for their own patients (clinicians), and for themselves (patients and families). These decision-makers want to know how likely it is that this intervention (apparently successful in this randomized trial) will be of benefit in their context, when administered by clinicians to patients in their organization, by them to their patients, or to them by their clinicians.

Two French statisticians, Schwartz and Lellouch, were the first to publish on the distinction between trials conducted under usual care conditions (which they termed 'pragmatic') and those conducted under idealized conditions (which they termed 'explanatory') (11, 12). They pointed out that pragmatic trials were perfectly designed to help choose between options for care in the real world, whereas explanatory trials were perfectly designed to test causal research hypotheses, for example, that an intervention causes a particular biological change.

There is a continuum rather than a dichotomy between explanatory and pragmatic trials. The pragmatic attitude favours design choices that maximize applicability of the trial's results to usual care settings, rely on unarguably important outcomes such as mortality and severe morbidity, and are tested in a wide range of participants (13).

The PRECIS tool

Recently a tool has been developed to assist trialists in understanding the continuum between pragmatic and explanatory attitudes when designing or interpreting a trial (8). The primary purpose of the tool is to help researchers assess the extent to which design decisions align with the trial's purpose, whether this be decision-making (pragmatic) or explanation (explanatory). The tool has ten dimensions based on trial design decisions. Table 2.1 shows the extreme positions of the pragmatic and explanatory continuum for these ten trial elements (14).

The PRECIS tool presents these ten trial elements as a graphical, ten-spoked 'wheel', with the explanatory end of the continuum represented by the hub and the pragmatic end of the continuum by the rim (Fig. 2.3). A highly pragmatic trial is out at the rim, whereas explanatory trials are nearer the hub. The advantage of this graph is that it quickly highlights inconsistencies in how the ten dimensions will be managed in a trial. This allows trialists to make adjustments, if possible and appropriate, to the design to obtain greater consistency with their trial's purpose.

Plotting mental health trials using the PRECIS tool

We now demonstrate how the tool works by plotting three of the trials described in the second half of this book, and use this to illustrate some of the design issues relevant to mental health researchers, and how choices may impact the pragmatic–explanatory attitude of their trial.

The trials we have summarized are described in depth in Chapters 9, 10, and 11 of this book. The COmmunity care for People with Schizophrenia in India (COPSI) trial was an individually randomized trial evaluating the effectiveness of augmenting facility-based care with community-based care, compared with facility-based care alone, for people living with schizophrenia and their caregivers (14).

The MANAS (MANashanti Sudhar Shodh, meaning 'project to promote mental health' in Konkani) trial, also undertaken in India, was a cluster trial evaluating the performance of collaborative stepped care (antidepressant medication prescribed by a doctor and a structured psychological intervention provided by a lay counsellor), compared with enhanced usual care for common mental disorders (15, 16).

Noknoy and colleagues report a cluster trial from Thailand in which they evaluated the effect of a three-session motivational enhancement therapy on alcohol consumption among hazardous drinkers, compared with the provision of written information (17).

A detailed PRECIS assessment of these three trials is provided in Table 2.2. Primary trial publications were supplemented by the information provided in the second half of the book, and by co-publications where available. This allowed a near-complete assessment of these trials. Usually, assessment is limited by incomplete reporting of trials, and in particular of the complex health interventions they evaluate. The recent Workgroup for Intervention Development and Evaluation Research (WIDER) guidelines (18) provide a useful structure for the reporting of complex health interventions, to assist those

Table 2.1 Trial elements illustrating the extremes of the pragmatic–explanatory continuum (24)

Element	Explanatory (or efficacy) trial	Pragmatic (or effectiveness or management) trial
the question	Can this Rx <u>work</u> under <u>ideal</u> circumstances?	Does this Rx <u>benefit</u> under <u>usual</u> circumstances?
participant eligibility	Strict: restricted to high-risk, highly responsive, highly compliant.	Free: everyone with the condition of interest.
experimental intervention	Inflexible, with strict instructions for every element. Both participants and practitioners are usually blind. Crossovers are prohibited.	Highly flexible, as it would be used in routine Health care. Nobody is blind. Crossovers are permitted
comparison intervention	Inflexible, with strict instructions (often employs a placebo). Both participants and practitioners are usually blind. Crossovers are prohibited.	Usual care for this condition in this setting. Nobody is blind. Crossovers are permitted.
practitioner expertise	Only practitioners and settings with previously documented high expertise	Full range of practitioners and settings in which a successful intervention would be applied.
participant compliance with interventions	Closely monitored, and may be a prerequisite for study entry. Both prophylactic strategies (to maintain) and 'rescue' strategies (to regain) high compliance are used.	Unobtrusive (or no) measurement of compliance. No special strategies to maintain or improve their compliance.
practitioner adherence to protocols	Close monitoring into how well clinicians and centers are adhering to the trial protocol and 'manual of procedures,' triggering vigorous interventions whenever deficient.	Unobtrusive (or no) measurement of practitioner adherence. No special strategies to maintain or improve their adherence.
follow-up intensity	Frequent, highly intense, with extensive data collection.	Usual intensity for this condition and setting, or restricted to administrative databases on mortality and utilization.
primary outcome	A restricted set of events, composite outcomes, or surrogate outcomes, often determined by blinded experts and adjudicators.	A broad set of events of importance to participants, determined in the routine course of health care.
primary analysis	Might try to justify excluding non-compliers or non-responders.	Never deviates from 'intention-to-treat' analysis of all participants who entered the trial.

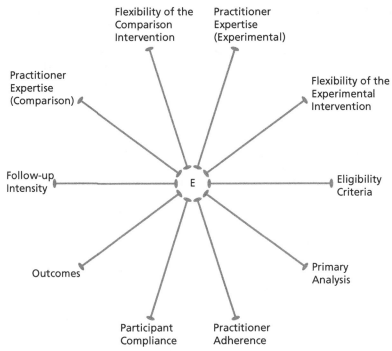

Fig. 2.3 The blank pragmatic–explanatory continuum indicator summary (PRECIS) 'wheel' (8). (Reproduced with permission from Thorpe KE, Zwarenstein M, Oxman AD, et al. A pragmatic-explanatory continuum indicator summary (PRECIS): a tool to help trial designers. J Clin Epidemiol. 2009 May; 62(5):464–75 © Elsevier inc. 2009).

who are trying to decide whether the trial's findings might be applicable to their setting, or to help those wishing to reproduce the intervention. The PRECIS wheel for each trial is depicted in Fig. 2.4.

Participant eligibility criteria

In all three trials the investigators aimed to enrol sites that were diverse and representative of usual care in their settings, in order to maximize generalizability. But in practice this proved challenging. In both the COPSI and alcohol trials, sites were purposively chosen; in the COPSI trial on the basis of being able to meet the fairly complex operational demands of the trial, and in the alcohol trial, because the investigators hoped that their enthusiastic nurses would optimize the intervention's chance of success. The MANAS trial encountered difficulties in selecting private practitioners to participate, because a large number declined or did not meet the eligibility criteria, with the result that those who did participate likely represented a group of practitioners unusually motivated to improving care for common mental disorders. While trials will always prove more attractive to practitioners and clinics who share an interest in the condition under study, generalizability can be enhanced by adopting a permissive attitude to the issue of enthusiastic and unenthusiastic health care workers.

Table 2.2 PRECIS assessment of three mental health trials

Trial	Assessment of domain
Domain: participant eligibility criteria	
COPSI	The trial was conducted in three diverse sites in India, including one that was rural and had no local access to mental health services prior to the trial. But sites were also selected based on their motivation to participate and ability to comply with the fairly complex nature of the trial. This is a moderately pragmatic approach. Eligibility criteria for individuals with schizophrenia were broad and thus pragmatic.
MANAS	This cluster trial included 12 primary care clinics and 12 general practices in India. While the primary care clinics appear fairly representative (and pragmatic), the selection of general practices eligible and willing to participate proved difficult, ultimately resulting in the selection of a group of GPs who were highly motivated and committed to improved mental health care. Thus this is a moderately pragmatic approach. Eligibility criteria for individuals with common mental disorders were broad and thus pragmatic.
Noknoy et al. (17)	The clinics were based in rural low-resourced primary care centres, but this pragmatic decision was compromised by enrolling only those with enthusiastic nursing staff, in order to optimize the intervention's chances of success. The trial enrolled patients with an AUDIT score ≥ 8 but had seven exclusion criteria, including alcohol dependence, co-morbid neurological or psychiatric disorders, and recent consumption of high amounts of alcohol per day. This is an explanatory approach.
Domain: experimental intervention flexibility	
COPSI	The intervention comprised supplementing usual facility care with a community-based intervention, co-ordinated by psychiatric social workers, and comprising an expected 22 home visits over a 1-year period, delivered by a community health worker. The intervention was closely monitored throughout the trial, and corrective efforts were made to improve compliance and fidelity. This is an explanatory approach.
MANAS	The intervention was collaborative stepped care comprising psycho-education and a structured psychological intervention provided by counsellors, and antidepressant medication prescribed by a doctor. Flexibility was permitted in that the counsellors and other staff were left to determine how the intervention was delivered. In fact uptake of the structured psychological intervention was low during the first phase of the trial (among primary care centres), leading to it being reserved for participants not responding to antidepressant therapy in the second phase of the trial (GPs). This is a pragmatic approach.
Noknoy et al. (17)	The intervention was a series of three 15-minute counselling sessions delivered by a trained nurse. Counselling sessions were not recorded or observed to assess the fidelity of the intervention, although nurses were asked to document them on structured records which could be reviewed by the research team. Nurses were also permitted to schedule the sessions according to the patient's availability. This is a moderately pragmatic approach.
Domain: experimental intervention practitioner expertise	
COPSI	The lay counsellors were trained to deliver the intervention during 6 weeks.

Table 2.2 (continued) PRECIS assessment of three mental health trials

Trial	Assessment of domain
MANAS	The lay counsellors had no health background prior to their involvement in the trial, and were trained over a period of 2 months, and received minimal supervision consistent with what would be reproducible during scale-up. This is a pragmatic approach.
Noknoy et al. (17)	The intervention was delivered by nurses trained during a single 6-hour session. This is a pragmatic approach.

Domain: comparison intervention(s)

COPSI	The comparator was facility-based care delivered by usual providers, and provided in the usual way. This is a very pragmatic approach.
MANAS	The comparator was enhanced usual care. Participants who screened positive were referred, together with their results, to the control group physicians, who were free to manage them as they saw fit. Control group physicians also received the manual prepared for the intervention clinic physicians but no training. Because these patients would not normally have been referred to a physician with the results of their assessments, this is an explanatory approach.
Noknoy et al. (17)	The comparator was the provision of written health information, developed as part of the intervention. This is a moderately explanatory approach.

Domain: comparison intervention(s) practitioner expertise

COPSI	Facility-based care was provided by the usual providers at control sites. This is a very pragmatic approach.
MANAS	The comparison intervention was provided by usual staff at the control sites. This is a very pragmatic approach.
Noknoy et al. (17)	The written health information was provided by the usual nurses at control group clinics. This is a very pragmatic approach.

Domain: follow-up intensity

COPSI	Outcomes were assessed at baseline, 6, and 12 months, and included interviews with caregivers. The frequency of assessments is typical of what would usually be offered to people with schizophrenia, but the extension of data collection to the caregiver and the extent of the data collected are more explanatory.
MANAS	Outcomes were assessed using interviews in the participants' homes at 2, 6, and 12 months. This is a moderately explanatory approach.
Noknoy et al. (17)	Follow-up comprised face-to-face interviews on three occasions, serum gamma-glutamyl transferase (GGT) at study entry and 6 months, and parallel interviews with collateral informants to corroborate the extent of alcohol consumption. These are all well beyond what would usually be available, meaning that this approach is very explanatory.

Domain: primary trial outcome

COPSI	The primary outcome was the symptoms of schizophrenia, assessed using the PANSS. This required an interview carried out by a mental health professional trained, certified, and supervised by experts, which is a very explanatory approach.

Table 2.2 (continued) PRECIS assessment of three mental health trials

Trial	Assessment of domain
MANAS	The primary outcome was the proportion of patients considered recovered from common mental disorders, assessed using the revised clinical interview schedule. This required an interview by a trained lay interviewer, which would otherwise not normally have been available, and is an explanatory approach.
Noknoy et al. (17)	The primary outcome was the volume of alcohol consumed in the previous week, measured in four ways, which would not usually be used to assess alcohol consumption.

Domain: participant compliance with 'prescribed' intervention

COPSI	Compliance with the intervention was high—intervention group participants received a mean of 18 community health worker (CHW) visits, and 90% received the predefined minimum 12 sessions. There was extensive supervision, which may have contributed to this high compliance. This is an explanatory approach.
MANAS	Compliance with the intervention was variable and typical of real-world settings, with limited uptake of the structured psychological intervention. This is a very pragmatic approach.
Noknoy et al. (17)	Compliance with the intervention was not described, and was thus assumed not to be extreme in either direction.

Domain: practitioner adherence to study protocol

COPSI	This was tightly regulated through supervision which assessed both compliance with the visit schedule and fidelity of the counselling provided. This is an explanatory approach as such supervision is unlikely to be reproducible in usual care.
MANAS	This was monitored through process indicators which captured antidepressant prescriptions and uptake of the psychological intervention, although it seems that this information was not used to 'rescue' low compliance, e.g. psychological intervention. This is a pragmatic approach.
Noknoy et al. (17)	Fidelity of the quality of the counselling was not assessed, but compliance with the counselling schedule was by research staff reviewing case report forms with nurses. This is an explanatory approach as this is unlikely to be reproducible in usual care.

Domain: analysis of primary outcome

COPSI	The primary analysis included all participants with at least one follow-up measurement, and all participants were analysed in trial arms as randomized. This is a pragmatic approach.
MANAS	The primary analysis excluded 20% of patients who were considered 'subthreshold' (those who screened positive using the General Health Questionnaire, but who were not considered to have a common mental disorder using the revised Clinical Interview Schedule). This is an explanatory approach as it restricts the effectiveness estimate to the group most likely to benefit from the intervention.
Noknoy et al. (17)	The primary analysis was conducted on all participants with outcome data, and all participants were analysed in trial arms as randomized. But 6/126 participants were excluded after randomization and the analysis adjusted for one of the baseline covariates found to be significantly different at baseline. This is an explanatory approach.

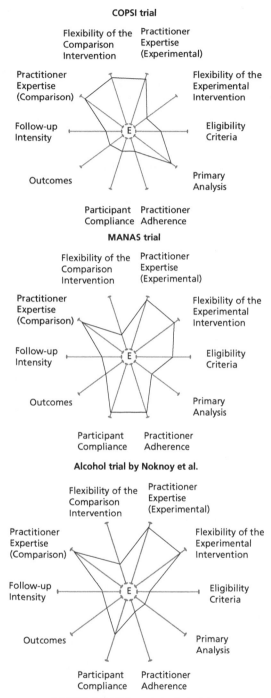

Fig. 2.4 PRECIS summary of COPSI, MANAS, and alcohol trials.

Eligibility criteria for individual participants in the COPSI and MANAS trials were broad and thus pragmatic in approach, whereas the use of extensive exclusion criteria in the alcohol trial is explanatory. In all three trials, participant exposure to the experimental or comparison interventions was dependent on research procedures used to identify those with the target condition. These procedures involved screening using a structured questionnaire containing validated screening tools (e.g. Alcohol Use Disorder Identification Test (AUDIT), revised clinical interview schedule, Positive and Negative Syndrome Scale (PANSS)) administered by trained lay workers. While this practice is typical of mental health trials, it is not typical of usual care. Researchers should be aware that this method of patient recruitment may have unintended consequences on determining the effectiveness of an intervention, by selecting patients most likely to benefit, and hence increasing the probability that the trial will show that the intervention is effective, but also simultaneously undermining its generalizability to usual care settings, as in the real world people referred for such interventions may not be so carefully assessed. A more pragmatic approach would be to allow clinicians at study sites to refer participants to the experimental or comparison intervention, and recruit participants for data collection independent of the care process. This would enhance generalizability by allowing the usual process of referral for care to be captured, but may mean that the effectiveness of the intervention is diluted by the inclusion of participants in the data collection who were not otherwise referred for the intervention by a clinician.

Experimental intervention flexibility

The trials demonstrate a range of approaches. In the COPSI trial community health workers were closely monitored and corrective action taken if they did not meet predefined quality standards. In the MANAS trial lay counsellors were free to vary the nature of the collaborative stepped-care intervention for participants.

Experimental practitioner expertise

All three trials scored towards the pragmatic end of the spectrum in this domain, primarily because of the shared focus on equipping non-specialized health workers to provide structured psychological interventions. In both the COPSI and MANAS trials, the lay health workers received between 6 and 8 weeks of training, similar to what would likely be provided in the event that these interventions were widely implemented. In the alcohol trial, usual nurses were equipped to provide the counselling during a one-off 6-hour training.

Comparison intervention

The choice of comparison intervention appeared constrained by the pronounced treatment gap in the trial settings for the conditions under study in the MANAS and alcohol trials, where control group participants could not be guaranteed even a basic level of care once identified. The accompanying ethical concern of detecting but not treating a common mental or alcohol use disorder was addressed by introducing aspects of the experimental intervention to the control group—what the MANAS investigators termed 'enhanced usual care' (see Chapter 8). This makes this aspect of these trials more explanatory.

Comparison intervention practitioner expertise

In all three trials, the comparison intervention was delivered by the staff who usually provide care in the trial settings, which is a very pragmatic approach.

Follow-up intensity

While the frequency of assessments for participants in all three trials was not excessive and could reasonably be expected to be similar to what would be offered to patients in usual care settings, the nature of these assessments was more explanatory in approach. Both the COPSI and alcohol trials included interviews with caregivers, which would normally not be offered in routine settings. The follow-up interviews in the MANAS trial occurred at the participants' homes. In all three trials, the volume of data collected was more extensive than would be typical outside of a trial setting, and included multiple instruments with which to assess participants' outcomes, economic and qualitative data, and even blood tests.

Primary trial outcome

Mental health lends itself to patient-important outcomes, which is consistent with a pragmatic approach. All three trials selected patient-important primary outcomes: symptoms of schizophrenia, recovery from common mental disorders, and volume of alcohol consumed in the last week. But adjudication of such outcomes requires specialized expertise not typically available in usual settings, making these domains more explanatory.

Participant compliance with 'prescribed' intervention

Participant compliance varied from excellent in the COPSI trial to variable in the MANAS trial. In real-world settings non-compliance is expected—the more this is permitted in a trial the more pragmatic and generalizable the results. It is important to distinguish upfront whether your intention is only to measure compliance with the intervention purely for descriptive purposes (pragmatic) or to feedback these measurements to improve compliance (explanatory).

Practitioner adherence to study protocol

The quality of psychological interventions may vary greatly in usual care, depending on the skill of the health worker responsible for delivering that intervention. Increasingly, researchers include an assessment of the fidelity of psychological interventions in trials. But in usual care settings, such assessments are rare. Researchers should be aware of the impact of what they do with the results of these assessments on the generalizability of their trial's findings. While using these assessments purely for descriptive purposes would be in keeping with a pragmatic approach, while contributing to an understanding of why the intervention did or did not work, sharing the results of these assessments with health workers for the purpose of improving their performance would shift this domain towards an explanatory approach. In the COPSI trial, intervention co-ordinators assessed the quality of several of the key home-based visits conducted by the community health workers, and provided feedback to ensure predefined quality standards were achieved. This is unlikely to be reproducible during scale-up of such an intervention and is a very explanatory approach.

Analysis of the primary outcome

The most pragmatic approach would be to include all participants; this makes no special provision for non-compliance, non-adherence, or practice variability, and analyses participants' data in the groups to which they were randomized (what was previously called an 'intention-to-treat' analysis). Example of analysis plans that would tend to make this domain more explanatory would be exclusion of participants post randomization (e.g. alcohol trial) or the restriction of the primary analysis to the sub-group of patients with the target condition (e.g. MANAS trial).

Conclusion

Most mental health interventions, and certainly all mental health programmes, qualify as complex interventions. The development and evaluation of complex health interventions presents numerous challenges to researchers, both in terms of committing adequate effort to their piloting before main-stage trial evaluation, and in the many design choices required in developing an appropriate protocol. It is important to understand how these choices align with the intention of the trial, whether this is primarily to determine causality, or to guide decision-making and applicability to settings beyond that of the trial. As yet, there is no alternative to randomization that matches its ability to control for the selection bias that occurs when those who receive an intervention differ from those who do not in ways that are likely to affect their outcomes. But the statistical method of randomization should be understood separately from the idealized and controlled conditions under which most trials are completed. Pragmatic trials favour design choices that maximize applicability of the trial's results to usual care settings, rely on unarguably important outcomes such as mortality and severe morbidity, and are tested in a wide range of participants. A mixed-methods approach, whereby trialists incorporate parallel qualitative and economic evaluations as well as provide detailed descriptions of the intervention, can further enhance applicability of such trials to real-world settings, as well as contribute to the understanding of how interventions do or do not work, so that they might be optimized and refined for future generations.

References

1 Patel V, Thornicroft G (2009) Packages of care for mental, neurological, and substance use disorders in low- and middle-income countries: PLoS Medicine Series, 6(10):e1000160.

2 Patel V, Simon G, Chowdhary N, Kaaya S, Araya R (2009) Packages of care for depression in low- and middle-income countries. PLoS Med, 6(10):e1000159.

3 World Health Organization (2013) mhGAP intervention guide for mental, neurological and substance use disorders in non-specialized health settings. <http://www.who.int/mental_health/evidence/mhGAP_intervention_guide/en/>.

4 Dua T, Barbui C, Clark N, Fleischmann A, Poznyak V, van Ommeren M, et al. (2011) Evidence-based guidelines for mental, neurological, and substance use disorders in

low- and middle-income countries: summary of WHO recommendations. PLoS Med, 8(11):e1001122.

5 Campbell M, Fitzpatrick R, Haines A, Kinmonth AL, Sandercock P, Spiegelhalter D, et al. (2000) Framework for design and evaluation of complex interventions to improve health. BMJ, 321(7262):694–6.

6 Medical Research Council (2008) Developing and evaluating complex interventions: new guidance. <http://www.mrc.ac.uk/Utilities/Documentrecord/index.htm?d=MRC004871>.

7 Craig P, Dieppe P, Macintyre S, Michie S, Nazareth I, Petticrew M (2008) Developing and evaluating complex interventions: the new Medical Research Council guidance. BMJ, 337:a1655.

8 Thorpe KE, Zwarenstein M, Oxman AD, Treweek S, Furberg CD, Altman DG, et al. (2009) A pragmatic–explanatory continuum indicator summary (PRECIS): a tool to help trial designers. J Clin Epidemiol, 62(5):464–75.

9 Scheltens T, Bots ML, Numans ME, Grobbee DE, Hoes AW (2007) Awareness, treatment and control of hypertension: the 'rule of halves' in an era of risk-based treatment of hypertension. J Hum Hypertens, 21(2):99–106.

10 Glasziou P, Chalmers I, Rawlins M, McCulloch P (2007) When are randomised trials unnecessary? Picking signal from noise. BMJ, 334(7589):349–51.

11 Schwartz D, Lellouch J (1967) Explanatory and pragmatic attitudes in therapeutical trials. J Chronic Dis, 20(8):637–48.

12 Schwartz D, Lellouch J (2009) Explanatory and pragmatic attitudes in therapeutical trials. J Clin Epidemiol, 62(5):499–505.

13 Zwarenstein M, Treweek S, Gagnier JJ, Altman DG, Tunis S, Haynes B, et al. (2008) Improving the reporting of pragmatic trials: an extension of the CONSORT statement. BMJ, 337:a2390.

14 Chatterjee S, Leese M, Koschorke M, McCrone P, Naik S, John S, et al. (2011) Collaborative community based care for people and their families living with schizophrenia in India: protocol for a randomised controlled trial. Trials, 12:12.

15 Patel VH, Kirkwood BR, Pednekar S, Araya R, King M, Chisholm D, et al. (2008) Improving the outcomes of primary care attenders with common mental disorders in developing countries: a cluster randomized controlled trial of a collaborative stepped care intervention in Goa, India. Trials, 9:4.

16 Patel V, Weiss HA, Chowdhary N, Naik S, Pednekar S, Chatterjee S, et al. (2010) Effectiveness of an intervention led by lay health counsellors for depressive and anxiety disorders in primary care in Goa, India (MANAS): a cluster randomised controlled trial. Lancet, 376(9758):2086–95.

17 Noknoy S, Rangsin R, Saengcharnchai P, Tantibhaedhyangkul U, McCambridge J (2010) RCT of effectiveness of motivational enhancement therapy delivered by nurses for hazardous drinkers in primary care units in Thailand. Alcohol Alcohol, 45(3):263–70.

18 Michie S, Fixsen D, Grimshaw JM, Eccles MP (2009) Specifying and reporting complex behaviour change interventions: the need for a scientific method. Implement Sci, 4:40.

19 Mayosi BM, Lawn JE, van Niekerk A, Bradshaw D, Abdool Karim SS, Coovadia HM, et al. (2012) Health in South Africa: changes and challenges since 2009. Lancet, 380(9858):2029–43.

20 Fairall LR, Bachmann MO, Louwagie GMC, van Vuuren C, Chikobvu P, Steyn D, et al. (2008) Effectiveness of antiretroviral treatment in a South African program: a cohort study. Arch Intern Med, 168(1):86–93.

21 Ingle SM, May M, Uebel K, Timmerman V, Kotze E, Bachmann M, et al. (2010) Outcomes in patients waiting for antiretroviral treatment in the Free State Province, South Africa: prospective linkage study. AIDS Lond Engl, 24(17):2717–25.

22 Colvin CJ, Fairall L, Lewin S, Georgeu D, Zwarenstein M, Bachmann MO, et al. (2010) Expanding access to ART in South Africa: the role of nurse-initiated treatment. South Afr Med J Suid-Afr Tydskr Vir Geneeskd, 100(4):210–12.

23 Fairall L, Bachmann MO, Lombard C, Timmerman V, Uebel K, Zwarenstein M, et al. (2012) Task shifting of antiretroviral treatment from doctors to primary-care nurses in South Africa (STRETCH): a pragmatic, parallel, cluster-randomised trial. Lancet, 380(9845):889–98.

24 Sackett DL (2011) Explanatory and pragmatic clinical trials: a primer and application to a recent asthma trial. Pol Arch Med Wewnętrznej, 121(7–8):259–63.

Chapter 3

Developing mental health interventions

Abhijit Nadkarni, Mary J. De Silva, and Vikram Patel

Introduction

In this chapter, we discuss why mental health interventions can be considered as 'complex interventions' and the need for a systematic framework for the development and evaluation of complex interventions. We describe the MRC framework, the most widely used framework for this purpose, and illustrate the steps that are followed to develop mental health interventions using the case study of PREMIUM, a research programme in India which is developing and evaluating psychological treatments for depression and alcohol use disorders (AUD). We also discuss two complementary frameworks (the Normalization Process Theory (NPT) and the Theory of Change (ToC)) which can strengthen the methodology for the development of complex interventions, enhancing the likelihood of their effectiveness and ultimate implementation.

What are complex interventions?

Complex interventions in health care are made up of a number of interconnected components, acting both independently and interdependently (1). Characteristics of interventions that make them complex include: multiple interactions between the components of the intervention; number and difficulty of behaviours required by those delivering or receiving the intervention; number of groups or organizational levels targeted by the intervention; number and variability of outcomes; and the degree of flexibility or tailoring of the intervention (1).

The Grand Challenges in Global Mental Health initiative aimed to identify research priorities that will make a substantial and immediate impact on the lives of people living with mental health problems (2). Virtually all of the leading priorities were for expanding access to evidence-based treatments for mental health problems, for example through integrating packages of care into routine primary health care, developing effective treatments for use by non-specialists, and providing effective and affordable community-based care and rehabilitation. Such interventions usually comprise biological, psychological, and social components delivered in various combinations. Each component might work independently by itself and also in combination with the other components to achieve a desired outcome. Besides fulfilling this fundamental

Table 3.1 Examples of interventions to address mental health problems

Intervention	Reason for complexity
Yuva Mitr: a multimodal community intervention programme for promoting health and wellbeing of youth in India (3)	◆ Multiple components, e.g. peer education programme, teacher training, and health information material ◆ Multiple groups or organizational levels targeted by the intervention, e.g. teachers, peers ◆ Multiple outcomes, e.g. mental health, violence
COPSI: a community-based intervention for people with chronic schizophrenia (4)	◆ Multiple components, e.g. psychiatric care and rehabilitation ◆ Multiple providers, e.g. psychiatrists, community-based workers and supervisors ◆ Multiple outcomes, e.g. adherence with drug treatment, symptoms, disability
MANAS: a lay counsellor-led intervention in primary care for people with depression and anxiety disorders (5)	◆ Multiple components, e.g. psychoeducation, interpersonal therapy, antidepressant therapy ◆ Variety of behaviours required by counsellors, e.g. liaison with primary care team, referral to specialist, engagement with supervision ◆ Number of providers, e.g. primary care doctor, counsellor, supervisor

characteristic of complex interventions, most mental health interventions also fulfil the criteria for complexity through a host of other factors which characterize complex interventions. Table 3.1 gives examples of some interventions that have been evaluated through RCTs, with reasons for why they are complex interventions.

To illustrate the point, let us look at the MANAS project, a collaborative stepped-care intervention led by lay counsellors for common mental disorders (depressive and anxiety disorders) in primary care in Goa, India (5). The effective implementation of the intervention required a collaborative approach between three key team members: the lay counsellor, the primary care physician, and a visiting psychiatrist. The locally recruited counsellors did not have health backgrounds. After a structured 2-month training course they acted as case-managers for patients with common mental disorders (CMD) and took overall responsibility for delivering all the non-drug treatments in close collaboration with the primary care physician and the psychiatrist. The intervention comprised multiple components, e.g. psychoeducation, antidepressant drug treatment, and interpersonal psychotherapy, delivered in a stepped manner (i.e. tailored to the needs of the individual patient). For example, psychoeducation was provided to all patients, while antidepressant drugs were recommended only for moderate or severe CMD. Referral to the clinical specialist was reserved for patients who were assessed as having a high suicide risk at any stage, were unresponsive to the earlier treatments, posed diagnostic dilemmas, had substantial co-morbidity, or for whom the primary care physician requested a consultation. Every facility team was supported by a psychiatrist who visited about once a month and was also available for consultation on the telephone to discuss cases.

As we can see here, the complexity of this intervention arises from a host of factors, which include: the interactions between specific components (psychoeducation, interpersonal therapy, antidepressants); the number of behaviours required by those delivering the intervention (e.g. referral to specialist, engaging with supervision) or receiving the intervention (e.g. regular attendance to treatment sessions, compliance with medications, adherence with strategies like breathing exercises); the number of providers (lay counsellors, primary care doctors, psychiatrists); and the degree of flexibility or tailoring of the intervention permitted (flexible number of sessions, intensity of intervention based on severity of symptoms, referral to specialist as per need). Similarly, as with most mental health interventions, there are multiple components dynamically interacting with each other with varying levels of complexity within the various component parts that make up the interventions.

The need for structured frameworks to design mental health interventions

The inherent complexity of mental health interventions makes their development and evaluation a complex process too. To an evaluator, complex interventions pose a number of methodological challenges which generally accompany any successful evaluation. In particular, complex interventions bring with them special challenges related to the 'difficulty of standardizing the design and delivery of the interventions, organizational and logistical difficulty of applying experimental methods to service or policy change, and the length and complexity of the causal chains linking intervention with outcome' (<http://www.mrc.ac.uk/complexinterventionsguidance>). Hence, a structured approach to the development and evaluation of complex interventions helps researchers to keep track of the research process and also ensures that the process is systematic, rigorous, and replicable. One could argue that while the development, piloting, evaluation, reporting, and implementation of a complex intervention is a lengthy process, the most important stage is the evaluation of the intervention. However, by forgoing adequate formative work necessary for the development of a complex intervention one might be dooming it for failure. As one example, consider an intervention that has been beautifully designed on paper but has very poor adherence in practice. To ensure that scarce resources are not wasted on evaluating interventions that might not work for lack of formative developmental work, one should first develop the intervention to the point where it can reasonably be expected to have a worthwhile effect, before devoting extensive time and resources on a substantial evaluation. Consequently, devotion of adequate time and resources with rigorous application of a structured framework, not just to the main evaluation but also to the development of the intervention, will result in a better designed intervention, that is easier to evaluate, more likely to be effective, and thus more likely to be worth implementing. Table 3.2 highlights some of the issues that may be covered in the formative and pilot work and possible methods of doing that.

Systematically conducted formative research prior to the definitive evaluation will also ensure that due consideration is given to the context in terms of the socioeconomic and cultural background, the health system, the nature of the problem that is being targeted, and the mechanisms by which the intervention works. Three primary

Table 3.2 Aims and methods of doing formative research

Aim of formative research	Method
Understanding the available evidence and identifying gaps that need to be addressed during intervention development	Identifying an appropriate and recent systematic review Conducting a new systematic review
Proposing a theory on how the intervention will potentially work	Identifying existing evidence through review of the literature Qualitative research involving experts in the field, intended recipients of the treatment, and potential delivery agents Treatment development workshops
Assessing acceptability and feasibility of the intervention	Qualitative research involving experts in the field, intended recipients of the treatment, and potential delivery agents n of 1 studies Case series
Fine-tuning the procedures for the evaluation	Case series Pilot RCT comparing the intervention against the control

questions are addressed in the development of an intervention, namely the feasibility (how logistically possible it is to deliver), acceptability (whether service users and providers find the intervention acceptable to receive and deliver), and scalability of the intervention (the extent to which the intervention could be delivered to a much larger population). A highly effective intervention is practically useless in the real world if it is not possible to deliver it, does not engage the target group (both the recipients and the delivery agents), and cannot improve access as it cannot be widely implemented.

Frameworks for the design and evaluation of complex interventions

The complex nature of mental health interventions leads to a host of challenges for researchers, in addition to the other routine difficulties that any successful evaluation of an intervention must overcome. These additional challenges include those related to the contextual fit of the intervention, as well as the length and complexity of the causal chains that link the intervention to the outcomes.

In 2000, the MRC published a *Framework for the Development and Evaluation of RCTs for Complex Interventions to Improve Health*, to help researchers to recognize and adopt appropriate methods to tackle such challenges (<http://www.mrc.ac.uk/Utilities/ Documentrecord/index.htm?d=MRC003372>). This framework had five phases which progressed sequentially: (1) 'preclinical' or theoretical (establish the theoretical basis that suggests that the intervention should have the effect(s) it is expected to); (2) phase I or modelling (delineating an intervention's components and how they interrelate and how active components of a complex package may relate to either surrogate or final outcomes); (3) phase II or exploratory trial (experiment with the intervention, varying different components to see what effect each has on the intervention as a whole); (4) phase III or main trial (evaluation of a complex intervention in the main RCT); and (5) phase IV or long-term surveillance (a separate study to establish the long-term and real-life effectiveness of the intervention) (6) (see Fig. 2.1 in Chapter 2).

Over the years, as this framework was increasingly implemented, its limitations became apparent. Some of these limitations included the linearity of the various phases of the model precluding iterative work, the apparent lack of evidence for many of the recommendations, the limited guidance on how to address the intervention's development and implementation phases, and the lack of attention to the social, political, or geographical context in which interventions were delivered (<http://www.mrc.ac.uk/complexinterventionsguidance>). As a consequence, an updated and extended revised version was developed and published in 2008 (7). Not only did this new framework emphasize the strengths of the original framework but it also addressed its limitations. What emerged was a considerably strengthened framework which was a more flexible and less linear model of the process, gave due weight to the development and implementation phases, and provided examples of successful approaches to the development and evaluation of a variety of complex interventions.

The main stages and the key functions and activities at each stage of the MRC framework are as follows (Fig. 3.1) (7): Development; Feasibility/piloting; Evaluation; and

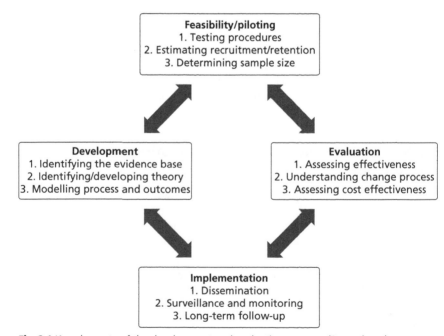

Fig. 3.1 Key elements of the development and evaluation process. (Reproduced with permission from the Medical Research Council, <http://www.mrc.ac.uk/complexinterventionsguidance>).

Box 3.1 The NPT framework

For successful implementation certain formative work needs to be done in the development phase. The NPT is a framework that allows researchers to think through such issues of implementation while designing a complex intervention and its evaluation, thus avoiding a situation where an effective intervention cannot be scaled up because of various contextual barriers. The components of the NPT are as follows:

1) Coherence (what does it mean to the participants?): in this component, the researcher tries to answer questions like 'Does the intervention have a clear purpose for all relevant participants?', 'What benefits will the intervention bring?', and 'Will the benefits be valued by potential participants?'

2) Cognitive participation (will participants commit to and engage with the intervention?): in this component, the researcher tries to answer questions like 'Will the participants see the need for the intervention?' and 'Will participants be prepared to invest time and energy in the intervention?'

3) Collective action (what will the participants have to do to make the intervention work?): in this component, the researcher tries to answer questions like 'What training will staff require to deliver the intervention?' and 'Is the intervention compatible with existing practices in the organization?'

Implementation. Each of these phases are described in more detail next, with the case study of an ongoing programme in India (PREMIUM) to illustrate the application of the first two phases. Further examples of these phases can be found in the case studies in the second part of this book. Detailed descriptions of the third phase are found in the descriptions of the trials also in the second part of the book, while examples of the final phase can be found in Chapter 16 (De Silva et al.). At the level of a large-scale implementation of an effective intervention another framework that speaks well with the MRC framework is the NPT (8), which identifies factors that affect the assimilation of complex interventions into routine practice. This in turn can inform the type of formative work that needs to be done in the pre-evaluation phases of the MRC framework (Box 3.1).

The development and feasibility/piloting phases of the MRC framework

In this section we describe the 'treatment development' and 'feasibility/piloting' phases of the revised MRC framework using the example of PREMIUM, a research project in India. PREMIUM aims to elaborate a psychological treatment development and evaluation methodology that will lead to new, culturally appropriate, feasible, acceptable, affordable, and effective psychological treatments for the target disorders of harmful drinking (HD) (in men) and Depressive Disorder in primary care. The methodology adopted in PREMIUM seeks to specifically address barriers to making psychological treatments accessible by ensuring that the treatments can be delivered by non-specialist health workers and that the treatment is culturally appropriate. The case study in this chapter focuses on the development of the treatment for HD in men.

Developing a complex intervention

This involves identifying the evidence base, identifying or developing appropriate theory (the likely process of change) by drawing on existing evidence and theory, supplemented if necessary by new primary research, and modelling process and outcomes to provide important information about the design of both the intervention and the evaluation.

Identifying the evidence base

The starting point for developing an intervention is to be fully aware of the relevant, existing evidence base. A systematic review of treatments for the target condition is a good place to begin. Sometimes one might find a recent high-quality review, but often you may need to conduct a systematic review that is specifically designed to answer questions relevant to the intervention being developed. Such a systematic review will help identify previous studies that provide empirical evidence for the same or a similar intervention as the one that is being developed and/or treatments for the same or similar disorder for which the intervention is being developed.

Identifying/developing appropriate theory

A theory is a set of assumptions, propositions, or accepted facts that attempts to provide a plausible explanation for a causal relationship between observed phenomenon, in this case, the intervention and outcomes. This implies that attention to the theory that drives an intervention is more likely to lead to an effective intervention rather than relying on a purely empirical or pragmatic approach. However, this is easier said than done in the case of complex interventions as the rationale behind how change will be achieved may not be clear at the outset. Hence, a vital task in the development stage is to develop a theoretical understanding of how the intervention will lead to the desired outcomes. This could be done by examining existing evidence and theory, and supplemented if necessary by new primary research. A ToC (see Fig. 3.2) may be very helpful at this stage in constructing a causal pathways map of how the intervention and its different components are expected to lead to the desired outcomes. Note that theory can be revised based on experiences gathered during the piloting phase and based on the results of the evaluation phase (consistent with the iterative nature of the revised MRC framework).

Modelling process and outcomes

Modelling a complex intervention prior to full evaluation helps to gain understanding of how the intervention works (for example through the independent and interactive effects of each component) and its possible effects (for example intermediate and final outcomes). Thus, modelling a complex intervention prior to a full-scale evaluation can provide important information about the various components of the intervention and their interrelationships and also helps to identify possible weaknesses in the intervention pathway which can then inform refinements in the intervention. Besides demonstrating how the intervention works, modelling helps to identify potential barriers to successful implementation of the intervention in the evaluation phase.

An example of modelling processes can be illustrated by the following example of the development of a guided self-help intervention for depression (9). Two systematic reviews were conducted and the results were synthesized with a consensus process which sought to interpret the evidence and address the ambiguities that remained. The results of the two reviews and consensus process were combined in a matrix, with each column of the matrix detailing one of the 'core components' of the intervention

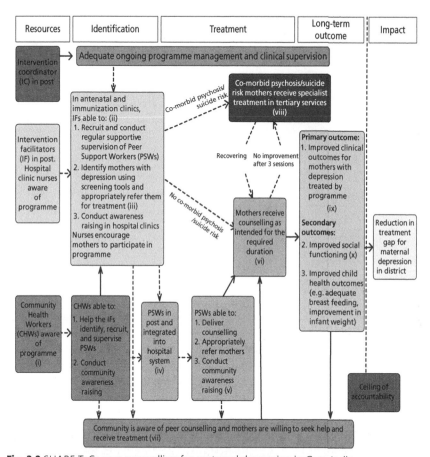

Fig. 3.2 SHARE ToC: peer counselling for maternal depression in Goa, India.

(1) Kakuma R, Minas H, van Ginneken N, Dal Poz MR, Desiraju K, Morris JE, et al. (2011) Human resources for mental health care: current situation and strategies for action. Lancet, **378**(9803):1654–63.

(2) Rahman A, Malik A, Sikander S, Roberts C, Creed F (2008) Cognitive behaviour therapy-based intervention by community health workers for mothers with depression and their infants in rural Pakistan: a cluster-randomised controlled trial. Lancet, **372**(9642):902–9.

(3) Yang L, Lo G, et al. (2012) Effects of labeling and interpersonal contact upon attitudes towards schizophrenia: implications for reducing mental illness stigma in urban China. Soc Psychiatry Psychiatr Epidemiol, **47**(9):1459–73.

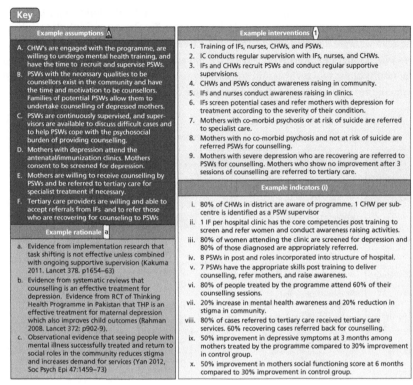

Fig. 3.2 (continued) SHARE ToC: peer counselling for maternal depression in Goa, India.

that the researchers wished to address, and the rows referring to the results from each of the three data sets (the two reviews and consensus process). This matrix was used as the platform for a discussion within the trial team to derive the final intervention to test. The ToC (described in the section 'The ToC approach for intervention development and evaluation') is also a useful framework to test the proposed causal pathways through modelling (see Box 3.2).

Box 3.2 What was done in PREMIUM?

Identifying the evidence base

Step 1

Objectives: To review the global evidence on effective psychological treatments for AUD to update the systematic reviews that formed the basis of the WHO mhGAP (2010) treatment recommendations.

Methods: Systematic review of published literature.

Summary results: Motivational Interviewing (MI) or Motivational Enhancement Therapy (MET) were the most commonly utilized psychological treatments for

Box 3.2 What was done in PREMIUM? (continued)

AUD. Some other effective treatment strategies that were identified included psychoeducation, cognitive behavioural techniques, social skills training, problem-solving, and maintenance of social supports.

Outcome: The systematic review findings were used to map effective psychological treatment strategies that would potentially inform the treatment development for PREMIUM.

Step 2

Objectives: To explore the explanatory models of AUD in South Asia and to examine the utility of these findings towards informing the contextual adaptation of the core psychological treatment.

Methods: Systematic review of the published literature.

Summary results: Causal attributions for alcohol use included psychosocial causes, peer influences, availability of disposable income, and functional use of alcohol to relieve physical stress. Alcohol consumption and AUD were perceived to result in adverse impacts on psychological health, occupational and social functioning, and family life.

Outcome: The findings were used to inform the selection of contextually appropriate psychological strategies as explanatory models influence help-seeking behaviour, acceptability of the treatment, subsequent concordance, and eventual patient satisfaction.

Step 3

Objectives: To understand the perceived cause of illness, perceived impact of illness, self-help coping strategies used, and expected outcomes, and to examine the utility of the findings to inform contextual adaptation of the identified core psychological treatment.

Methods: A qualitative study was conducted in patients with AUD and family members of those with AUD.

Summary results: Alcohol consumption and AUD are seen to be mainly caused by psychosocial stress, with other factors being peer influences, availability of disposable income, and drinking for pleasure. They are perceived to result in a range of adverse impacts on social life, family life, personal health, and family finances. Various coping strategies were used by men with AUD and their significant others, for example avoidance, substitution, distraction, religious activities, support from AA/friends/family, restricting means to buy alcohol, and anger management. Reduction/cessation in drinking, improved family relationships, improved emotional/physical wellbeing, and better occupational functioning were the most desired treatment outcomes.

Outcome: The findings were used to inform the selection of contextually appropriate psychological strategies as well as to adapt and refine the core psychological treatment.

Developing a theory/modelling process and outcomes

Box 3.2 What was done in PREMIUM? (continued)

Step 4

Objectives: To prioritize the psychological treatment strategies identified through steps 1–3 in terms of acceptability, feasibility, effectiveness, and safety for delivery by non-specialist health workers.

Methods: A survey administered to a panel of mental health experts and non-specialist health workers in which they rated each psychological treatment strategy along four dimensions, viz. 1) acceptability, 2) feasibility, 3) effectiveness, and 4) risk of harm when delivered by non-specialist health workers on a five-point Likert scale.

Summary results: Psychological treatment strategies like problem-solving, social skills training, and personalized feedback were endorsed as acceptable, feasible, effective, and safe to be delivered by non-specialist health workers.

Outcome: This resulted in the identification of psychological strategies that were perceived to be acceptable, feasible, effective, and safe when delivered by non-specialist health workers in under-resourced settings, thus narrowing down the treatment strategies for the next stage of treatment development.

Step 5

Objectives: To develop a model that assembled the prioritized strategies into a coherent psychological treatment.

Methods: Treatment development workshops with international experts and Indian clinical experts (psychiatrists, psychologists, and psychiatric social workers).

Summary results: MET was selected as the core psychological treatment around which other appropriate strategies like problem-solving could be used. The emerging treatment was arranged in four sessions. The first session covered psychoeducation, personalized feedback, and motivational enhancement. The second session covered problem-solving skills, social skills training, vocational counselling, and enlisting social support. During the third session, based on the patient's needs, strategies could be selected from a menu which offered relaxation skills, physical exercise, recreational activities, and religious and spiritual practices. The final session would focus on relapse prevention strategies and linking the patient to the existing support groups. MET was a cross-cutting strategy that would be employed throughout the psychological treatment delivery.

Outcome: A theoretical model for the new intervention began to emerge which would then be refined in subsequent stages.

Feasibility and piloting

Evaluations of interventions are often compromised because of barriers related to the acceptability of the intervention, adherence with the intervention, delivery of the intervention, recruitment of and retention of participants, and inadequate effect sizes. The aims of this phase of the framework include testing procedures and the intervention for their acceptability, estimating the likely rates of recruitment and retention of subjects, and the calculation of appropriate sample sizes. To achieve these aims a mixture of qualitative (e.g. to understand acceptability of the intervention) and quantitative (e.g. to estimate retention rates) methods is needed. Depending on the results, a series of studies may be required to progressively refine the intervention as well as the design of the definitive evaluation. In the final step before the definitive trial, a pilot study is carried out. Typically, a pilot study could be designed as a smaller controlled study (with or without the element of randomization) or as a cohort study of individuals who are offered the intervention (i.e. without a control group). Thus, a pilot study is usually a smaller version of the planned definitive evaluation and should usually involve a mixture of qualitative and quantitative methods (See box 3.3).

Box 3.3 What was done in PREMIUM?

Step 1

Objectives: To document the delivery barriers and facilitators; elaborate the psychological treatment techniques; define how the additional strategies, identified in the earlier states of PREMIUM, could be added to the core treatment (MET); and identify additional strategies or techniques that needed to be incorporated into the treatment.

Methods: Two case series were conducted sequentially. In the first case series, mental health specialists delivered MET to patients with AUD identified in primary care settings. In the second case series, lay counsellors delivered the intervention in primary care.

Summary results: Although the core treatment prescribed four treatment sessions, for several patients the therapeutic work reached a saturation point after two sessions. In addition, the core treatment had a limited role of psychoeducation and different clients expressed different unmet needs.

Outcomes: Adaptations and additions to the core treatment to make it more acceptable and feasible to deliver. This new treatment was named Counselling for Alcohol Problems (CAP).

Step 2

Objectives: To evaluate and compare the acceptability of CAP delivered face to face or over the telephone by lay counsellors in a primary health care setting;

To identify the barriers to the delivery of CAP by lay counsellors using these two delivery methods and evaluate strategies to address these; and

To generate preliminary information for the RCT by evaluating the procedures for recruitment of participants in the trials, evaluating the acceptability and feasibility of outcome and process measures, and estimating the likely rates of recruitment and drop-outs.

Methods: A pilot study conducted in two stages. Stage 1 was a treatment cohort with a before and after design. Stage 2 was a single blind, parallel group, exploratory two-arm RCT.

Box 3.3 What was done in PREMIUM? (continued)

Summary results: Face to face delivery at home emerged as the primary mode of delivery to ensure retention in treatment. Alcohol dependence was identified as the disorder to target along with harmful drinking, as this condition was the most visible alcohol-related problem in the primary health care clinic (PHC) (and thus, addressing the condition enhanced the acceptability of the counselling), and patients with dependence accounted for only a third of the total AUD case load and had similar rates of retention in treatment as harmful drinking. The process indicators (e.g. numbers of screen positives, numbers entering treatment) suggested that a 1-year period would be adequate to recruit the requisite sample size for the evaluation phase. At the time of writing this chapter, the phase II pilot study was in progress.

Outcome: The final psychological treatment which emphasized procedures for enhancing treatment completion and planned discharge; the procedures and tools for recruitment, informed consent, randomization, and outcome evaluation; and the planning of the implementation of the definitive trial.

Evaluating a complex intervention

Complex interventions can be evaluated using a range of randomized controlled study designs and an appropriate one needs to be selected based on the research questions and the context. Along with evaluating the efficacy/effectiveness of the intervention, it is useful to conduct a process evaluation and an economic analysis. The process evaluation provides an understanding of why an intervention succeeds (or fails) and an economic evaluation helps make the results more meaningful for decision-makers. Details of these methods and case studies can be found in other chapters of this book. In some circumstances, when an experimental approach is not feasible, for example because the intervention applies to the whole population, or because large-scale implementation is already under way, alternative non-experimental designs may be considered (see Chapter 16).

Implementation and beyond

The research process does not end after an intervention is proven to be effective. It is important that the intervention is successfully implemented so that its advantages are accrued by larger sections of the population for whom it was originally developed. Addressing the questions (Box 3.1 on NPT) during the early phases of intervention development promises an intervention that is more likely to be scaled up. Examples of some strategies for a potentially successful implementation plan include: involving stakeholders in the choice of question and design of the research; provision of evidence in an integrated and graded way; taking account of context; identifying and generating evidence for key elements relevant to decision-making, such as benefits, harms, and costs; making recommendations as specific as possible; and using a multifaceted approach involving a mixture of interactive dissemination meetings, audit, feedback, reminders, and local consensus processes.

Successful implementation needs to be supplemented by measures to monitor rare or long-term impacts through routine data sources and record linkage, or by recontacting study participants. The ToC (described in the section 'The ToC approach for intervention development and evaluation') may be a useful framework to hang the above methods onto, to assist in planning and evaluating the scale-up of an intervention. Implementation of complex interventions is described in greater detail in Chapter 16.

The ToC approach for intervention development and evaluation

While the MRC framework provides extremely useful guidance on how to develop and evaluate complex interventions, implementing complex interventions within a health service setting, such as is the case for most global mental health trials, provides additional challenges that the MRC framework has been criticized for not adequately addressing. In addition, conducting trials in low-resource settings poses additional challenges which the MRC framework was not originally designed to address (see Table 3.3).

In addition, the MRC framework has been criticized for its 'lack of specific theory-driven approaches to design and evaluation' (10). Prospective, theoretically driven process of intervention design and evaluation is required in order to understand not just whether, but how and why an intervention has a particular effect, and which parts of a

Table 3.3 Challenges to using the MRC framework in health service trials, particularly in low-resource settings

MRC framework	Health service trials, particularly in low-resource settings
Medical focus	Drug plus psychological and social interventions
Patient focused	Health care provider/health system focus
HIC focused	LAMIC focused with added complexity such as medicine stock-outs, staff shortages, and lack of training and awareness. This means that the interventions delivered in LAMIC are often more complex than those in HIC, as they involve health system strengthening before the intervention can begin to be delivered
Control over setting	Little control over setting, e.g. changes to policy context and contextual factors which may interact with interventions
High research capacity	Low research capacity: evaluation may interact with intervention
Implementation	Sustainability and scalability of intervention need to be considered in the light of unstable funding and limited resources

Adapted from <http://www.actconsortium.org/pages/guidance-notes.html>

complex intervention have the greatest impact on outcomes. Integrating ToC into the MRC framework may provide a solution.

What is ToC?

ToC is 'a theory of how and why an initiative works' which can be empirically tested. It is developed in collaboration with stakeholders and modified throughout the intervention development and evaluation process through an 'ongoing process of reflection to explore change and how it happens' (11, 12). It is visually represented in a causal pathways map which illustrates how an intervention is expected to achieve its impact within the constraints of the setting in which it is implemented (see Fig. 3.2 for an example of a ToC map of a peer-led counselling intervention for maternal depression developed in Goa, India).

Unlike logic models or driver diagrams which are either linear or cyclical in nature and aim to present a simplified model of action, ToC seeks to reflect the complexity of the causal pathways through which the intervention leads to real-world impact. ToC is not a sociological or psychological theory of *why* change occurs, such as Complexity Theory (13) and the Theory of Planned Behaviour (14), but a framework that describes *how* the intervention affects change. These sociological or psychological theories could be inserted at key points in the ToC to explain why particular links happen. A ToC approach is complementary to other frameworks that seek to reduce the chance of implementation failure, such as NPT (8) (Box 3.1). While NPT provides a framework detailing *what* questions should be asked to design an intervention that is more likely to be 'normalized' into routine practice, ToC provides an explanation for *how* those questions can be answered.

Developing a ToC

At the start of the intervention development phase, ToC uses a participatory approach by bringing together a range of stakeholders (for example health service planners, health care workers, and service users) to develop a ToC map and to encourage stakeholder buy-in to the project (15). This could take the form of a series of workshops, interviews, or focus groups, with the choice of method based upon what is locally feasible and acceptable (16).

Stakeholders first agree on the real-world impact they want to achieve. They then identify the causal pathways through which this change can be achieved in that context using the available resources. These are articulated as a series of outcomes, the order of which can be adjusted as the pathway develops. Determining what contextual conditions are necessary to achieve the outcomes, what resources are required to implement the interventions, and how the programme gains the commitment of those resources are crucial outputs of the process.

Key components of the ToC map include:

1 identifying the *interventions* needed to move from one *outcome* in the causal pathway to the next;

2 articulating the evidence for each link in the pathway (*rationale*). The rationale may be drawn from a range of sources including research evidence, behaviour change theories, and local knowledge, or from primary research conducted as part of the intervention feasibility and piloting stage. Drawing on diverse

sources of knowledge should yield a more plausible intervention with an increased chance of achieving its goal of improving the outcomes of those who receive it;

3   highlighting the key *assumptions* that set out the conditions that the causal pathway needs to achieve impact. Through this process, potential barriers and interventions needed to overcome these barriers can be identified so that the ultimate outcome can be achieved;

4   identifying *indicators* for each outcome in the pathway to evaluate whether each stage of the pathway leading to the final impact is achieved.

All these components are displayed graphically on a ToC map, often with an accompanying narrative that describes the pathways and key assumptions (as shown in Fig. 3.2). Further guidance and resources on how to develop a ToC are available via the Centre for Theory of Change (<http://www.theoryofchange.org/>).

Refining a ToC

Before an intervention is implemented, key aspects of the ToC should be tested in the feasibility and piloting phase of the MRC framework. This involves turning the assumptions articulated in the ToC into research questions to test in formative research. This may help reduce implementation failure as weak links in the causal pathway are tested and strengthened if necessary, leading to a revision of the intervention. The ToC is then modified to reflect changes resulting from the feasibility and piloting phase and a revised ToC is taken forward for formal testing in the evaluation phase. Developing a ToC must be a continual process of reflection and adaptation as barriers to implementation arise and new evidence comes to light, requiring the pathway to be changed and strengthened.

Evaluating a ToC

The evaluation of a complex intervention using a ToC approach involves identifying at least one indicator for every outcome within that framework to measure whether it has been achieved. Indicators must be specific enough to describe what change is necessary in the outcome to move up the causal pathway (e.g. how many people need to be trained with the appropriate level of competency in order to deliver the intervention as intended).

Evaluation using a ToC framework involves measuring indicators at all stages of implementation, not just an intervention's primary and secondary outcomes. This includes a wider range of input, process, output, and outcome indicators than may normally be measured, with a clear focus on measuring whether key stages in the causal pathway are achieved. ToC allows for multiple outcomes of the intervention to be prespecified within a theoretical framework, thereby explicitly evaluating the multiple outcomes that complex interventions may lead to. As a result, an evaluation based on a ToC will require a number of different methods to capture all of the indicators.

Disseminating a ToC

Experience of implementation and evidence gathered from the evaluation is combined to revise the ToC and produce the final 'story' of how the intervention worked in a particular setting. This provides a comprehensive description of the intervention which can be disseminated to a variety of audiences, providing information on the active components of the intervention that need to be adapted for use in other settings. The MRC guidance calls for more detailed and standardized descriptions of complex interventions in published reports to facilitate exchange of knowledge and encourage

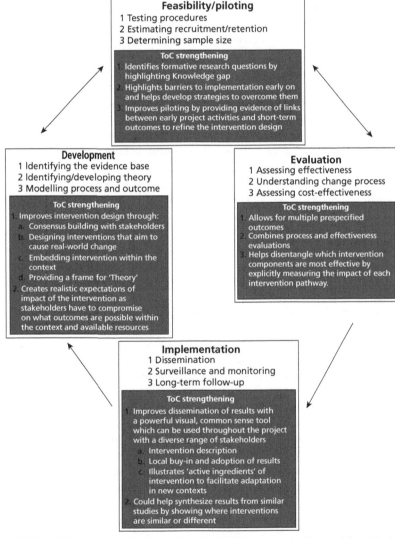

Fig. 3.3 How ToC can be used to strengthen the MRC framework. (Adapted from Craig 2008 (17)).

synthesis of results from similar studies (17, 18). ToC may be a useful tool to meet this challenge.

Using ToC has a number of benefits, which improve the existing MRC framework for complex interventions, and include:

1 helping a diverse range of stakeholders reach a realistic consensus on what is to be achieved, how, using what resources, and under what constraints;

2 ensuring the intervention has the buy-in of stakeholders from the start and embedding the design in a real-world context, which increases the likelihood that it will be effective and subsequently scaled up;

3 providing an overarching theoretical framework incorporating formative, process, and impact evaluation research questions;

4 providing information about how and why an intervention works in addition to whether it works;

5 facilitating timely and informative information about the progress of the project which can be understood by a diverse range of audiences.

Figure 3.3 illustrates how using ToC strengthens each phase in the MRC framework. Used in conjunction with the MRC framework, ToC may be a useful tool to improve the design and evaluation of complex interventions, increasing the likelihood that the intervention will be ultimately effective, sustainable and scalable.

Conclusion

In this chapter we discussed the nature of complex interventions and how mental health interventions are complex. We then described the need for a structured framework for developing and testing complex interventions and described the MRC framework, one of the most widely used frameworks for this purpose. Finally we focused on the treatment development phase of the MRC framework and illustrated the various steps in this phase using the example of a research project from Goa, India. Complex interventions are made up of a number of interconnected components, acting both independently and interdependently, a characteristic commonly seen in mental health interventions. Using a structured framework like the MRC framework and complementing it with other frameworks like the NPT and ToC helps to address the host of challenges inherent to the development, evaluation, and implementation of mental health interventions.

References

1 **Medical Research Council** (2000) A framework for development and evaluation of RCTs for complex interventions to improve health. London: Medical Research Council.

2 **Collins PY, Patel V, Joestl S, March D, Insel TR, Daar AS, et al.** (2011) Grand challenges in global mental health. Nature, **475**:27–30.

3 **Balaji M, Andrews T, Andrew G, Patel V** (2011) The acceptability, feasibility, and effectiveness of a population-based intervention to promote youth health: an exploratory study in Goa, India. J Adolesc Health, **48**:453–60.

4 **Chatterjee S, Patel V, Chatterjee A, Weiss HA** (2003) Evaluation of a community-based rehabilitation model for chronic schizophrenia in rural India. Br J Psychiatry, **182**:57–62.

5 Patel V, Weiss HA, Chowdhary N, Naik S, Pednekar S, Chatterjee S, et al. (2010) Effectiveness of an intervention led by lay health counsellors for depressive and anxiety disorders in primary care in Goa, India (MANAS): a cluster randomised controlled trial. Lancet, **376**:2086–95.

6 Campbell M, Fitzpatrick R, Haines A, Kinmonth AL, Sandercock P, Spiegelhalter D, et al. (2000) Framework for design and evaluation of complex interventions to improve health. BMJ, **13**:694–6.

7 Craig P, Dieppe P, Macintyre S, Michie S, Nazareth I, Petticrew M (2008) Developing and evaluating complex interventions: the new Medical Research Council guidance. BMJ, **337**:a1655.

8 Murray E, Treweek S, Pope C, MacFarlane A, Ballini L, Dowrick C, et al. (2010) Normalisation process theory: a framework for developing, evaluating and implementing complex interventions. BMC Med, **8**:63.

9 Lovell K, Bower P, Richards D, Barkham M, Sibbald B, Roberts C, et al. (2008) Developing guided self-help for depression using the Medical Research Council complex interventions framework: a description of the modelling phase and results of an exploratory randomised controlled trial. BMC Psychiatry, **8**:91.

10 Anderson R (2008) New MRC guidance on evaluating complex interventions. BMJ, **337**:a1937.

11 Weiss C (1995) Nothing as practical as good theory: exploring theory-based evaluation for comprehensive community initiatives for children and families. In: Connell JP (ed.) New approaches to evaluating community initiatives: concepts, methods, and contexts. Washington, DC: Aspen Institute.

12 James C (2011) Theory of Change review. A report commissioned by Comic Relief. London: Comic Relief.

13 Kernick D (2006) Wanted—new methodologies for health service research. Is complexity theory the answer? Family Practice, **23**:385–90.

14 Ajzen I (1991) The theory of planned behavior. Organ Behav Hum Decis Process, **50**:179–211.

15 Taplin D, Clark H, Collins E, Colby D (2013) Theory of Change technical papers: a series of papers to support development of theories of change based on practice in the field. New York: ActKnowledge.

16 Mason P, Barnes M (2007) Constructing Theories of Change: methods and sources. Evaluation, **13**:151–70.

17 Craig P, Dieppe P, Macintyre S, Nazareth I, Petticrew I (2008) Developing and evaluating complex interventions: the new Medical Research Council guidance. BMJ, **337**:a1655.

18 Campbell NC, Murray E, Darbyshire J, Emery J, Farmer A, Griffiths F, et al. (2007) Designing and evaluating complex interventions to improve health care. BMJ, **334**:455–9.

Chapter 4

Design issues in global mental health trials in low-resource settings

Helen Weiss

Introduction

The goal of a trial in mental health, as in other fields of medicine, is to provide the gold-standard evidence of whether a specific intervention is effective in a specified population. The intervention may be a new medication or new psychotherapy technique, or may be a package of interventions. In this chapter we describe design issues for trials in global mental health, focusing on RCTs, and discuss how a trial that is well designed and analysed will minimize the chance of drawing an incorrect conclusion about how well an intervention works.

Framing the question

Stating the research hypothesis

The first step in a research study is to define the *research hypothesis*. This will usually arise from an identified gap in knowledge, often arising from previous research. A clearly defined research hypothesis is essential in formulating research, and there are several frameworks that can be used to clearly define the hypothesis, such as the PICOT criteria (Box 4.1).

An example from a trial of treating depression in primary care in Chile (1) is as follows:

Population: among low-income women with major depression attending primary care in Chile.

Intervention: a stepped-care programme (comprising 3-month, multicomponent intervention led by a non-medical health worker, which included a psychoeducational group intervention, structured and systematic follow-up, and drug treatment for patients with severe depression) is effective.

Comparison: compared with usual care (received all services normally available in the primary care clinic, including antidepressant medication or referral for specialty treatment).

Outcomes: in reducing depression as measured using the Hamilton Depression Rating Scale (HDRS).

Time: at 6 months follow-up.

Box 4.1 PICOT criteria

P: Population (patients)—define the specific population you are interested in
I: Intervention—define the intervention or package of interventions
C: Comparison—define the alternative that will be given to those in the comparison arm
O: Outcome of interest—define how the outcome will be measured
T: Time—define the period over which you will evaluate the intervention

---

Defining outcomes

Guidance on the design of randomized clinical trials is provided by the CONSORT statements (2, 3). These recommend only a single primary outcome. A key reason to focus on relatively few primary and secondary outcomes is to reduce the burden on the trial participant, and to maximize the quality of the data, which can diminish if participants are required to complete long questionnaires. However, it is sometimes appropriate to have multiple outcomes. These may include alternative scales to measure the outcome, or an absolute, as well as a relative, cut-off. For example, in the Chilean depression treatment trial (1), the primary analyses included two measures of the HDRS— (1) 'improvement' as defined by a > 50% reduction in HDRS score at 3 and 6 months, respectively, and (2) 'recovery' as defined by an HDRS score below 8. The authors also combined the two endpoints (3 and 6 months).

A recent review of RCTs of depression treatment with multiple outcomes showed that authors often reported more outcomes than those defined in the protocol (4). If several outcomes are shown, this can be problematic, as it becomes likely that at least one analysis will show a statistically significant effect.

Multiple outcomes of interest are also common in trials to treat long-term mental health conditions because a single measure may not sufficiently characterize the treatment effect on a broad set of domains (4). For example, a trial of depression treatment included a composite outcome of recovery (defined as 8 weeks with partial or full remission) or recovering (4 weeks with low levels of symptoms) (5).

Effectiveness versus efficacy trials

Intervention trials in mental health often involve complex health care systems, perhaps including better diagnosis, management, and referral to specialized services. However, many trials of pharmacological or psychotherapeutic interventions occur in secondary care, among highly selected patients. If an intervention is found to be effective in one of these tightly controlled 'efficacy' trials, it may need to be evaluated in a more pragmatic effectiveness trial to assess the impact of the intervention in 'real-life' circumstances. For example, intramuscular olanzapine is one of the drugs recommended by the National Institute for Health and Care Excellence (NICE) for treating violence, based on efficacy trials which found that intramuscular olanzapine was safe and efficacious in treating acute agitation in people with schizophrenia, mania, and dementia (6). These trials had strict exclusion criteria (excluding people with co-morbid alcohol or drug dependence, those with violence towards others, and those who needed restraints) and were sponsored and authorized by the drug industry. A further, pragmatic trial was conducted in a psychiatric hospital in Vellore, South India, to assess the effectiveness of using intramuscular olanzapine versus a commonly used, relatively inexpensive, and effective intervention of combined haloperidol and promethazine (7). This trial took place in the real-life setting of an emergency department of a psychiatric unit with little interference to normal clinical practice. The trial outcomes were chosen by the team, independently of industry sponsorship. The consent procedures also allowed a responsible relative to give consent if the patient lacks capacity to consent.

Trial design

Randomization

Randomization is the central principle in trial design. In an RCT, participants are allocated randomly to the intervention group, using a random number generator. When done correctly, this will minimize systematic differences between treatment groups in known or unknown factors that may affect the outcome (confounders). In the absence of randomization, the two groups may differ in terms of key characteristics associated with the outcome. For example, a non-randomized trial in India recruited people with schizophrenia into a study in which they received either yoga therapy or treatment as usual (including routine pharmacotherapy), to assess the effect of yoga therapy on cognitive function (8). The yoga therapy was delivered at an outpatient clinic of the hospital where patients were recruited. If patients were eligible and able to attend the yoga therapy sessions, they did so, and if patients could not attend the yoga therapy sessions (e.g. through preference or inability to travel or take time off work), they received treatment as usual. At the end of the trial, the patients in the yoga therapy arm had significantly better cognitive function outcomes. However, given differences between the two groups in factors such as education level and more severe illness, one cannot be sure that the difference was due to the yoga therapy.

Unit of randomization

A key design issue is the unit of randomization. The effectiveness trial of intramuscular olanzapine in India was an individually randomized trial (7). Consecutive patients were assessed for eligibility, and those for whom consent was obtained were randomized. The trial of the effectiveness of a stepped-care programme in Chile was also individually randomized (1). In this trial, patients were recruited at three primary care clinics, and randomization was stratified by clinic—i.e. a separate randomization list was computer-generated for each clinic, to avoid imbalances in numbers attending each clinic by arm.

Many trials of complex interventions in global mental health lend themselves to interventions at a primary care, or community, level. For example, the trial may involve screening patients for CMD, or educating primary care clinicians to better recognize and manage care of mental disorders. In these cases, the primary care clinic would be the unit of randomization, not the individual patient. Sometimes, whole communities are randomized, rather than primary care clinics. For example, in a trial to assess the effectiveness of cognitive-behaviour therapy delivered by community health workers on maternal depression in Pakistan, the unit of randomization was a Union Cluster, which is the smallest administrative unit in Pakistan, with a population of around 15,000–20,000 (9). This is because the intervention was being delivered by a community health worker, called a Lady Health Worker (LHW). Each LHW works within a Union Cluster and is responsible for about 100 households in her village. Supervision of the LHWs takes place at the Union Cluster, and hence it made sense to randomize Union Clusters and to train all the LHWs within a Cluster in the same way. The MANAS trial is another example of a cluster randomized trial of treatment for CMD in Goa, India (10). In this trial, the intervention was to involve a lay health counsellor in a primary care clinic. This meant that the unit of randomization had to be the clinic, rather than individual level.

Cluster randomized trials require a larger number of patients than an individually randomized trial. This is because patients within a cluster are likely to be more similar to each other in terms of the outcome measure, compared with patients in a different cluster. This means that the usual assumption of independence between individuals does not hold and the clustering effect needs to be taken into account in the design and analysis of the trial (11). As cluster randomized trials tend to have fewer randomization units (clusters) than individually randomized trials, it is important to try to minimize imbalance between the arms. This can be done by stratifying clusters based on known factors associated with the outcome, or a process such as minimization or restricted randomization, which is a process by which only allocations that satisfy certain predetermined criteria of balance are eligible. Further details are given in Hayes and Moulton (11). For example, the MANAS trial included only 24 clusters, and these were randomized within predefined strata of clinic type (public vs private), presence/absence of a visiting psychiatrist, and clinic size.

Allocation concealment

Once the randomization process has been conducted, it is important that no bias occurs in allocating patients to arms. This means that the person allocating the participant should have no knowledge of which arm the next participant will be allocated to. Allocation concealment refers to the method used to implement the randomization sequence. For example, in the Chilean depression trial, allocations were kept in opaque numbered sealed envelopes in each clinic, and were opened by an individual who had not recruited patients. This method is commonly called 'SNOSE' (sequentially numbered, opaque sealed envelopes) and is a cheap and effective method to preserve allocation concealment (12). With cluster randomized trials, the allocation is made in advance of the trial, so allocation concealment is less of an issue.

Parallel arm trials, non-inferiority, and equivalence trials

Most RCTs aim to determine whether one intervention is superior to another. These may be parallel arm trials, in which each group of participants is exposed to only one intervention. Typically, one group will be randomized to receive a standard of care, or control. The control may be enhanced usual care, a standard treatment, or a placebo (if ethically acceptable). In a two-arm trial, there is one intervention of interest (e.g. a stepped-care counselling intervention or an experimental drug), but trials may also be three-armed (e.g. with two separate interventions against the control group).

It is also possible to design a trial that aims to determine whether the intervention of interest is therapeutically similar to the control condition (equivalence trial), or whether the intervention is no worse than the control condition (non-inferiority trial). In these trials, a prestated margin of non-inferiority is chosen (13). The intervention will be recommended if it is similar or better than the control condition, but not if it is worse by more than the margin of non-inferiority. For example, a three-arm non-inferiority trial design was used to evaluate whether internet-based cognitive behaviour therapy (iCBT) guided by a technician was as effective as when guided by a clinician (14). Participants in both groups received access to an iCBT programme for depression comprising six online lessons, weekly homework assignments, and weekly supportive contact over a treatment period of 8 weeks. There was also a delayed treatment group. Participants in the clinician-assisted group also received access to a moderated online discussion forum. The main outcome measures were the Beck Depression Inventory (BDI-II) and the Patient Health Questionnaire-9 Item (PHQ-9). At post-treatment, both treatment groups reduced scores on the BDI-II ($p < 0.001$) and PHQ-9 ($p < 0.001$) compared to the delayed treatment group but did not differ from each other. The trial provided support for large-scale trials to determine the clinical effectiveness and acceptability of technician-assisted iCBT programmes for depression.

Cross-over and stepped-wedge designs

An alternative to the parallel arm trial is the cross-over design, in which each participant (or cluster, for cluster randomized trials) receives two treatments, one after the other, usually in random order so that the effects of any time-trends are controlled for. There is often a 'wash-out period' between the two treatment periods, to avoid carry-over effects of the first treatment received into the second period. An important advantage of the cross-over design is that comparison can be made within individuals (or clusters) rather than between individuals/clusters. This reduces the sample size needed for the trial, but there are some disadvantages to this trial. It increases the length of the study as both interventions need to be administered to all participants, and because interventions often take time to have a full effect, each participant/cluster needs to remain in each arm for long enough for the full effect to be observed. For example, a recent trial in Malaysia used a cross-over design to evaluate the effect of Talbinah food (barley soup cooked with milk and sweetened with honey) on mood and depression among institutionalized elderly people (15). Participants were randomized to receive the intervention or control (usual food) for 3 weeks, followed by a 1-week 'wash-out period' and then 3 weeks on the alternative diet (Fig. 4.1).

An alternative design, applicable to cluster-randomized trials, is the stepped-wedge design. In this design, all the clusters commence the trial in the control arm. The intervention is then introduced gradually at regular intervals, either one cluster at a time or in small groups of clusters. At the end of the trial, the intervention is in place in all the

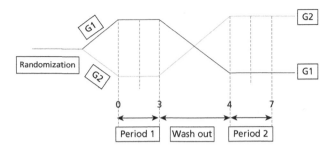

Fig. 4.1 Study design for a cross-over trial of the effect of Talbinah food on mood and depression among institutionalized elderly people in Malaysia (15).

Notes: Week 0: baseline assessment; Week 3: end of period I; Week 4: end of wash-out period; Week 7: end of period 2. GDS-R, DASS, and POMS scales were scored at weeks 0, 3, 4, and 7. Nutritional status assessments (weight, height, MUAC, CC, and SGA) were done at weeks 0, 3, 4, and 7. Two-day food-weighing record was done once during each period.

Abbreviations: GDS-R, Geriatric Depression Scale-Residential; DASS, Depression Anxiety and Stress Scale; POMS, Profile of Mood States; MUAC, mid upper arm circumference; CC, calf circumference; SGA, subjective global assessment. (Reproduced with permission from Badrasawi MM, Shahar S, Abd Manaf Z, Haron H. Effect of Talbinah food consumption on depressive symptoms among elderly individuals in long term care facilities, randomized clinical trial. Clin Interv Aging, 2013; 8:279–85).

clusters. The order in which the intervention is introduced is randomized. This design can be used to address ethical issues where there is already considerable evidence that the intervention may have a beneficial effect, and assigning some communities to the control arm for the duration of the trial may be unacceptable. Stepped-wedge trials are relatively rare in mental health, but could provide a pragmatic public health intervention for community-level interventions likely to have a beneficial effect. One example is a recent trial of the evaluation of a care programme to improve the detection and treatment of depression in nursing homes (16). Sixteen dementia units and 17 somatic units were enrolled and randomized to one of five groups. A multidisciplinary care programme (Act in Case of Depression (AiD)) was implemented at one of five time points (Fig. 4.2), approximately 4 months apart.

Alternative trial designs

A particular problem with mental health trials can be that the trial population is not representative of a wider target population, because many clinical trials demonstrating higher success rates have typically enrolled highly selected and motivated staff and patients. Modifications of the traditional trial designs can help address these issues of non-adherence, biased patient selection, and attrition (loss to follow-up) (17). These include 'fixed adaptive designs' in which patients are randomized to treatment arms that allow treatment changes to adapt to intermediate patient outcomes (including the stepped-care intervention in the MANAS trial (10)), or 'patient preference' trials, in which participants decide if they are to be randomized to the interventions, or allowed

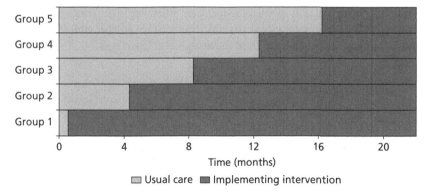

Fig. 4.2 Design for a stepped-care trial of the evaluation of a care programme to improve the detection and treatment of depression in nursing homes in the Netherlands (16). (Reprinted from *The Lancet*, 29;381 (9885), Leontjevas R, Gerritsen DL, Smalbrugge M, Teerenstra S, Vernooij-Dassen MJ, Koopmans RT, A structural multidisciplinary approach to depression management in nursing-home residents: a multicentre, stepped-wedge cluster-randomised trial, 2255–64. Copyright (2013), with permission from Elsevier)

to select the intervention assignment. These may be particularly relevant for mental health trials where participants have a strong treatment preference. Relatively few trials have used these methods, and there is no conclusive evidence as to whether there is any effect of patient preference on treatment outcome, but it is clear that the characteristics of patients who do not consent to randomization differ from those who refuse, contributing to patient selection bias (18).

Choice of comparison condition

The selection of an appropriate comparison condition is one of the key design elements for an RCT, especially for behavioural interventions where, unlike pharmaceutical interventions, there is no placebo drug (19, 20). The principle of having a control condition in an RCT is to evaluate the intervention condition against the care that would be given in the absence of the intervention (i.e. standard or usual care), thus maintaining the internal validity of the trial. The control condition may vary from no treatment to an active alternative treatment. Commonly used control conditions in global mental health trials include existing-practice control groups (largely equivalent to 'treatment as usual', or 'usual care'). A variant is 'Enhanced Usual Care', in which usual care is systematically improved by the research protocol to overcome ethical or methodological problems. For example, in the MANAS trial in which primary care clinics were randomized to a collaborative stepped-care intervention for CMD, or a comparison arm, it was necessary to screen all potential participants for CMD as the screening result formed part of the eligibility criteria (21). It was therefore necessary to screen participants in the comparison arm of the trial, but it would then be unethical to conceal screening results from the physicians. Consequently, physicians in comparison arm practices received screening results and could choose to initiate treatment. This enhancement to usual care in the control practices may have reduced the difference in outcomes between intervention and control practices, but was ethically necessary. Further ethical considerations in the choice of comparison group are discussed in Chapter 8.

Masking of providers and participants

The term masking (or 'blinding') refers to keeping trial participants, investigators, and outcome assessors unaware of the allocation that has been assigned. The purpose of masking is to minimize bias in assessing the effect of the intervention. For example, if participants know that they have received a new treatment, this may result in improved perceptions and reports of the treatment effect. Knowledge of treatment allocation can also affect adherence to the intervention and loss to follow-up. Similarly, if investigators are not masked, this may affect how they deliver the intervention. However, in many trials it may not be possible to mask the investigators and participants. For example, in many trials, especially cluster randomized trials, both patients and investigators will be aware of their allocation if the intervention includes additional components compared to the comparison arm (such as the stepped-care programmes evaluated in several of the trials mentioned in this chapter (1, 9, 10)). This may be unavoidable, but it is important that an independent team is used to assess the outcomes for the study, and that this team remain masked to the allocation arm. For example, in the Chilean depression trial, the outcome interviews at 3 and 6 months were conducted by an independent clinician masked to treatment allocation, and in the MANAS trial, masking of the research assessor who conducted the outcome interviews was maximized by: undertaking assessments at home; randomly allocating unique identification numbers to patients so that there was no association between their number and the identity of the facility; outcome assessment being done by an independent institution whose team did not know the randomization allocation; and undertaking the primary outcome assessment before all other assessments.

Validity and reliability

It is very important in randomized trials with mental health outcomes to ensure that the measurements of the outcome and exposures are valid and reliable, i.e. that the scale used is an accurate measure of the true outcome of interest. This may involve some pilot work prior to the trial to assess the performance of a particular measure. For example, a study in Singapore was conducted to assess the internal validity and reliability of the Geriatric Depression Screening Scale (GDS-15) (22) (Box 4.2).

In this study, the authors aimed to assess the validity of the English, Chinese, and Malay versions of the GDS-15 scale against the 'gold standard' structured clinical interview (SCID) to make Diagnostic and Statistical Manual of Mental Disorders, Fourth Edition (DSM-IV) diagnosis of major depressive disorder (MDD). The GDS-15 was administered by face-to-face interviews with trained and experienced nurses in the languages and dialects preferred by the respondents. The SCID was administered by a medically qualified researcher with training in psychiatric assessment, who was masked to the results of the GDS-15. The validity was assessed by estimating the sensitivity, specificity, positive predictive value, and negative predictive

---

Box 4.2 Validity and reliability in mental health trials

Reliability: the degree to which results from a measurement tool can be replicated. Lack of reliability can arise from divergences between observers or measurement instruments, measurement error, or instability of the attribute being measured.

Internal validity: the extent to which differences identified between randomized groups are a result of the intervention being tested. Internal validity depends on good design, conduct, and analysis of the trial to minimize biases and confounding.

External validity: the extent to which the results of a trial provide a correct basis for generalizations to other study populations.

---

value of the GDS-15 against the SCID and selecting the cut-off that had optimal characteristics (cut-off of 4/5). In addition, the authors assessed the reliability of the GDS-15 using the Cronbach's alpha coefficient, and interrater reliability among seven interviewers.

The results of RCTs are used to guide treatment guidelines and, prior to conducting a new trial of a given intervention, it is important to systematically review previous trials of the intervention. This review should include assessment factors that will affect whether these previous results are generalizable to the new setting. Issues that affect this generalizability (or external validity) include the trial setting, eligibility criteria, participation rate, loss to follow-up, severity of baseline disease, appropriateness/relevance of the control condition, and other aspects of trial design (23).

Sample size

The aim of a sample size calculation is to estimate an appropriate size of a trial that will provide sufficient power to answer the research question, but will not be larger than necessary (to avoid logistical and financial problems). Detailed descriptions of conducting sample size calculations for individual and cluster randomized trials are widely available (24–26), and we will only review the key concepts here.

1 *Null hypothesis:* this will typically be that there is no difference between the two arms of the trial.

2 *Type I error (α-level):* this is the strength of the evidence required to reject the null hypothesis. An α-level of 0.05 (5%) is typically used.

3 *Type II error (1-power):* this is the probability that we would like to have of achieving this level of significance, i.e. the probability of rejecting the null hypothesis when it is false.

4 *Effect size:* for binary outcomes, we will typically compare the proportion with the outcome in the two arms. The estimated proportions need to be provided in the sample size calculation. For continuous outcomes, the comparison is the difference in means in the two groups, divided by the standard deviation (Cohen's d).

5 *Coefficient of variation (for cluster randomized trials only)*: for a cluster randomized trial, one has to allow for between-cluster variability in the outcome measurement. This means that the sample size to detect a given effect size will be larger than for an individually randomized trial (26).

For a two-arm RCT with a quantitative endpoint, the objective is to compare the mean of the outcome variable in the intervention and control arms. The null hypothesis is that there is no difference in the mean, and the total sample size is given by the formula:

$$N = 2 \times \left(\frac{z_{1-\frac{\alpha}{2}} + z_{1-\beta}}{\delta} \right)^2 \sigma^2$$

where N is the total sample size, z is the Z value obtained from the standard normal distribution, α is the type I error, β is the power (1-type II error), δ is the true difference in means between the two arms, and σ^2 is the true population variance (27).

For example, in the Chilean depression trial, the researchers designed the study to have 80% power to detect a 2.5-point difference in mean HDRS score, with a standard deviation of 7 points and 5% significance. So $\delta = 2.5$, $\alpha = 0.05$, $\beta = 0.8$, $\sigma = 7$, giving a sample size $N = 248$ (1).

For binary outcomes, the formula is based on the proportion in each arm with the primary outcome, as follows:

$$\frac{\pi_0(1-\pi_0) + \pi_1(1-\pi_1)}{\pi_1 - \pi_0^2}$$

where π_0 and π_1 are the true proportions in the presence and absence of the intervention, respectively.

Note that these formulae are for individually randomized, superiority trials. For cluster randomized trials, the formula changes to incorporate the between-cluster coefficient of variation of the true proportion or means in the two arms (11, 26). Non-inferiority and equivalence trials seek to determine whether the intervention is not worse than the control condition, and the sample size calculation is based on a pr-estated margin of non-inferiority (28). We recommend that researchers consult a statistician when planning a trial to ensure that the trial will be adequately powered.

Data monitoring, management, and analysis

Data monitoring

Most funding bodies require randomized trials to set up an independent data and safety monitoring board (DSMB). The purpose of such a committee is to ensure the safety of participants and the validity and integrity of the data, and members must have the expertise required to monitor the trial and not be involved in the day-to-day management. The US National Institutes of Health issued guidelines in the late 1990s to require DSMBs for phase III trials (29), and a specific policy for the National Institutes of Mental Health was published in 2007 (30, 31). The DSMB performs the following roles: (1) monitoring of the integrity of the trial, including adherence to the study protocol, and the recruitment, randomization, retention, adherence, and follow-up of trial participants; (2) review of predefined serious or unexpected adverse reactions among trial participants; and (3) holding the randomization code for the trial, enabling them to conduct preplanned interim analyses to evaluate the evidence for an intervention effect (32). The Board can then recommend to the investigators whether there are monitoring or safety concerns, whether there is evidence to stop the trial before the original end-date, or to discontinue one of the trial arms.

Stopping a trial early may occur because the intervention is working either particularly well or badly. For example, a trial to evaluate the efficacy and tolerability of a once-monthly aripiprazole intramuscular depot as maintenance therapy for patients with schizophrenia was terminated early because a preplanned interim analysis showed that the primary outcome measure (time to exacerbation of psychotic symptoms/impending relapse) was significantly delayed in the aripiprazole-intramuscular-depot treatment arm compared with the placebo arm (10% vs 40%; $p < 0.0001$) (33). Early stopping of the trial has immediate implications for trial participants in the control arm, as they should then be offered the intervention, and also policy implications. In this case, the results of this trial led to Food and Drug Administration (FDA) approval for the 1-monthly injectable drug for patients with schizophrenia in March 2013, a year after the trial was halted. This decision would have been delayed had the trial continued to its original endpoint. However, there are potential problems with stopping trials early as this can lead to erroneous results, and expert statistical advice is needed when planning interim analyses (27).

Data management

Achieving high quality data is an essential step in conducting a rigorous RCT. Briefly, trial data management is the process of collection, cleaning, and management of trial data, in compliance with principles of Good Clinical Practice (GCP) or regulatory standards, as appropriate. The main objective of data management is to minimize any errors or missing data, and to deliver a data set ready for statistical analysis. A data management plan is frequently required to be submitted to funding bodies as part of the research proposal.

The data management plan will typically include the following elements:

- types of data to be collected and methods to be used (qualitative, quantitative, medical records, interviewer-collected, etc.);
- methods for data management and storage (including data entry, back-up, data cleaning);
- data security (methods to preserve confidentiality of data, data access);
- data sharing (suitability for sharing with potential new users, governance of future data access).

Typically, the data themselves can be divided into process indicators and outcome measures. Process indicators are the measures that monitor adherence to the protocol, for example the recruitment and retention rates, delivery and fidelity to the intervention, adherence, and loss to follow-up. These data should be reviewed regularly by the trial investigators to ensure that the trial is implemented to the highest possible quality. Outcome measures should usually be collected be a team independent of the intervention delivery, and will include assessment of the primary and secondary outcomes of the trial.

Many trials now use hand-held computers (tablets, personal data assistants, etc.) for direct data entry whilst interviewing participants. These methods have the advantages of allowing real-time data quality checks and analyses, but need investment in programming of the computers to function smoothly, including incorporating comprehensive consistency checks, considerable piloting to ensure that the quality of data is sufficient, and ongoing training and monitoring of research staff. The trial may also need to comply with GCP principles, ensuring, for example, an audit trail so that all changes to the database are recorded. For trials that use paper-based questionnaires, the data entry can be a time-consuming process, and steps must be taken to minimize data entry errors and comply with GCP. For example, data should be entered twice by two independent data entry clerks, and compared (validated) to ensure accuracy. Data cleaning programs also need to be run, to ensure internal consistency of the data.

Data analysis

In this chapter we give an outline of the main steps and principles of analysing trials. Details of statistical methods are covered in textbooks on medical statistics (24, 27), and as analysis of trials can often be complex, we strongly advise involving a medical statistician at an early stage of planning the trial.

The first step in data analysis should be to draft an analysis plan, ideally when the study is being initially designed, in order to ensure that the design incorporates the elements (e.g. baseline measures of the outcome) that may be needed in the analysis. Each specific objective should be tied to planned analyses.

Following appropriate data management and cleaning, the data should be exported to a statistical analysis package for analysis. We recommend that the CONSORT Guidelines for reporting the results of trials are followed (2, 3, 28). For example, this includes a flowchart to show the numbers screened, eligible, excluded, and recruited. The numbers randomized to each arm are also shown, with details of numbers lost to follow-up, and included in the final analysis.

Analyses should include a comparison of baseline characteristics of participants by arm in order to describe the trial population and to assess whether there is balance in key characteristics between arms. For continuous variables that follow a normal distribution, the data can be summarized as a mean and standard deviation; otherwise a median and interquartile range is preferable. For categorical variables, the number and proportion of participants in that category should be shown, by arm. Although a common error is to show a p-value to compare baseline characteristics by arm in a randomized trial. This is incorrect, as we know that any differences have occurred by chance, by definition, through the randomization process.

Intention-to-treat analyses and missing outcome data

The key strength of an RCT is to be able to assess causal relationships, through avoiding confounding—i.e. the only difference between the two groups of participants at baseline should be the intervention condition. The best way to preserve this benefit of randomization is to analyse data as 'intention-to-treat' (ITT). The principle of ITT analyses is that participants are analysed in the groups to which they have been randomized. This means that participants are analysed in their randomization group, regardless of whether or not they received or adhered to the intervention, and also participants who are lost to follow-up should also be included. The latter issue is often a problem, as participants who are lost (e.g. because of death, moving away, withdrawal) will usually not have outcome data. A full ITT analysis will use statistical methods to impute the missing outcome data, but if the proportion with missing data is small, a 'complete case' analysis can be performed, in which analyses are restricted to participants who do have observed outcome data. This is a common approach, but it may cause bias if the outcome is related to the probability of being lost to follow-up—and this is often the case in mental health intervention trials. For example, in the MANAS randomized trial of treatment for CMD, 13% of participants were not seen at the 6-month endpoint (10). These 'lost-to-follow-up' participants were more likely to be young and male, than those seen at the endpoint. The primary analysis included only participants seen at follow-up, but a secondary (sensitivity) analysis was conducted to impute outcomes for those missing, using their baseline characteristics. In this example, results were similar for the complete case and imputed analysis. Analyses by level of adherence to the protocol can also be informative, but it is important to note that these 'per protocol' analyses are non-randomized comparisons and subject to bias.

Effect modification and mediating factors

The overall effect of the intervention will be captured in the primary analysis of the trial, but further analyses are often useful to understand the mechanisms by which the intervention works, and to identify sub-groups of participants who may respond particularly well or poorly to the intervention.

Moderators are variables that affect the intervention effect, i.e. the effect of the intervention on the trial outcome is modified (altered) depending on the value of the moderating variable. For example, a cluster randomized trial among children affected by war in Sri Lanka (34) was conducted to test the hypothesis that a 15-session CBT intervention delivered in schools by non-specialized personnel would lead to improved child mental health outcomes. The researchers stated a priori that they were interested in examining moderators (gender and age) that had previously been shown to moderate the effects of similar interventions for children affected by armed conflict. The trial showed that overall there was no effect of the intervention, but significant effects were seen among younger children, and among boys for some outcomes. This indicates that age, and to some extent gender, modified the intervention effect in this trial.

Mediators are factors that are on the causal pathway between the intervention and the trial outcome. In the Sri Lankan trial, the authors identified coping behaviour as a potential mediator of the intervention effect. This was because the intervention aimed to enhance coping behaviours, which in turn were expected to directly improve trial outcomes. However, in this trial there was no evidence that outcomes differed by coping behaviour, suggesting that this did not act as a mediator in this study.

Conclusion

In this chapter we have outlined the key principles in design and analysis of trials for mental health. We have focused on randomized trials as these are the gold-standard trial design, as this design minimizes confounding due to other factors and enables us to draw conclusions about the effectiveness of the intervention. Other key principles of trial design include a clearly stated, testable research hypothesis, well-defined outcomes, appropriate choice of the control condition, masking of providers and participants where possible, and appropriate analysis plans.

References

1 Araya R, Rojas G, Fritsch R, Gaete J, Rojas M, Simon G, et al. (2003) Treating depression in primary care in low-income women in Santiago, Chile: a randomised controlled trial. Lancet, 361(9362):995–1000.

2 Campbell MK, Elbourne DR, Altman DG (2004) CONSORT statement: extension to cluster randomised trials. BMJ, 328(7441):702–8.

3 Schulz KF, Altman DG, Moher D (2011) CONSORT 2010 statement: updated guidelines for reporting parallel group randomised trials. Int J Surg, 9(8):672–7.

4 Tyler KM, Normand SL, Horton NJ (2011) The use and abuse of multiple outcomes in randomized controlled depression trials. Contemp Clin Trials, 32(2):299–304.

5 Goldberg JF, Perlis RH, Ghaemi SN, Calabrese JR, Bowden CL, Wisniewski S, et al. (2007) Adjunctive antidepressant use and symptomatic recovery among bipolar depressed patients with concomitant manic symptoms: findings from the STEP-BD. Am J Psychiatry, 164(9):1348–55.

6 National Collaborating Centre for Nursing and Supportive Care (UK) (2005) Violence: clinical practice guidelines. The short-term management of disturbed/violent behaviour in in-patient psychiatric settings and emergency departments. London: Royal College of Nursing.

7 Raveendran NS, Tharyan P, Alexander J, Adams CE (2007) Rapid tranquillisation in psychiatric emergency settings in India: pragmatic randomised controlled trial of intramuscular olanzapine versus intramuscular haloperidol plus promethazine. BMJ, 335(7625):865.

8 Bhatia T, Agarwal A, Shah G, Wood J, Richard J, Gur RE, et al. (2012) Adjunctive cognitive remediation for schizophrenia using yoga: an open, non-randomized trial. Acta Neuropsychiatr, 24(2):91–100.

9 Rahman A, Malik A, Sikander S, Roberts C, Creed F (2008) Cognitive behaviour therapy-based intervention by community health workers for mothers with depression and their infants in rural Pakistan: a cluster-randomised controlled trial. Lancet, 372(9642):902–9.

10 Patel V, Weiss HA, Chowdhary N, Naik S, Pednekar S, Chatterjee S, et al. (2010) Effectiveness of an intervention led by lay health counsellors for depressive and anxiety disorders in primary care in Goa, India (MANAS): a cluster randomised controlled trial. Lancet, 376(9758):2086–95.

11 Hayes R, Moulton L (2009) Cluster randomised trials. London: Chapman & Hall.

12 Doig GS, Simpson F (2005) Randomization and allocation concealment: a practical guide for researchers. J Crit Care, **20**(2):187–91; discussion 91–3.

13 Piaggio G, Elbourne DR, Altman DG, Pocock SJ, Evans SJ (2006) Reporting of noninferiority and equivalence randomized trials: an extension of the CONSORT statement. JAMA, **295**(10):1152–60.

14 Titov N, Andrews G, Davies M, McIntyre K, Robinson E, Solley K (2010) Internet treatment for depression: a randomized controlled trial comparing clinician vs. technician assistance. PLoS One, **5**(6):e10939.

15 Badrasawi MM, Shahar S, Abd Manaf Z, Haron H (2013) Effect of Talbinah food consumption on depressive symptoms among elderly individuals in long term care facilities, randomized clinical trial. Clin Interv Aging, **8**:279–85.

16 Leontjevas R, Gerritsen DL, Smalbrugge M, Teerenstra S, Vernooij-Dassen MJ, Koopmans RT (2013) A structural multidisciplinary approach to depression management in nursing-home residents: a multicentre, stepped-wedge cluster-randomised trial. Lancet, **381**(9885):2255–64.

17 TenHave TR, Coyne J, Salzer M, Katz I (2003) Research to improve the quality of care for depression: alternatives to the simple randomized clinical trial. Gen Hosp Psychiatry, **25**(2):115–23.

18 Howard L, Thornicroft G (2006) Patient preference randomised controlled trials in mental health research. Br J Psychiatry, **188**:303–4.

19 Freedland KE, Mohr DC, Davidson KW, Schwartz JE (2011) Usual and unusual care: existing practice control groups in randomized controlled trials of behavioral interventions. Psychosom Med, **73**(4):323–35.

20 Mohr DC, Spring B, Freedland KE, Beckner V, Arean P, Hollon SD, et al. (2009) The selection and design of control conditions for randomized controlled trials of psychological interventions. Psychother Psychosom, **78**(5):275–84.

21 Patel VH, Kirkwood BR, Pednekar S, Araya R, King M, Chisholm D, et al. (2008) Improving the outcomes of primary care attenders with common mental disorders in developing countries: a cluster randomized controlled trial of a collaborative stepped care intervention in Goa, India. Trials, **9**:4.

22 Nyunt MS, Fones C, Niti M, Ng TP (2009) Criterion-based validity and reliability of the Geriatric Depression Screening Scale (GDS-15) in a large validation sample of community-living Asian older adults. Aging Ment Health, **13**(3):376–82.

23 Rothwell PM (2006) Factors that can affect the external validity of randomised controlled trials. PLoS Clin Trials, **1**(1):e9.

24 Kirkwood BR, Sterne JAC (2003) Essential medical statistics. Oxford: Blackwell Publishing.

25 Zhong B (2009) How to calculate sample size in randomized controlled trial? J Thorac Dis, **1**(1):51–4.

26 Hayes RJ, Bennett S (1999) Simple sample size calculation for cluster-randomized trials. Int J Epidemiol, **28**(2):319–26.

27 Pocock SJ (1983) Clinical trials: a practical approach. London: Wiley.

28 Piaggio G, Elbourne DR, Pocock SJ, Evans SJ, Altman DG (2012) Reporting of noninferiority and equivalence randomized trials: extension of the CONSORT 2010 statement. JAMA, **308**(24):2594–604.

29 National Institutes of Health (1998) NIH policy for data and safety monitoring. <http://grants.nih.gov/grants/guide/notice-files/not98-084.html>.

30 NIMH Collaborative HIV/STD Prevention Trial (2007) Role of the data safety and monitoring board in an international trial. AIDS, **21**(2):S99–102.

31 National Institutes of Health (2007) NIMH policy on data and safety monitoring in extramural investigator-initiated clinical trials. <http://www.nimh.nih.gov/funding/grant-writing-and-application-process/nimh-policy-on-data-and-safety-monitoring-in-extramural-investigator-initiated-clinical-trials.shtml>.

32 Leon AC (2012) Independent data and safety monitoring in psychiatric intervention research. J Clin Psychiatry, **73**(2):e257–63.

33 Kane JM, Sanchez R, Perry PP, Jin N, Johnson BR, Forbes RA, et al. (2012) Aripiprazole intramuscular depot as maintenance treatment in patients with schizophrenia: a 52-week, multicenter, randomized, double-blind, placebo-controlled study. J Clin Psychiatry, **73**(5):617–24.

34 Tol WA, Komproe IH, Jordans MJ, Vallipuram A, Sipsma H, Sivayokan S, et al. (2012) Outcomes and moderators of a preventive school-based mental health intervention for children affected by war in Sri Lanka: a cluster randomized trial. World Psychiatry, **11**(2):114–22.

Chapter 5

Defining relevant outcomes

Paul Bolton and Judith Bass

Introduction

While mental health problems can cause mortality, currently the main purpose of mental health services is to reduce morbidity and improve client wellbeing. In terms of mental health outcomes this translates into two priority types of outcome measures for both services and trials—reduction in burden of mental health symptoms and improvement in ability to function, particularly with respect to fulfilling one's roles within family and community.

Reduced function, particularly in tasks for daily living, is the main change by which mental and psychosocial problems adversely affect both the people who have these problems and those around them. Inability to do tasks for oneself and all the other tasks that form one's role as a father/mother/parent/community member results in tasks not being done or having to be done by others. Loss of non-task functions like socializing also affect the quality of life of the family and community. Therefore, outcomes related to function and specifically to the ability to perform locally relevant activities (as defined by culture and circumstances) are a major means of evaluating the negative impact of mental health and psychosocial problems, while improvement in this area can be considered one of the most important expected outcomes of mental health and psychosocial programmes.

The burden of mental health symptoms can include functional deficits, but, as used in this chapter, the term mainly refers to changes in thoughts and emotions that are distressing to the patient and those around them and that contribute to functional deficits. Deficits in this context refer to reduced ability to engage in activities of daily living related to caring for oneself and others in the family, and participating in the community. As in physical health, symptoms tend to occur in patterns which together constitute disorders. One of the major debates in global mental health has been around the cross-cultural applicability of mental disorder descriptions used in western countries (and therefore outcomes and instruments based on them)—the extent to which individual symptoms and how they group together vary according to culture and circumstances (1). Dealing with this issue is one of the content areas of this chapter, with examples drawn from our work specifically with vulnerable and trauma-affected populations.

In addition to the outcome measures of function and symptoms, which should be common to all outcome assessments, additional outcomes commonly assessed in mental health treatment trials include:

- questions about exposure to potentially traumatic events (PTEs) or other stressful circumstances that contribute to mental health problems;
- coping and social support information;
- health care or other service utilization;
- economic outcomes;
- stigma; and
- risky behaviours, including the use and abuse of drugs and other substances.

This chapter describes outcomes related to all of these categories, with emphasis on function and mental health symptoms. Trials may also include outcome measures that specifically reflect other issues specific to the population and their situation, the specific concerns of researchers or service providers, or the type of intervention being studied. There are no fixed rules about which types of outcome to employ except that function and mental health symptoms should always be included. As most mental health interventions target mental health symptoms, the main focus of this chapter is to describe an approach to deciding which symptom outcomes to assess in a trial and how to define these outcomes.

Data sources for deciding outcomes

Four sources of information inform the decision of which outcomes to use and how to measure them:

1 *Existing literature.* This includes literature on the population being studied and similar populations describing their important mental health issues. Studies of the prevalence of problems are helpful in deciding on priorities but are uncommon for populations in LAMIC. Qualitative or anthropologic studies are particularly useful where they describe the population's priority problems from their own viewpoint. This is particularly helpful when working with a new population or one that has undergone recent changes (such as conflict, displacement, or disaster).

The literature review should also include studies on what has been found effective for the proposed outcomes. Emphasis should be on reviewing studies among the same populations and those facing similar challenges, noting which outcomes improved and which did not.

2 *Experts.* These include experts on the study population and/or similar populations. They can provide valuable advice on the types of outcomes likely to be important and amenable to locally feasible interventions.

3 *Local stakeholders.* These include existing local providers of physical care, mental health care providers including government, non-government organizations (NGOs), and other professional organizations, and other prominent people and organizations that have an interest in the community's welfare and knowledge about their problems (i.e. traditional healers, religious figures, and local leaders).

4 *Local population.* Any discussion of relevant outcomes raises the question 'relevant for whom?' Views taken from the literature and other stakeholders are important

but must be weighed against the views of the local population. Researchers should not assume that the views of local stakeholders and prominent people will be representative of those of the general population. Stakeholders often come from different backgrounds or circumstances than many of the study population and may hold different views and priorities, which is why we recommend that members of the study population be consulted separately. Understanding their views is critical if the intervention is to engage their cooperation during and after the trial. Trials focused on outcomes that the population either do not understand or do not consider important are less likely to engage their interest or result in services that people will access.

Of these four data sources, the first three are straightforward. The literature is organized into searchable databases and stakeholders and experts are accustomed to formulating their views on request and require no special methods to interview. Obtaining the population's views is more difficult, particularly from those who are not accustomed to being interviewed. Collecting data that reflects what the study population thinks requires systematic open-ended interviewing methods. Therefore, in this chapter, we will focus on collecting information from the population. There are many open-ended interviewing methods, both individual and group, and describing the various options is beyond the scope of this chapter. Instead we describe one approach to using qualitative open-interview methods to assess population views and how (in combination with the other three data sources) this information can be used to inform the selection of outcomes and the design of outcome measures. Much of the material presented here draws from a manual of research methods which readers can access for further details.[1]

Understanding population priorities

Qualitative methods are designed to investigate how local people understand their own situation, with emphasis on understanding local concepts and language usage. These methods are particularly useful for obtaining local input on decisions related to relevant outcomes. Here we list some of the ways in which these methods can inform outcome selection, along with brief examples:

1 *Identifying priority mental health problems among local people.* A 2007 qualitative assessment of violence-affected populations in Aceh, Indonesia, found that anxiety and depression and not post-traumatic stress were the major problems faced by the population following exposure to extreme stressors (2).

2 *Identifying relevant co-occurring psychosocial problems.* A 2008 qualitative study of formerly trafficked girls in Cambodia found that the social consequences (i.e. rejection by former friends, family, community, and society at large) were important consequences of having been abused (3). In 2012, survivors of sexual violence in the Democratic Republic of Congo described fear and hopelessness as well as abandonment by their husbands, reportedly because of fear of disease, as co-occurring psychosocial issues (4).

[1] <http://www.jhsph.edu/research/centers-and-institutes/center-for-refugee-and-disaster-response/response_service/AMHR/dime/index.html>

3   *Understanding local perceptions of what constitute important areas of function related to daily living, as the basis for a local function measure.* A study of new mothers in the capital of the Democratic Republic of Congo identified specific functions
related to taking care of their baby, including washing the baby and washing the
diapers, that helped to identify women who were having difficulties functioning in
their roles as mothers (5).

One way the authors have used qualitative methods to explore these issues is through
rapid studies that combine three qualitative methods: free listing, key informant interviews, and focus groups. The study begins with free listing interviews among respondents representing a broad spectrum of the population (by gender, age, socioeconomic
status, ethnicity, geography, and any other variables that may significantly affect responses). When the focus is on identifying priority problems (for example) respondents are asked to name and briefly describe all the problems affecting local people.
Emphasis is on identifying as many potentially important problems as possible that
could serve as intervention targets. 'Potentially important' refers to problems that are
frequently mentioned by respondents (suggesting that they are priority issues), and are
potentially amenable to interventions. For mental health the focus is on identifying
problems that are mental health related, defined as those related to thinking, feeling,
and/or relationships.

Once potentially important problems are identified in the free lists they are then
investigated in more detail in key informant interviews. Here persons from the population who are particularly knowledgeable about the selected problems are interviewed
in detail about those problems.[2] Local perceptions of functioning are also explored by
free listing interviews (usually at the same interview) by asking respondents to identify
activities that people regularly do. This is then followed by focus groups of men and
women, usually separately, to identify activities not included in the Free Lists and to
review and prioritize the Free List activity results.

The processes for using data from these qualitative interviews to inform the selection, adaptation, and testing of specific outcome measures, along with examples, are
now discussed.

Development of specific outcome measures

Assessment of function—local measures

Like mental health instruments, many of the available function assessment instruments
were created in western countries. Others, like the WHO Disability Assessment Schedule (DAS) (6), were developed specifically for cross-cultural use. The WHODAS 2.0 (6)
and short-form health survey (SF-36) (7) have been found to have good psychometric
properties across many populations (for examples of studies see 8–11). However, being
fixed instruments, they do not necessarily include or reflect specific priority activities
of local people. Priority activities can vary by culture, situation, age, and gender and are
often tied to interpretations and expectations of specific roles different individuals have

---

[2]   These persons are identified at the end of the free list interviews: interviewees are asked to
name local persons who are knowledgeable about the problems they have identified.

within their families and communities. The variation in activities of daily living requires the development of locally defined function assessments for different situations and/or cultures. This locally defined function instrument can be used alongside the standard function instruments to assess both broad functional categories comparable across cultures (using standard instruments) and activities of local importance (using locally defined measures). Examples of standard instruments like the WHODAS 2.0 and the SF-36 are well described elsewhere (6, 7) and so are not described further here.

Locally defined function instruments developed by the authors have generally focused on activities that local people do to care for, or contribute to, the wellbeing of themselves, their families, and their communities. As mentioned previously, for each community the local function instrument is based on qualitative interviews with a representative sample of the population to be studied, using both free listing interviews and focus group discussions. Qualitative interviewing methods are a useful data source for this type of information because of their emphasis on not leading respondents, making it more likely that responses will really reflect local priorities.

Free list interviews are the first activity. For function free lists, men and women are separately asked to describe all the tasks and activities that men/women regularly do. This may include specific reference to activities done to care for themselves, their family, and their community in order to focus on activities that affect others and that are important aspects of their regular family and community roles. This can be done by asking each respondent to list separately the activities referring to care for self, family, and community (i.e. three lists for each person). All respondents' responses for each free list are then combined into a single composite (or summary) list, ordered according to how many respondents mentioned each activity. This is done separately for men and women. Focus group discussions are then convened, with participants selected in the same way as the free list respondents, with separate groups for men and women. Each group is asked the same function free list questions, as well as sharing the results of the previously completed free lists which focus group respondents review and comment on.

The interviewers and study coordinator together review the free list and focus group data. For each of the categories of self, family, and community activities they select the most frequently mentioned activities that also meet the following four criteria:

1 *Inability to do the activity will clearly affect others*

This criterion is optional as programmes may decide that activities that clearly affect individuals are priorities regardless of their impact on others. On the other hand, if there are many activities reported and not all need be included in the instrument, priority should be given to those that affect the most people. For example, in a study in Rwanda, 'praying' was frequently mentioned as an activity that people did to care for themselves. However, it was not included as a function question because it was not clear that inability to pray would adversely affect others. On the other hand, 'washing oneself' was included, as it was clear that if a person were unable to do this, others would have to do it for them (12).

2 *The activity is not actually the same as (or part of) another activity on the list*

This is best explained by an example. In Uganda some men listed 'sending children to school' as an important activity in caring for the family. But their descriptions made it clear that their major activity was to earn enough money to pay the fees. 'Sending children to school' was therefore removed since it was covered under the 'earning money' activity already listed. Avoiding this issue is done by reviewing the short description of each activity collected as part of the free listing interview of what the person actually does (in this case, earning money) rather than considering only the end result (that children go to school).

3 *The activity is clearly done by a large majority of the study population*

The qualitative study should identify specific tasks that people often do. As with any specific task, there will be some people who do not do that task. For example, caring for one's children is a very important task for women in most countries, but may not apply to women who do not yet have children. If the study population consisted of many unmarried women this might not be a useful item for a function instrument. This issue led to the decision to generate separate function assessments for men and women, since they divide important tasks between them in most cultures.

4 *The activity is done frequently, such as daily or at least monthly*

Tasks that are important but are done rarely are less likely to show change when assessed as an outcome for a trial. Therefore, although important and done by many, they are not included in most outcome measures. For example, burying the dead would not be included except in circumstances of high mortality.

The most frequently mentioned activities in each category (self, family, and community) that meet these four criteria constitute the local function assessment section. The number of activities chosen for each category depends on the desired length of the instrument and the number of activities that are frequently mentioned. For example, if only three self-care activities were mentioned by more than a few respondents or agreed to by focus group participants, then only those three would be included.

The purpose of the local function instrument is to assess important activities that someone who belongs to the study population would regularly do. If the study population includes people who are experiencing ongoing trauma or living in an insecure environment, the nature of these activities may be different than for a non-trauma-affected population or populations living in a stable environment. For this reason, it is important to ensure that the free list and focus group data used to create the function items are generated from respondents who are the same or similar to the trial study population.

Mental health and psychosocial problems

Investigation of how local people perceive and prioritize their mental health and psychosocial problems is important in deciding which problem(s) to address and therefore which outcomes to use. Most often this decision is based on input from researchers or other outside expert(s), based on a review of available literature and their own experiences, both of which are often derived from work with other populations. While this input is important, those deciding which mental health and psychosocial problems to address tend to focus on the most dramatic or negative experiences of the population and to address problems likely to arise from those experiences or the problems they expect to be most important based on work with other populations. For example, when working with populations affected by traumatic experiences it is commonly assumed that PTSD is the major mental health problem, based on many survey studies that have found PTSD to be prevalent in such populations.

Once a problem has been identified and selected researchers should not assume that the problem will be expressed in similar ways across populations; that symptoms, causes, and effects will generally be the same. While quantitative surveys in non-western cultures appear to confirm the existence and similarity of the common mental disorders of depression, anxiety, and PTSD across cultures, these studies have generally used questionnaires based on symptoms found among western populations. Since questionnaires use closed and/or leading questions (i.e. multiple choice or yes/no response options), a respondent need not understand the question (or recognize the symptom) in order to respond. This raises doubt about whether the results of such interviews alone really constitute evidence for the local existence of a problem and how it is manifested. Standard questionnaires based on already identified mental health and psychosocial problems also do not provide an effective means of identifying whether there are other problems or symptoms that are locally important but not included in the questionnaires.

Qualitative methods provide a more open and less leading approach to identifying the important mental health problems of a given population at a given point in time. If the priority problems described by local people based on non-leading interviewing methods match those given by other populations (or from western psychiatry) there is a much greater likelihood that those same problems really do occur locally. A variety of qualitative study methods can be used to identify and describe priority mental health and psychosocial problems. Here we describe a process that the authors have used in multiple countries and contexts which parallels the approach described for assessment of function.

The qualitative study methods include free listing to identify key mental health and psychosocial problems and key informant interviews to provide detailed descriptions of the problems (i.e. symptoms and signs, causes, and effects), what people currently do about the problems, and what people believe should be done. This provides the basis by which the local descriptions can be compared with descriptions from western-based psychiatry or elsewhere. (These interviews also provide information on selecting appropriate and acceptable interventions for the trial, although this is beyond the scope of this chapter.)

The qualitative data are used to answer the following questions as the basis for deciding what problems (and therefore outcomes) should be studied:

1 *Does the suspected problem(s) occur in the population?*

Implementing organizations and research teams normally begin their work with preliminary assumptions about the types of problems that exist among the study population. Qualitative open-ended interviewing methods allow the implementing organizations and researchers to learn from the local population if these suspected problems really are relevant in the local context, and if there are other problems that deserve investigation. This is because open-ended non-leading interviews that produce descriptions of problems similar to those of other groups are better indicators that the population truly has that problem, compared with responses to lists of leading questions on a questionnaire.

2 *What does the problem 'look like' locally?*

Open-ended interviewing methods allow the study team to understand the local pres-entation of mental health and psychosocial issues, using the terminology and idioms of the target population themselves. For example, a qualitative study conducted in 2006 with trauma-affected populations in Tamaulipas, Mexico, identified locally relevant terms for mental health and psychosocial issues, such as: (1) *depresión* for feeling im-potence or hopelessness, crying all the time, picking fights with others, thinking of suicide; (2) *nervios* for symptoms related to fear and anxiety, such as hypervigilance, re-experiencing, dissociation, avoidance; and (3) *se queden traumados* for problems with interpersonal relationships as a result of a basic lack of trust, a pervasive sense of fear and withdrawal from relationships, as well as problems with drinking and taking drugs (13).

In our experience with trauma-affected populations in low-income countries, quali-tative study respondents almost always describe most of the established symptoms of major depression and anxiety and many of those of PTSD. However, there is always some variation in the local symptoms and how they are expressed. For example, we rarely see depression, anxiety, and PTSD symptoms grouped into the same discrete syndromes as we found in the Mexico example; more commonly they occur in different combinations which vary by culture and situation.

3 *Do local people consider it a problem?*

Even if the mental health or psychosocial 'problem' occurs in the population and is rec-ognized in ways similar to other populations, it may not necessarily be considered to be a problem. This is particularly important where people might recognize the symptoms, but may not think that they are problematic for the people experiencing them. For example, in some communities, hearing voices is considered to be in communication with spirits or the dead rather than a symptom of psychosis.

4 *Do people consider the selected problem(s) to be a priority?*

Populations in need of assistance programmes tend to have many problems. If a pro-gramme is seen to be addressing a minor issue, or an issue affecting only a few people, local people may not consider it worthy of support. For example, when investigating the problems among adolescents in internally displaced persons camps in northern Uganda, depression, anxiety, and behavioural problems associated with life in the camps were higher priority issues than the mental health effects of past traumas (14). Based on these results, an intervention trial was designed around interventions that addressed the priority issues (15) which then became the trial outcomes, rather than focusing on trauma-based issues such as PTSD which were present but a lower priority.

Developing mental health and psychosocial symptom outcome measures

Our experience is that the above questions should be investigated and the answers should guide the selection of the primary mental health and psychosocial outcomes for the trial. Having selected which outcomes to prioritize, the next issue is how to assess them; i.e. how to construct measures for these outcomes. If the descriptions of the problems from the qualitative study are consistent with specific western mental health and psychosocial concepts, this is preliminary evidence that these concepts are locally valid/applicable, and that existing instruments based on these concepts might be adapted for local use. For example, if the free list and key informant respondents describe a depression-like problem with most of the signs and symptoms identified in the DSM and International Classification of Diseases (ICD) diagnostic manuals for depression disorders, then it is appropriate to use an existing screener or assessment tool for depression disorders. Existing instruments are then reviewed and those whose content most closely matches that of the qualitative data are selected. When the local description generally matches a predefined disorder but additional important symptoms from the qualitative study are not in the standard instrument, questions on these symptoms should be added to the standard instrument using the existing question format.

Typically, the selected instrument will also include symptoms that did not emerge in the qualitative data. These symptoms are generally retained. The rationale for this is that qualitative methods are effective tools for understanding local concerns, and particularly for identifying new local concepts, but they are not appropriate for determining which content to exclude. The fact that an issue or concept does not appear in the interviews or is mentioned only rarely is not proof that the issue/concept is not important. The weak exclusionary power of the qualitative study is due to small sample sizes and reliance on convenience or non-random sampling which increases the likelihood of non-representative samples.

The final result, after assessment tools are selected and local symptoms are added, is an expanded version of the existing instrument. An instrument is selected and adapted in this way for each of the priority problems identified in the qualitative study (e.g. if depression and post-trauma symptoms were both identified as priority problems, then both a depression instrument and an instrument measuring post-trauma symptoms would be adapted).

An example of this process is the instrument development process that the authors conducted in Kurdistan, Iraq. Informants from a qualitative study of male and female torture survivors described combinations of symptoms highly consistent with the following mental disorders described in other countries: *generalized anxiety disorder, major depression, PTSD,* and *traumatic grief,* as well as less-structured psychosocial problems related to poor relationships within the family and marginalization from the wider Kurdish society (16). Based on these findings we selected as outcome measures three existing questionnaires that together reflected most of the symptoms respondents described: the Hopkins Symptom Checklist for *anxiety* and *depression* (HSCL-25) (17, 18), the symptom section of the Harvard Trauma Questionnaire (HTQ) (19) for *PTSD,* and the Inventory of Traumatic Grief (20). These standard questionnaires were further adapted with the addition of several local depression-related, PTSD-related, and traumatic grief items.

There are a wide range of pre-existing assessment tools used worldwide to assess various mental health and psychosocial problems. Each tool has its own strengths and weaknesses, and most have been validated among at least some populations. Some instruments are freely available, while others require permission of the creators and/ or a paid licence. Literature and internet searches on the mental health problem(s) to be addressed will provide the names of the most common instruments as well as (in the case of the published literature) the populations for which the instruments have been validated and used. A review of published articles related to the identified mental health and psychosocial problems among the population to be studied (or similar populations) will identify researchers who can be contacted for suggestions on measures and assessments.

Other potentially relevant assessments and outcomes

In addition to function and mental health symptoms outcome measures, additional outcome measures may be added depending on local priorities, the nature of the study population, or pre-existing concerns of researchers or service providers. Some of the more common examples are now briefly described.

Risky behaviours including substance abuse

Many studies have documented co-morbidity between substance abuse and other mental health problems (e.g. 21). Identifying appropriate outcome measures can be done using the same process for function and symptoms: i.e, on the basis of compatibility of local qualitative data on substance abuse with existing measures. Measures typically refer to both the types of abuse and frequency. One substance abuse measure that has been developed for cross-cultural use is the Alcohol, Smoking, and Substance Involvement Screening Test (ASSIST) (22).

Trauma exposure assessments

Most surveys of trauma-affected populations include questions about the types of PTEs the respondents have witnessed and/or experienced. There are many indexes of PTEs in the literature which could be adapted using similar methods as described for the function and symptom scales (i.e. by matching information and wording from the qualitative study to existing items on a PTE index or by adding specific context-relevant PTEs). If an existing instrument does not match any of the data from the qualitative studies, the study team may opt to generate their own index that includes experiences that were directly mentioned in the qualitative study. For example, in Thailand with a study involving Burmese victims of torture and trauma, items such as 'Forced labour' and 'To be sold/trafficked' were included in the section evaluating exposure to PTEs (23).

The trauma-experience section is not used as an outcome measure, but these data can be used to investigate the degree and/or number of incidents a person has witnessed and/or experienced and their correlation with the person's psychological wellbeing and level of improvement during the trial.

Coping behaviours and degree of social support

Standard measures that ask about general coping activities (such as playing sports or praying) or levels of social support (such as number of close friends) may be relevant as outcome measures for some intervention trials that include activities around building social capital and/or improving positive coping practices. Examples of standard questionnaires for measuring coping strategies are the Brief COPE (24) and the Cross-Cultural Coping Scale (25). The Medical Outcomes Study (MOS) Social Support Survey (26), the Interpersonal Support Evaluation List (27), and the Multidimensional Scale of Perceived Social Support (28) are all examples of standard measures of social support that have been adapted to different populations. A simple checklist may also be used to find out which strategies or types of social support have been used by the study participant over a defined period of time (last month, year, ever, etc.). Items in the checklist can be derived from interviews with local informants regarding what is available. It can also include items derived from the qualitative study. This includes data from the key informant interviews referring to what people currently do to address their problems.

Stigma

In many cultures stigma can be a major barrier to seeking care and treatment for those with metal health problems. Stigma refers to the discrimination that society exerts on persons, as well as the feelings that this attitude and behaviour causes in the person experiencing the discrimination. Instruments (and interventions) to address stigma may address one or both meanings. There are many types of stigma-related measures (for a comprehensive review see 29). Some examples of instruments that measure the discrimination that society exerts on persons are the Key Informant Questionnaire (30) and a vignette-based questionnaire (31). There are also instruments aimed at measuring both the discrimination that society exerts on persons and the subjective feelings of discrimination. These include the Explanatory Model Interview Catalogue (EMIC) (32) and the Perceived Devaluation–Discrimination Questionnaire (33), among others.

As with trauma exposure, stigma may not be a specific trial outcome (unless the intervention targets stigma-related issues). However, data on discrimination and perceived stigma can still be used to investigate reasons why certain individuals drop-out of treatment or do not use the services that are provided, as well as the correlation of perceived stigma with the person's psychological wellbeing. As with mental health and function scales, processes should be in place to evaluate the reliability and validity of any adapted stigma- or discrimination-specific scale within the local context (see, for example, 34).

Service utilization outcomes

While most trials focus on testing interventions to reduce the burden of mental health problems, some interventions also aim to increase use of other health services. For example, there is evidence that HIV-infected people with severe depression symptoms are less likely to initiate antiretroviral treatment even if they are eligible, or, once initiated, have lower adherence rates to treatment protocols than individuals without significant depression symptoms (35, 36). Mental health interventions that seek to improve use of services should include service use questions as study outcomes. Questions can include a list of services used, the frequency of use, and in-depth questions about service content and quality.

Economic outcomes

Most populations in LAMIC with significant mental health problems also have many other problems including poverty. Little is known about how improvements in mental health affect poverty but, given the strong link between mental health problems and impairment in functioning, it seems likely that mental health problems would make it more difficult to engage in economic activities. Our own trials of mental health interventions have found improvements in locally defined tasks involving providing financially for one's family.

The use of poverty indicators as outcomes for mental health trials is not yet common. Agreed-upon indicators and approaches to assessing levels of poverty for use in trials are still being developed. The choice of economic outcomes depends on the study context (i.e. what type of work is available in that area), the level of detail required (i.e. total days worked in a defined period of time, total amount of money earned, etc.), and the extent to which changes are expected (i.e. if the outcomes are to be assessed after a short period of time, then less change will be expected than after longer term follow-up). Examples of economic indicators include asset indices (i.e. what types of things people own), food consumption measures, hours worked, and money earned. Examples can be found on the World Bank's websites for the Living Standards Measurement Study[3] and the Core Welfare Indicators Questionnaire[4].

Conclusion

Defining relevant outcomes for mental health and related intervention trials requires consultation with experts and stakeholders, but also with the population for whom the services are being provided. This latter group is not often consulted systematically, but doing so is necessary to ensure that their priorities are being addressed within the study objectives and outcomes, and that instruments measure the outcomes accurately. This will increase the likelihood that a service found to be effective will be sustained after the trial is completed. Otherwise there is a risk that once a trial is over services will not be supported or used because they were never a priority for the population.

Finally, changes in the types of outcomes assessed in these trials are not static. Once the intervention is over these changes may continue to accumulate or decline with time. Wherever possible it is important to measure outcomes over extended periods, at specific intervals after the intervention is completed (e.g. 6 or 12 months or even later). Outcomes that measure amount of change, such as symptom or function scale scores, will be more sensitive to tracking long-term impacts of interventions as opposed to outcomes that only measure the presence/absence of a problem or activity.

---

[3] <http://econ.worldbank.org/WBSITE/EXTERNAL/EXTDEC/EXTRESEARCH/EXTLSMS/0,,contentMDK:21610833~pagePK:64168427~piPK:64168435~theSitePK:3358997,00.html>

[4] <http://web.worldbank.org/WBSITE/EXTERNAL/COUNTRIES/AFRICAEXT/EXTPUBREP/EXTSTATINAFR/0,,contentMDK:21104598~menuPK:3091968~pagePK:64168445~piPK:64168309~theSitePK:824043,00.html>

References

1 Bass J, Bolton P, Murray L (2007) Do not forget culture when studying mental health. Lancet, **370**:918–19.

2 Poudyal B, Bass J, Subyantoro T, Jonathan A, Erni T, Bolton P (2009) Assessment of the psychosocial and mental health needs of the violence-affected populations in Birueuen, Aceh: a qualitative study. Torture, **19**(3):218–26.

3 Bolton P, Nadelman S, Wallace T (2008) Qualitative assessment of trafficked girls in Cambodia. Report for World Vision International, Boston, MA.

4 Bass JK, Annan J, Murray SM, Kaysen D, Griffiths S, Cetinoglu T, et al. (2013) Controlled trial of psychotherapy for sexual violence survivors in DR Congo. N Engl J Med, **368**:2182–91.

5 Bass JK, Ryder RW, Lammers MC, Mukaba TN, Bolton PA (2008) Postpartum depression in Kinshasa, Democratic Republic of Congo: validation of a concept using a mixed-methods cross-cultural approach. Trop Med Int Health, **13**:1534–42.

6 World Health Organization (2012) WHO Disability Assessment Schedule 2.0. <http://www.who.int/classifications/icf/whodasii/en/index.html>

7 Ware JE Jr, Sherbourne CD (1992) The MOS 36-item short-form health survey (SF-36): I. Conceptual framework and item selection. Med Care, **30**(6):473–83.

8 Buist-Bouwman MA, Ormel J, De Graaf R, Vilagut G, Alonso J, Van Sonderen E, et al. (2008) Psychometric properties of the World Health Organization Disability Assessment Schedule used in the European Study of the Epidemiology of Mental Disorders. Int J Meth Psychiatric Res, **17**(4):185–97.

9 Hoopman R, Terwee CB, Devillé W, Knol DL, Aaronson NK (2009) Evaluation of the psychometric properties of the SF-36 health survey for use among Turkish and Moroccan ethnic minority populations in the Netherlands. Qual Life Res, **18**(6):753–64.

10 Lam ETP, Lam CLK, Lo YYC, Gandek B (2008) Psychometrics and population norm of the Chinese (HK) SF-36 Health Survey : version 2. HK Pract, **30**(4):185–98.

11 Luciano JV, Ayuso-Mateos JL, Fernández A, Serrano-Blanco A, Roca M, Haro JM (2010) Psychometric properties of the twelve item World Health Organization Disability Assessment Schedule II (WHO-DAS II) in Spanish primary care patients with a first major depressive episode. J Affect Dis, **121**(1):52–8.

12 Bolton P, Tang A (2002) An alternative approach to cross-cultural function assessment. Soc Psychiatry Psychiatr Epidemiol, **37**(11):537–42.

13 Betancourt T, Gray A, Bolton P (2006) Qualitative assessment of trauma affected populations in Tamaulipas, Mexico. Report for the USAID Victims of Torture Fund, Boston, MA.

14 Betancourt TS, Speelman L, Onyango G, Bolton P (2009) A qualitative study of mental health problems among children displaced by war in northern Uganda. Transcult Psychiatry, **46**(2):238–56.

15 Bolton P, Bass J, Betancourt T, Speelman L, Onyango G, Clougherty KF, et al. (2007) Interventions for depression symptoms among adolescent survivors of war and displacement in northern Uganda: a randomized controlled trial. JAMA, **298**(5):519–27.

16 Bolton P, Michalopoulos L, Ahmed AM, Murray LK, Bass J (2013) The mental health and psychosocial problems of survivors of torture and genocide in Kurdistan, northern Iraq: a brief qualitative study. Torture, **23**(1):1–14.

17 Hesbacher PT, Rickels K, Morris RJ, Newman H, Rosenfeld H (1980) Psychiatric illness in family practice. J Clin Psychiatry, **41**(1):6–10.

18 Winokur A, Winokur DF, Rickels K, Cox DS (1984) Symptoms of emotional distress in a family planning service: stability over a four-week period. Br J Psychiatry, **144**:395–9.

19 Mollica RF, Caspi-Yavin Y, Bollini P, Truong T, Tor S, Lavelle J (1992) The Harvard Trauma Questionnaire. Validating a cross-cultural instrument for measuring torture, trauma, and posttraumatic stress disorder in Indochinese refugees. J Nerv Ment Dis, **180**(2):111–16.

20 Prigerson HG, Shear MK, Jacobs SC, Reynolds CF 3rd, Maciejewski PK, Davidson JR, et al. (1999) Consensus criteria for traumatic grief. A preliminary empirical test. Br J Psychiatry, 174:67–73.

21 Conway KP, Compton W, Stinson FS, Grant BF (2006) Lifetime comorbidity of DSM-IV mood and anxiety disorders and specific drug use disorders: results from the National Epidemiologic Survey on Alcohol and Related Conditions. J Clin Psychiatry, **67**:247–57.

22 World Health Organization (2012) ASSIST project—Alcohol, Smoking and Substance Involvement Screening Test. <http://www.who.int/substance_abuse/activities/assist/en/index.html>.

23 Lee C, Robinson C, Bolton P (2011) Qualitative assessment of displaced persons in Mae Sot, Thailand affected by torture and related violence in Burma. Report for the USAID Victims of Torture Fund, Boston, MA.

24 Carver CS (1997) You want to measure coping but your protocol's too long: consider the Brief COPE. Int J Behav Med, **4**(1):92–100.

25 Kuo BCH, Roysircar G, Newby-Clark IR (2006) Development of the cross-cultural coping scale: collective, avoidance, and engagement coping. Meas Eval Couns Dev, **39**(3):161–81.

26 Sherbourne CD, Stewart AL (1991) The MOS social support survey. Soc Sci Med, **32**(6):705–14.

27 Cohen S, Hoberman HM (1983) Positive events and social supports as buffers of life change stress. J Appl Soc Psychol, **13**(2):99–125.

28 Zimet GD, Dahlem NW, Zimet SG, Farley GK (1988) The multidimensional scale of perceived social support. J Pers Assess, **52**(1): 30–41.

29 Link BG, Yang LH, Phelan JC, Collins PY (2004) Measuring mental illness stigma. Schizophr Bull, **30**(3):511–41.

30 Wig N, Suleiman M, Routledge R, Srinivasa Murthy R, Ladrido-Ignacio L, Ibrahim H, et al. (1980) Community reactions to mental disorders—a key informant study in three developing countries. Acta Psychiatr Scand **61**(2):111–26.

31 Link BG, Phelan JC, Bresnahan M, Stueve A, Pescosolido BA (1999) Public conceptions of mental illness: labels, causes, dangerousness, and social distance. Am J Public Health, **89**(9):1328–33.

32 Weiss MG. (1997) Explanatory Model Interview Catalogue (EMIC): Framework for comparative study of illness. Transcult Psychiatry **34**:235–263.

33 Link BG, Cullen FT, Frank J, Wozniak JF (1987) The social rejection of former mental patients: understanding why labels matter. Am J Sociol, **92**(6):1461–500.

34 Brohan E, Clement S, Rose D, Sartorius N, Slade M, Thornicroft G (2013) Development and psychometric evaluation of the discrimination and stigma scale (DISC). Psychiatry Res, **208**(1):33–40.

35 Gonzalez JS, Batchelder AW, Psaros C, Safren SA (2011) Depression and HIV/AIDS treatment nonadherence: a review and meta analysis. J Acquir Immune Defic Syndr, **58**(2):181–7.

36 Blashill AJ, Perry N, Safren SA (2011) Mental health: a focus on stress, coping, and mental illness as it relates to treatment retention, adherence, and other health outcomes. Curr HIV/AIDS Rep, **8**(4):215–22.

Chapter 6

Economic evaluations in global mental health

Iris Mosweu and Paul McCrone

Introduction

Mental health disorders are common and contribute substantially to the burden of disease in LAMIC, but somehow fail to attract appropriate policy attention and funding (1–5). Neuropsychiatric conditions account for about 10% of the burden in LAMIC, while AUD contribute close to 4% (4, 6, 7). The consequences of mental health disorders are marked and not only affect the patient, but also can have negative impacts on families, health and social systems, employers, and society more generally. Even though a relatively small proportion of health budgets are allocated for these conditions, the economic burden is quite substantial (4, 8, 9). Mental disorders are responsible for increased health and social care costs, poor quality of life, increased risk of disability, reduced work-hours, possible loss of employment, and high risk of mortality (9, 10). Mental illness is even more devastating when it co-exists with chronic life-threatening ailments such as diabetes and HIV. People with these physical conditions are highly susceptible to anxiety, depression, suicide, and alcohol and drug abuse, and such co-morbidity also has debilitating effects on quality of life, costs, and clinical outcomes (11–13). In addition, mental illness has been reported to have a negative interaction with poverty, which, though not established whether it is causal or not, consequently can lead to stagnation of development (14).

Despite this high disease burden, the majority of health care resources are still largely targeted at communicable diseases, while the allocation of mental health is < 1% of the health budget in many LAMIC (5, 15–17). Shortages in human resources and services for mental health care persist and, where available, they are likely to be inequitably distributed (18). The 'treatment gap' for mental health disorders differs across LAMIC (19) and some (20) suggest that this variation may stem from differences in the magnitude of 'Group 1 burden' (i.e. resulting from HIV, malaria, tuberculosis, maternal and perinatal ailments, and poor nutrition). High burden in these areas results in most countries allocating the highest proportion of their health budget to these conditions and it is unlikely that evidence regarding the cost-effectiveness of specific interventions for their treatment compared to the cost-effectiveness of treatments for mental health problems is particularly influential (20).

There have been calls to prioritize mental health in LAMIC, and efforts are being made globally to ensure that mental health services are integrated into primary care and availed to those in need of them (21, 22). WHO's mhGAP is one such initiative, aiming to support LAMIC in making efforts to 'scale up' mental health services (23). Similarly, research has been carried out to determine the possible costs of scaling up an essential mental health package in LAMIC (15). Albeit a fundamental step in ensuring access, scaling up mental health services does not come without challenges, including deciding on the type of services to prioritize, user discrimination, shortage of resources, and establishing how to allocate resources. Integrating mental health services into primary health care is a means to an end, and more needs to be put in place to ensure its success (14, 23).

Decisions regarding the introduction and scaling up of mental health services in all countries require information on effectiveness and, due to scarce resources, also cost-effectiveness. This is arguably most important in countries with fewer resources and yet it is in these countries that economic evaluation is least used. Other considerations to factor into decisions about prioritizing mental health include affordability, equity, and non-health benefits. The purpose of this chapter is to describe key methods used in economic evaluation and to provide examples of how these have been used in LAMIC.

Although quite modest, evidence in most LAMIC suggests that a significant amount of resources need to be injected into health systems in order to scale up to provide a core package of mental health (an additional $0.20/capita per year for low-income countries and $0.30 for middle-income) (15), but this additional cost appears quite reasonable when compared to that required to address other conditions contributing to the high global burden of disease (15). Nevertheless, affordability is a crucial consideration in addition to that of cost-effectiveness (which does not necessarily mean cost savings) and this may be particularly so in LAMIC.

Types of economic evaluation

In all health systems, mental health disorders compete for finite resources with other health conditions, and economic evaluation can be used to identify health interventions that proffer good 'value for money'. Economic evaluation has gained increasing support as a guiding principle in promoting allocative efficiency and for evaluating costs and effects of interventions in health systems. Its results contribute to informing policy decisions for selecting services and interventions that produce the greatest benefit for the available budget (8, 24, 25).

In general, economic evaluation compares two or more alternative courses of action and takes one of several five forms. All measure costs in monetary terms but differ in the approach to outcome measurement. Examples of the methods described here will be provided later in this chapter. A *cost-minimization analysis (CMA)* only seeks to identify the intervention with the least costs, as it is normally preceded by knowledge that outcomes are identical. These are similar to cost-offset studies that compare costs incurred with costs saved, while ignoring the user's outcomes (i.e. not even assuming identical outcomes as with CMA) and hence are not usually regarded as formal economic evaluations (25–29).

Cost-consequences analysis (CCA) considers costs alongside multiple clinical outcomes, in recognition of the broader picture of the impact of the intervention. CCA allows decision-makers to form their own judgement of the relative importance of competing alternatives and because of the multiplicity of outcome measures does not require the formal synthesis of these with costs.

Cost-effectiveness analysis (CEA) is a frequently used method, and this formally links costs and a single outcome measure to provide a measure of relative cost-effectiveness known as the incremental cost-effectiveness ratio (ICER). The ICER is a measure of the cost per additional unit of health gain produced by one intervention compared with another. In this approach, benefits are valued using condition-specific or service-specific measures such as symptom changes, depression-free days, or life years gained. The equation for ICER is:

$$ICER = (C1 - C2)/(E1 - E2)$$

where C1 and E1 are the cost and effect in the intervention or treatment group, while C2 and E2 are the cost and effect in the control care group.

CEA can only be performed if the effects of interventions under review can be measured on the same scale, in which case the use of life years saved or disability days avoided are more desirable. Higher ICERs indicate lower cost-effectiveness.

Cost-utility analysis (CUA) is the newest approach to economic evaluation and involves measuring outcomes in terms of generic (i.e. not condition-specific) measures, solving the problem of multiple outcomes. In some countries the most common approach is to use quality-adjusted life years (QALYs), where time in a health state, or over a follow-up period in a study, is adjusted according to an index of quality of life anchored by 1 representing full health and 0 representing death. Such an index can be derived from the EQ-5D or SF-36 but requires a set of 'utility weights' to be available. While QALYs are useful, this is mainly so in countries that have decided to adopt their use in official decision-making strategies, such as in England.

In LAMIC it is far more common to use disability-adjusted life-years (DALYs). These were designed by the World Bank and WHO in 1993 to measure the global burden of disease (29, 30). The rudimentary concept behind DALYs is to think of health benefits in terms of a reduction in disease burden. DALYs incorporate age-weights and signify a year of life at full health that is lost, and are generally represented by 'DALYs averted', which have similarities to QALYs but where a disability index scores 0 to represent no disability and 1 for total disability. QALYs and DALYs originate from different disciplines; they measure and interpret disease weights differently, which subsequently leads to dissimilar results, and therefore the question of whether one is better than the other seems irrelevant. An important issue in this discussion relates to the weights used in the calculation of these measures, since they are normally adjusted to account for life expectancy of those affected. Concerns about fairness (i.e. they favour the young over the old) have been raised over time, with some arguing that using DALYs may be at odds with equity principles (31). The debate on the appropriateness of QALYs in assessing benefits of health interventions found its way into the mental health area, with suggestions that commonly used generic measures of health such as the EQ-5D may be unsuitable and unresponsive to changes in mental health conditions such as schizophrenia and other complex conditions (e.g. dementia). As such, there is on-going work to develop relevant QALYs in mental health (32–34).

Finally, *cost-benefit analysis (CBA)* attaches monetary values to benefits, making it easier to estimate a net benefit of a particular intervention in health with investments in other sectors, such as education. Willingness-to-pay (WTP) and the human capital approach (HCA) are two methods used for measuring health effects in monetary terms. However, both are problematic—the former due to the complexity of asking for hypothetical values to be placed on health outcomes and the latter because of its focus on employment gains rather than other outcomes.

The type of economic evaluation to undertake is mainly determined by the specific research question being asked. In this chapter we concentrate on CEA, as it appears to be the most commonly used method, even in LAMIC (35). A CEA can be carried out alongside a clinical trial or by using simulation models (27–29, 36). Whatever approach is used, an economic evaluation requires the collection of service use, cost and effectiveness data, which are then combined to determine the cost-effectiveness of different options.

Cost-of-illness studies

Burden of disease or cost of illness (COI) studies translate the societal impact of disease into costs. These studies are useful in priority-setting, budget justification, and resource allocation in health systems (37, 38). However, there is an on-going debate on the usefulness of COI studies, with critics questioning the value in identifying areas of high expenditure which does not necessarily prove inefficiency or wastefulness in a health system (39). Another argument suggests that COI studies have the potential to divert policy-makers' attention away from conditions/areas where the economic burden is more limited. CEA seems to be favoured over COI because of the former's comparative advantage in contributing to allocative efficiency in health systems compared with the latter (39).

In a recent example of a COI study from Thailand, Phanthunane and colleagues estimated the economic burden of schizophrenia (40). This study used data from a survey conducted among patients and carers attending mental health hospitals in 2008 and from this the authors estimated the costs associated with hospital outpatient and inpatient care, medication, patient travel time, and the indirect costs linked to productivity losses both for patients and their families. The study estimated that the costs of schizophrenia amounted to US $925 million per annum in Thailand, or US $2600 per person. Loss of employment, absenteeism, and presenteeism accounted for the highest proportion (61%) of costs. Within hospital costs, hospital admissions accounted for 50%. Although the authors aimed to adopt a societal perspective in their costing, the exclusion of some intangible and other indirect costs such as those associated with contacts with the criminal justice system may have led to an underestimation of costs.

Evidence on cost-effectiveness of services in LAMIC

There is a paucity of evidence regarding the cost-effectiveness of health interventions in LAMIC compared to developed countries and this is particularly so for mental disorders (35, 41). In places where such evaluations have taken place, it is not clear if the results of these studies are being used to inform resource allocation priorities or not. However, results from existing studies are encouraging and provide a persuasive economic case for mental health interventions, especially for common disorders, in LAMIC (42–47).

Available cost-effectiveness studies in LAMIC have concentrated more on evaluating packages of care rather than the traditional comparative analysis of individual services or interventions, (44–46). Studies that have evaluated such packages of care have reported favourable cost-effectiveness thresholds (42, 46). For example, the results of an economic evaluation of a 'task-shifting' intervention for common mental disorders in India, which used community lay workers to provide front-line care, reported a high probability of cost-effectiveness at relatively low thresholds for unit improvements in outcome (42). The authors concluded that there may be a persuasive case for using community lay workers, since this appeared to be dominant (i.e. improves health outcomes and lowers costs) when time costs are added to the analysis.

In Nigeria, Gureje and colleagues (46) undertook a CEA of a package of selected interventions for common neuropsychiatric disorders. The study identified different interventions that produced the best health and social benefit for patients, within the budget, and together they produced one extra year of life for less than the average per capita income of Nigeria, and this was deemed to indicate cost-effectiveness according to WHO guidelines for cost-effective interventions (47).

Gureje and colleagues had access to costs collected for the WHO CHOICE (*CHO*osing *I*nterventions that are *C*ost-*E*ffective) project (46). These data are from a regional database and the authors were concerned about their generalizability at country-level, and hence engaged in a process of contextualization. This involved identifying conditions responsible for the highest mental health burden in Nigeria, followed by adapting the WHO database figures to the local context for demographic data, epidemiological figures, effectiveness, health use, and costs associated with certain mental health conditions in Nigeria. Experts fed into this process by suggesting expected service use, and an exercise of validating individual unit costs for relevant services was undertaken. Although this was not a traditional costing exercise which would be undertaken in similar circumstances, the use of local data provides reasonable estimates for Nigeria. The authors make important observations relating to the challenges of adopting traditional economic evaluation methodologies in LAMIC, where some data are not readily available, and the lack of health structures to implement the intervention(s) being evaluated.

Many studies have focused on interventions for depression, probably because this is the most common mental health disorder in LAMIC, accounting for approximately 65 million DALYs lost globally. One study (45) used a simulation (Markov) model to assess the *value of investing* in group psychotherapy (with booster sessions to deal with recurrence) for depressed patients in Uganda. The study reported that the intervention resulted in I $1150 per QALY gained (falling below Uganda's gross domestic product (GDP) per capita), compared to no intervention. Although it was thus deemed to be cost-effective, the major limitation of this study relates to the use of some data (model parameters) from HIC, which introduces a certain amount of uncertainty in the model. Uncertainty was dealt with through the use of deterministic sensitivity analysis (one- and two-way, which is less robust compared to probability sensitivity analysis (PSA)), which investigates the joint uncertainty of all model parameters and variables.

Two Chilean studies (37, 44) have assessed the cost-effectiveness of an intervention for depressed women in a primary care setting. Araya and colleagues (37) used data from an RCT and based the ICER on a cost per depression-free day, while Siskind and colleagues (44) used a Markov model to evaluate stepped care compared to no intervention. The latter used QALYs in the denominator of the ICER and extrapolated beyond the observed period to calculate lifetime costs and effects. The two studies found conflicting results, with Siskind and colleagues reporting an ICER of I $113 per QALY gained and Araya and colleagues reporting higher health system costs, but with an incremental cost per depression-free day of US $1.04. These results demonstrate clearly how context-specific economic evaluation can be, which is why in most cases generalizability (to other settings) can be problematic. However, a key message here is that stepped care is cost-effective in both the short and long term.

Comparisons have also been made of drug treatments and psychological therapies for depression. One such study conducted alongside a randomized trial in India established that fluoxetine improved clinical outcomes and represented good value for money in a general health care setting, albeit in the short term (43). To cost the interventions, the authors used an adapted version of the Client Services Receipt inventory, originally designed to collect health and social service use for mental health patients in the UK, but flexible to use in various contexts (48). Using this service use measure data relating to hospital use, medication, and informal care for the all study participants were collected (43). Productivity losses for both patients and their carers were also estimated and so was travel time to the clinic and waiting time. In the absence of pre-existing unit costs, Patel and colleagues applied a micro-costing strategy to estimate these, a method more comprehensive compared to the one used in (46). These were then attached to service use data to estimate costs per month (after relevant price adjustments).

WHO, through CHOICE, has contributed substantially to the evidence regarding mental health care in LAMIC (15, 47, 49–51). WHO CHOICE was developed in 1998 and designed to provide economic evidence on a range of health interventions. Through this initiative, a standard method for CEA has been created, including the production of regional databases of a summary of cost-effectiveness of varying interventions. Evidence from the WHO CHOICE initiative presents results for predefined regions of the WHO, and instead of using patient-level data, the work adopts a population-level CEA, which is argued to be more consistent and 'generalized' (52).

In another (population) model, Chisholm and colleagues (51) evaluated the cost-effectiveness of multiple depression interventions in 14 WHO epidemiological subregions and attempted to estimate how these could decrease the burden of disease associated with depression. The study used a state transition model to evaluate depression interventions used in primary care to estimate DALYs averted by the use of antidepressants and/or psychotherapy compared to a do-nothing scenario over a period of 10 years. Model parameters, including effectiveness rates and costs, were obtained from a variety of sources, with some costs being derived from primary data. Uncertainty was dealt with by the use of one-way sensitivity analyses, best- and worst case scenarios, as well as probabilistic sensitivity analysis. Although this model is based on a WHO subregion, estimated costs and effects can be adapted for specific country-level analyses. The study reports a potential reduction of the disease burden of between 10 and 30%, and acceptable cost-effectiveness thresholds (each DALY averted costing less than the annual average per capita income) for pharmacotherapy, including older antidepressants with or without collaborative care.

Despite heterogeneity among the studies, there is overwhelming evidence of the value in investing in mental health interventions and services in developing countries. Economic studies carried out in LAMIC do not seem to explicitly follow the traditional scientific techniques of economic evaluation, which may consequently compromise the robustness of the analysis. There is some variation in methods used in different studies relating to outcome measures (QALYs, life years, or DALYs), perspective, type of analysis, type of modelling study, sensitivity analyses (deterministic or probabilistic), cost-effectiveness thresholds applied, and indeed the interventions themselves (packages, behavioural, drugs, etc.). The variability in interventions has the potential to hinder the interpretation and conclusion of results, as well as their generalizability. However, evaluations from HIC may not always be generalizable to LAMIC due to different service structures and associated costs.

Earlier reviews of economic evidence of interventions for mental health (24, 53) found that studies conducted then were methodologically poor, primarily because of a limited understanding of economic evaluation and failure to include health economists, which consequently resulted in failure to adhere to rudimentary principles in the area.

Specific issues associated with undertaking economic evaluation in LAMIC

Although economic evaluation is quite pragmatic and has been identified as a guiding principle for effective resource allocation, it is not without challenges, especially in LAMIC where the adoption of its techniques has been limited. In general, studies in HIC tend to use more advanced methods of economic evaluation and this is often due to requirements of research funding bodies. NICE in England is responsible for considering both the effectiveness and cost-effectiveness of treatments and then making recommendations based on the combined evidence. NICE consequently provides guidelines and recommendations for economic evaluations, which provide an impetus for economic evidence submitted for review to meet certain criteria.

The WHO CHOICE initiative came close to creating standardized methods for economic evaluations in LAMIC, but the regional databases of unit costs are not updated annually. Those who use them have to adjust for inflation, which may be a limitation as these costs may be affected by other factors. WHO also recommends the use of gross national product (GNP) for cost-effectiveness thresholds, but whether or not policymakers in LAMIC have made these formal in their specific countries is unclear. There are, however, other initiatives in LAMIC such as the mhGAP, which aims to support LAMIC in scaling up mental health services, which are expected to adopt cost-effective ways of diagnosing and managing mental health conditions (23). Alongside this initiative, WHO has also designed a costing tool that aims to identify resource gaps, assess affordability, as well as estimate resources required for scaling up mental health in LAMIC (23). The lack of cost-effectiveness thresholds guidance in most LAMIC combined with other issues related to the adoption of economic evaluation techniques in those settings presents researchers with particular challenges.

Demand for economic evaluations

Existing evidence from LAMIC suggests that results of economic evaluations are not widely used in decision-making, priority setting, and resource allocation (41). It is therefore not surprising that guidance regarding the conduct and design of economic evaluations is not generally available. It seems as though most of the studies in these countries are primarily funded by donors, hence indicating the influence that may be yielded by these institutions in research and possibly decision-making.

Availability of unit cost data

The numerator of the ICER represents incremental costs of interventions under evaluation, and these costs are calculated based on the quantity of health and social care services used by participants and relevant unit costs. One of the challenges in economic evaluation is deciding which services/costs to include, and this is especially challenging in LAMIC, where measurement may be problematic and unit costs of specific health services are not readily available. Although the inclusion of some services such as hospital costs is explicit, others such as productivity costs, informal care costs, costs to the criminal justice system, and out-of-pocket payments for health services, transport, and traditional healers may not be so obvious, and hence likely to be left out. Researchers tasked with undertaking economic evaluations therefore have to embark on a lengthy (and sometimes costly) exercise of calculating unit costs of services accessed by respondents in their study, or using proxy measures that may have limited validity.

Lack of formally established cost-effectiveness thresholds

ICERs reveal the extra cost incurred by an intervention to produce a unit improvement in outcome. This then needs to be compared to a threshold to determine whether it represents good value for money. In England, NICE recommends the use of QALYs, and cost-effectiveness is achieved if the cost per QALY is below £20,000–£30,000. Other countries that have adopted the QALY measure have their own threshold values. In the US, a value of $50,000 was recommended by the Panel on Cost-Effectiveness in Health and Medicine in 1996 (54), but some have challenged the relevance of this figure and its consistency with current societal preferences in the US (55).

The above thresholds are to a certain extent arbitrary, but they do have common resonance. In LAMIC the situation is less clear. WHO uses a more general criterion based on using DALYs. The Commission on Macroeconomics and Health through the WHO CHOICE project has recommended the use of GDP, since it is a readily available indicator, to derive the following three categories of cost-effectiveness: *highly cost-effective* (less than GDP per capita), *cost-effective* (between one and three times GDP per capita), and *not cost-effective* (more than three times GDP per capita). However, having a threshold is really only useful if data on cost-effectiveness in relation to the thresholds are used for decision-making purposes.

LAMIC are increasingly recognizing the importance of incorporating cost-effectiveness in priority setting in health care, which is evident from the growth in designing, undertaking, and using the evidence from economic analyses to influence both clinical and policy decision-making (56, 57). Brazil and Thailand established Health Technology Assessment structures as part of their Ministries of Health (58, 59). These not only focus on health systems research, but also conduct economic appraisals with the aid of methodological guidelines for economic evaluation created solely for this purpose (58). In South Africa there is evidence of a fragmented use of results from economic evaluations to set priorities and inform policy, albeit no formal guidelines (56).

Conclusion

Some, if not all, of the issues described in this chapter can be dealt with only if policy-makers in LAMIC take an interest in economic evaluation and decide to use it in evaluating individual interventions, and ultimately in priority setting and budget allocation. There is enough evidence globally indicating that a modest investment in interventions that proffer good value for money can potentially reduce the burden of mental health disorders. However, there is a paucity of similar evidence in prevention interventions and services in the developing world. While health economics studies tend to focus on the cost elements of service supply, its techniques can also be applied in promotion, prevention, and early interventions for suicide, anxiety, depression, psychosis, and conditions caused by alcohol and drug abuse. Investment in these may produce better cost-effective results compared to treatment interventions (46, 60, 61). Stigma is another important area in mental health as its presence in a society increases social isolation, whilst also prohibiting access to treatment. Investment in a social marketing campaign aimed at reducing stigma has produced cost-effective results (62), indicating that changing society's attitudes towards mental illness can proffer great economic benefits for the wider society.

Economic evaluation should, however, be seen as a means to an end. Assessing cost-effectiveness will be meaningless if access to services and interventions is restricted. Evidence from LAMIC suggests that there are challenges with access to mental health services associated with poverty, stigma, and health financing. Many LAMIC have no social welfare programmes or national health insurance, which leaves most of the burden on patients and their families. Out-of-pocket payments are still common and exemptions for the poor and vulnerable are not often in place. Stigma can potentially deter access to treatment, especially in communities where having a mental health condition is seen as a sign of mental weakness, or entangled with other cultural issues.

Economic evaluation studies in themselves are time-consuming and context-specific, and in some instances can be costly, which implies that investing in such studies and not using their results to inform health policy and resource allocation would in itself be an inefficient use of resources. The adoption of economic evaluation in health systems should be preceded by policy-makers' awareness of or training in the benefits of economic evaluation in priority setting and resource allocation.

References

1 World Health Organization (2001) The world health report 2001—mental health: new understanding, new hope. Geneva: WHO.

2 Lund C, Tomlinson M, De Silva M, Fekadu A, Shidhaye R, Jordans M, et al. (2012) PRIME: a programme to reduce the treatment gap for mental disorders in five low- and middle-income countries. PLoS Med, 9(12):e1001359.

3 Patel V, Araya R, Chatterjee S, Chisholm D, Cohen A, De Silva M, et al. (2007) Treatment and prevention of mental disorders in low-income and middle-income countries. Lancet, 370(9591):991–1005.

4 Lopez A, Mathers CD, Essati M, Jamison DT, Murray CJL (2006) Global burden of disease and risk factors. Washington, DC: World Bank.

5 Tomlinson M, Lund C (2012) Why does mental health not get the attention it deserves? An application of the Shiffman and Smith framework. PLoS Med, 9(2):e1001178.

6 Prince M, Patel V, Saxena S, Maj M, Maselko J, Phillips MR, et al. (2007) No health without mental health. Lancet, 370(9590):859–77.

7 World Health Organization (2008) Global burden of disease: 2004 update. Geneva: WHO.

8 Knapp M, (ed.) (1995) The economic evaluation of mental health care. Bury St Edmunds: Arena.

9 Kirigia J, Sambo L (2003) Cost of mental and behavioural disorders in Kenya. Ann Gen Hosp Psychiatry, 2(1):7.

10 Lund C, Myer L, Stein DJ, Williams DR, Flisher AJ (2013) Mental illness and lost income among adult South Africans. Soc Psychiatry Psychiatr Epidemiol, 48(5):845–51.

11 Molosankwe I, Patel A, José G, Knapp M, McDaid D (2012) Economic aspects of the association between diabetes and depression: a systematic review. J Affect Disord, 142(Suppl):S42–55.

12 World Health Organization (2008) HIV/AIDS and mental health Report. Geneva: WHO.

13 Lawler K, Mosepele M, Ratcliffe S, Seloilwe E, Steele K, Nthobatsang R, et al. (2010) Neurocognitive impairment among HIV-positive individuals in Botswana: a pilot study. J Int AIDS Soc, 13:15.

14 Lund C, De Silva M, Plagerson S, Cooper S, Chisholm D, Das J, et al. (2011) Poverty and mental disorders: breaking the cycle in low-income and middle-income countries. Lancet, 378(9801):1502–14.

15 Chisholm D, Lund C, Saxena S (2007) Cost of scaling up mental healthcare in low- and middle-income countries. Br J Psychiatry, 191:528–35.

16 Patel V. (2007) Mental health in low- and middle-income countries. Br Med Bull, 81–2:81–96.

17 Araya R. (2009) Invited commentary on . . . Mental health research priorities in low- and middle-income countries. Br J Psychiatry, 195(4):364–5.

18 Saxena S, Thornicroft G, Knapp M, Whiteford H (2007) Resources for mental health: scarcity, inequity, and inefficiency. Lancet, 370(9590):878–89.

19 Kohn R, Saxena S, Levav I, Saracenso B (2004) The treatment gap in mental health care. Bull World Health Organ, 82:858–66.

20 McBain R, Salhi C, Morris JE, Salomon JA, Betancourt TS (2012) Disease burden and mental health system capacity: WHO Atlas study of 117 low- and middle-income countries. Br J Psychiatry, 201(6):444–50.

21 Lund C, Petersen I, Kleintjes S, Bhana A (2012) Mental health services in South Africa: taking stock. Afr J Psychiatry (Johannesbg), 15(6):402–5.

22 World Health Organization (2008) Integrating mental health into primary care: a global perspective. Geneva: WHO.

23 World Health Organization (2010) mhGAP intervention guide for mental, neurological and substance use disorders in non-specialized health settings. Geneva: WHO.

24 Singh B, Hawthorne G, Vos T (2001) The role of economic evaluation in mental health care. Aust N Z J Psychiatry, 35(1):104–17.

25 Drummond M, Sculpher MJ, Torrance GW, O'Brien BJ, Stoddart GL (eds) (2005) Methods for the economic evaluation of health care programmes, 3rd edn, p. 379. New York: Oxford University Press.

26 Reed SD, Bakhai A, Briggs AH, Califf RM, Cohen DJ, Drummond MF, et al. (2005) Conducting economic evaluations alongside multinational clinical trials: toward a research consensus. Am Heart J, 149(3):434–43.

27 Briggs A, Claxton K, Sculpher M (2007) Decision modelling for health economic evaluation. Oxford: Oxford University Press.

28 Glick H, Doshi JA, Sonnad SS, Polsky D (2010) Economic evaluation in clinical trials. Oxford: Oxford University Press.

29 Gray AM, Clarke PM, Wolstenholme JL, Wordsworth S (2011) Applied methods of cost-effectiveness analysis in healthcare. Oxford: Oxford University Press.

30 Sassi F. (2006) Calculating QALYs, comparing QALY and DALY calculations. Health Policy Plan, 21(5):402–8.

31 Robberstad B. (2005) QALYs vs DALYs vs LYs gained: what are the differences, and what difference do they make for health care priority setting? Norsk Epidemiologi, 15(2): 183–91.

32 Brazier J. (2008) Measuring and valuing mental health for use in economic evaluation. J Health Serv Res Policy, 13(3):70–75.

33 Mulhern B, Rowen D, Brazier J, Smith S, Romeo R, Tait R, et al. (2013) Development of DEMQOL-U and DEMQOL-PROXY-U: generation of preference-based indices from DEMQOL and DEMQOL-PROXY for use in economic evaluation. Health Technol Assess, 17(5):v–xv, 1–140.

34 Mangalore R, Knapp M (2007) Cost of schizophrenia in England. J Ment Health Policy Econ, 10(1):23–41.

35 Hoque ME, Kahn JA, Hossain SS, Gazi R, Rashid H, Koehlmoos TP, et al. (2011) A systematic review of economic evaluations of health and health-related interventions in Bangladesh. Cost Eff Resour Alloc, 9:12.

36 Petrou S, Gray A (2011) Economic evaluation using decision analytical modelling: design, conduct, analysis, and reporting. BMJ, 342:d1766.

37 Araya R, Flynn T, Rojas G, Fritsch R, Simon G (2006) Cost-effectiveness of a primary care treatment program for depression in low-income women in Santiago, Chile. Am J Psychiatry, 163(8):1379–87.

38 Rice DP (2000) Cost of illness studies: what is good about them? Inj Prev, 6:177–9.

39 Byford S, Torgerson DJ, Raftery J (2000) Cost of illness studies. BMJ, 320:1335.1.

40 Phanthunane P, Whiteford H, Vos T, Bertram M (2012) Economic burden of schizophrenia: empirical analyses from a survey in Thailand. J Ment Health Policy Econ, 15(1): 25–32.

41 McDaid D, Knapp M, Raja S (2008) Barriers in the mind: promoting an economic case for mental health in low- and middle-income countries. World Psychiatry, 7(2):79–86.

42 Buttorff C, Hock RS, Weiss HA, Naik S, Araya R, Kirkwood BR, et al. (2012) Economic evaluation of a task-shifting intervention for common mental disorders in India. Bull World Health Organ, 90(11):813–21.

43 Patel V, Chisholm D, Rabe-Hesketh S, Dias-Saxena F, Andrew G, Mann A (2003) Efficacy and cost-effectiveness of drug and psychological treatments for common mental disorders in general health care in Goa, India: a randomised, controlled trial. Lancet, 361(9351): 33–9.

44 Siskind D, Araya R, Kim J (2010) Cost-effectiveness of improved primary care treatment of depression in women in Chile. Br J Psychiatry, 197(4):291–6.

45 Siskind D, Baingana F, Kim J. (2008) Cost-effectiveness of group psychotherapy for depression in Uganda. J Ment Health Policy Econ, 11(3):127–33.

46 Gureje O, Chisholm D, Kola L, Lasebikan V, Saxena B (2007) Cost-effectiveness of an essential mental health intervention package in Nigeria. World Psychiatry, 6(1):42–8.

47 Chisholm D (2005) Choosing cost-effective interventions in psychiatry: results from the CHOICE programme of the World Health Organization. World Psychiatry, 4(1):37–44.

48 Beecham J, Knapp M (2001) Costing psychiatric interventions. In: Thornicroft G (ed.) Measuring mental health needs. London: Gaskell.

49 Chisholm D (2005) Cost-effectiveness of first-line antiepileptic drug treatments in the developing world: a population-level analysis. Epilepsia, 46(5):751–9.

50 Chisholm D, Rehm J, Van Ommeren M, Monteiro M (2004) Reducing the global burden of hazardous alcohol use: a comparative cost-effectiveness analysis. J Stud Alcohol, 65(6):782–93.

51 Chisholm D, Sanderson K, Ayuso-Mateos J (2004) Reducing the global burden of depression: population-level analysis of intervention cost-effectiveness in 14 world regions. Br J Psychiatry, 184:393–403.

52 Acharya A, Adam T, Baltussen R, Evans D, Hutubessy R, Murray CJL, et al. (2003) Making choices in health: WHO Guide to Cost-Effectiveness Analysis. Geneva: WHO.

53 Evers S, Van Wijk A, Ament AJ (1997) Economic evaluation of mental health care interventions. A review. Health Econ, 6(2):161–77.

54 Weinstein M, Siegel JE, Gold MR, Kamlet MS, Russell LB (1996) Recommendations of the Panel on Cost-effectiveness in Health and Medicine. JAMA, 276(15):1253–8.

55 Braithwaite RS, Meltzer DO, King JT Jr, Leslie D, Roberts MS (2008) What does the value of modern medicine say about the $50,000 per quality-adjusted life-year decision rule? Med Care, 46(4):349–56.

56 Doherty J (2010) Cost-effectiveness analysis for priority-setting in South Africa—what are the possibilities? S Afr Med J, 100(12):816–21.

57 Doherty J (2009) Health policy analysis institutes: landscaping and learning from experience, South Africa. The case of the Health Economics Unit in South Africa. <http://www. who.int/alliance-hpsr/projects/witwatersrand_evidence/en/index.html>.

58 Tantivess S, Teerawattananon Y, Mills A (2009) Strengthening cost-effectiveness analysis in Thailand through the establishment of the health intervention and technology assessment program. Pharmacoeconomics, 27(11):931–45.

59 Vanni T, Luz PM, Ribeiro RA, Novaes HM, Polanczyk CA (2009) Avaliação econômica em saúde: aplicações em doenças infecciosas. Cadernos de Saúde Pública, 25(12):2543–52.

60 Mihalopoulos C, Vos T, Pirkis J, Carter R (2011) The economic analysis of prevention in mental health programs. Annu Rev Clin Psychol, 7:169–201.

61 Knapp M, McDaid D, Parsonage M (2011) Mental health promotion and mental illness prevention: the economic case. London: Department of Health.

62 Evans-Lacko S, Henderson C, Thornicroft G, McCrone P (2013) Economic evaluation of the anti-stigma social marketing campaign in England 2009–2011. Br J Psychiatry Suppl, 55:s95–101.

Chapter 7

Working with vulnerable populations

Examples from trials with children and families in adversity due to war and HIV/AIDS

Theresa S. Betancourt, William Beardslee, Catherine Kirk, Katrina Hann, Moses Zombo, Christine Mushashi, Fredrick Kanyanganzi, Morris Munyana, and Justin I. Bizimana

Introduction

This chapter discusses key issues to consider when conducting clinical trials with vulnerable children, youths, and families, with particular attention paid to groups affected by communal violence/war and families affected by HIV/AIDS. Across these contexts, there is an overlap of several forms of adversity and vulnerability which require careful attention from researchers. We also discuss ethical practices with vulnerable groups including the use of qualitative methods to enhance understanding of local perspectives and language around mental health problems and resilience, planning for appropriate referral networks before commencing research with vulnerable populations, adapting intervention trials to the needs of vulnerable populations, and applications of community-based participatory research (CBPR), such as inclusion of Community Advisory Boards (CABs). Such practices can be used to raise community awareness and increase community engagement in addressing mental health services needs in vulnerable populations, improve the sensitive implementation of clinical trials, and also facilitate the translation of findings in promoting practice and policy change. The chapter draws on examples from work in Sub-Saharan Africa and includes examples from our own research as well as that of other research teams working in diverse settings. We conclude with a series of recommendations for advancing research practices sensitive to the situation of vulnerable populations.

Commonly accepted definitions of *vulnerable populations* in clinical trials refer to groups susceptible to coercion or undue influence in research. These groups, as outlined in the US Department of Health and Human Services Regulations (45 CFR 46.111(b)) (1) include children, wards of the state, prisoners, pregnant women and fetuses, persons who are mentally disabled or otherwise cognitively impaired, and economically or educationally disadvantaged persons. Subsequently, many national and international regulatory bodies require that special consideration be given to protecting the welfare of these groups. Research is critically needed to design the best possible prevention and treatment approaches to advance the health and wellbeing of vulnerable populations, yet the conduct of such research must be carefully planned and executed, with priority attention given to ethical practice. Unfortunately recent history is rife with examples of research that has been conducted with little attention to strong ethical practice, particularly among minority communities and in LAMIC (2–5).

To illuminate some of these issues, we draw from research focused on the two exceptions to recent improvements in child health globally: populations affected by communal violence/war, and populations affected by HIV/AIDS (6, 7), with particular attention to work with children and work with economically disadvantaged populations. In these contexts, there is an overlap of several forms of adversity that must be considered in the design and implementation of clinical trials and other forms of mental health services research.

The reality of concentrated adversity in low-resource settings: HIV/AIDS, communal violence/war, and their co-existence

Populations affected by HIV/AIDS

HIV and AIDS have dramatically altered the lives of children and families worldwide. The pandemic's effect on child development and wellbeing has been especially profound. In the most-affected countries, such as Botswana and Zimbabwe, AIDS-related causes are now the leading contributors to death of children under the age of five (8). Globally, approximately 3.3 million children under the age of 15 are living with HIV and more than 230,000 died of AIDS in 2011 (9). As of 2009, 16.6 million children had lost one or both of their caregivers to AIDS (10). In many parts of the globe, young people, particularly young women, are at great risk of contracting the virus through sexual activity as well as sexual exploitation and abuse. Recent estimates indicate that 39% of all new HIV infections—approximately 2700 every day—are among young people between the ages of 15 and 24 (9).

HIV and AIDS also have broad effects on family functioning and mental health, making family-based work an important opportunity for prevention and intervention research. For instance, misinformation and fear in families affected by HIV may lead to painful interactions between parents and children, such as children being afraid to touch or kiss their caregivers, or to share their food. For parents, impairment and the attention directed at medical care and follow-up can mean less time for children and, in many families, children may begin to take on increasing responsibilities in the household in order to help the family survive. Family dynamics due to HIV may also bring additional negative consequences for child mental health. Research to date has demonstrated that families affected by HIV are characterized by higher levels of family violence, stigma, and parental mental health problems (11–18). These and other dynamics contribute to a higher risk of mental health problems in children affected by HIV/AIDS (19, 20).

Despite these risks, mental health needs of HIV-affected children often receive little attention as families struggle to address immediate medical concerns and the subsequent economic and social consequences of HIV (21–24). Preventive interventions that reduce the risk of mental health problems in HIV-affected children, including behavioural problems, may also prevent future HIV infection by decreasing HIV risk behaviour (25–29). Family-based interventions can improve quality of life for HIV-affected families (30), yet few evidence-based programmes exist to prevent mental health problems in HIV-affected children. Even fewer family-based interventions have been developed for use in Sub-Saharan Africa despite the region's high HIV prevalence (31, 32). Addressing misinformation and fear and strengthening caregiver–child relationships can have important preventive benefits for children in HIV/AIDS-affected families and can improve overall family functioning and health outcomes (30). As access to HIV testing and treatment becomes increasingly available in Sub-Saharan Africa, preventive programmes to support children and families identified as at high risk for mental health problems have the potential to be systematically integrated into the services provided to HIV-affected families (33).

Child health and wellbeing in regions affected by armed conflict

More than one billion children worldwide live in areas affected by armed conflict. Of these children, 30% are below the age of five (34). War-related violence has contributed to the displacement of an estimated 18 million children as of 2006, including 5.8 million child refugees and 8.8 million children internally displaced within their own countries (34, 35). Nearly half of all forcibly displaced individuals globally are children (36). Like HIV/AIDs-affected children, families affected by war and those living as refugees—both under active displacement and resettlement—face a massive reconfiguration of family roles and responsibilities as well as post-conflict stressors, such as food and housing insecurity, which exacerbate risks for mental health problems already elevated due to war-related violence exposure and loss.

In conflict-affected settings, deaths caused by war extend beyond violent killings or injuries; they set off a cascade of conditions threatening to caregiver and child mental health that are worsened by armed conflict. These factors include economic insecurity, weakened community structures, insufficient social services, poor access to education, destruction of local economies, and declines in health infrastructure (37). Of the many tragedies of war, growing attention has been paid to the involvement of children in armed conflict. It is estimated today that approximately 250,000 boys and girls under the age of 18 are involved in more than 15 active armed conflicts (38–41). Children associated with armed forces and armed groups often witness extreme violence and may also take part in committing atrocities. In some cases, children and youths may be forced to commit acts of violence against their own family or community members in direct attempts to sever ties between young people and their loved ones, making it difficult for them to run away from the armed group, fearing they will not be accepted back home.

All war-affected children, and child soldiers in particular, often live for years in environments that are frightening, unsafe, and marked by repeated abuse, neglect, and trauma. Studies have shown that children involved with armed forces and armed groups exhibit high rates of mental health problems (42), and the ability of former child soldiers to navigate reintegration in post-conflict settings may also be thwarted by community stigma and difficulties in interpersonal relationships (43–46). Case studies profiled in this chapter outline several sensitivities that must be considered when conducting clinical trials with children, youths, and families from such vulnerable backgrounds. Very few evidence-based mental health interventions have been adapted and tested among war-affected youth, and implementation research on the topic is altogether non-existent. Although research in high-income countries has identified common treatment elements important for improving mental health and functioning in violence-affected youth, these treatments have been largely untested in low-resource settings.

In many regions of the world, the effects of armed conflict and HIV/AIDS overlap, presenting a situation of compounded adversity. For instance, of the 25 countries with the highest proportion of children orphaned by AIDS, approximately one-third have been affected by armed conflict in recent years. Additionally, UNICEF estimates that two-thirds of all children without access to primary school globally live in regions affected by armed conflict (34).

Preparing to work in vulnerable communities

A basic principle of best practice in research with vulnerable groups is to consider the potential issues that may arise in mental health services research with such groups, to anticipate the risk situations that may arise, and to plan for referrals that will be necessary for appropriate responses. For example, interviews with participants may reveal a risk of harm situation due to ongoing abuse or suicidality. In this manner, risk of harm cases might be defined as situations that involve life and death situations or harm to the physical integrity of study participants. Such instances might refer to risk of suicide; risk of physical or sexual abuse; risk of harming another person; or risk of being a victim of a serious crime.

In conducting mental health research with vulnerable populations, a research team should anticipate coming into contact with a significant number of vulnerable youths and caregivers who will require appropriate responses to ensure participant safety in such instances, and referrals potentially to a higher level of care; this is particularly true in mental health services research and research with vulnerable populations where participants are often asked to share very sensitive and personal information (47–50) but live in settings where access to mental health services is poor. In our experience, these referrals on average are about 5% of a study population (46, 51, 52), but they involve serious cases that require serious responses. In our research in Sierra Leone alone, we have uncovered cases of young girls whose 'caregivers' were refusing consent. Upon further investigation, these individuals turned out to be unrelated adults in the community who had the girls involved in prostitution and wanted to deny access to group counselling and services being offered in the intervention research as it threatened their exploitative relationship. In such cases, the research team worked closely with the biological parents to ensure that the girls were removed from these exploitative situations and that social workers conducted follow-up case management.

In order to anticipate risk of harm situations and ensure adequate follow-up in our research in both Sierra Leone and Rwanda, we have developed risk of harm protocols that provide study staff with structured approaches to addressing high-risk situations, while ensuring safety and appropriate referral to available services. According to the protocol, those considered as being a risk to themselves or others or at risk of immediate harm due to abuse and neglect were referred for appropriate mental health care, social work services, and/or other appropriate authorities. A crucial part of the protocol is networking in advance with those who can provide such services to subjects who are identified as needing them. To anticipate and address the vulnerabilities, a research team may not always be located within service-rich environments. Indeed, in low-resource settings, few communities and even health systems may have awareness of the contributions of mental health to overall child and adolescent health and wellbeing, and few have the capacity to screen for or treat these conditions. Nonetheless, it is critical to anticipate and plan for referrals to other forms of supports and to consider other resources that may exist outside of formal services. For instance, in Rwanda, community health workers and local village leaders have been important in ensuring the safety and wellbeing of participants at risk of harm.

In practice, the use of a risk of harm protocol ensures that research team members are knowledgeable and prepared to respond to crises immediately, sensitively, and professionally. See the appendix for an example of a mental health risk of harm protocol used in collaborative research with Partners in Health (PIH) in Rwanda. The protocol describes instances that necessitate intervention by the study team should an indication of risk of harm be detected; outlines steps to take to activate the safety plan; and discusses appropriate responses to cases of varying severity. Emmanuel's story in the following case study highlights how the risk of harm protocol can ensure a research participant's safety.

Case study: Emmanuel

Emmanuel is a 15-year-old boy who lost both his parents to AIDS just months after he was born. Emmanuel is HIV-positive and now lives with his elderly grandmother in a rural area of eastern Rwanda. Despite the challenges early in life, Emmanuel has a positive relationship with his grandmother and they described having many characteristics of *kwizerana*, a local term to describe a strong, unified family. While overall a well-behaved child, Emmanuel frequently drinks *urwarwa*, a locally made alcohol from bananas, as a way to have fun. However, Emmanuel suffers from maltreatment and stigma in his community and feels isolated from his peers. Emmanuel has had thoughts of ending his life to escape stigma from neighbours who do not want him around their children because he is HIV-positive.

He dropped out of school as a result of stigma and harsh treatment from other children. Feeling as though there were no other options to escape the harassment, he planned to drown himself in the nearby river or disappear to Rwanda's capital city of Kigali. The field team spoke to Emmanuel's grandmother who was deeply worried about Emmanuel's suicidal thoughts. He had told her before that he wanted to commit suicide, or run away so no one would ever see him again. In addition to concerns about suicide, Emmanuel had not been adhering well to his antiretroviral therapy. He skipped doses when he was drinking, and sometimes went days without taking any medications; his grandmother even told him it was okay to not take his medicine if he was drinking *urwarwa* because it could interact with his HIV medication.

His *accompagnateur*, a community health worker who is tasked with visiting HIV-positive community members daily to provide medications, was not helping him to access medicines. As a result, he sometimes spent several days without taking any medication. As an additional hurdle to accessing services, the family is not currently covered by health insurance as they wait for their premium to be paid since they fall into a category of vulnerable families that qualify for free *mutuelle de santé*, Rwanda's community-based health insurance. Without health insurance, service costs are prohibitively high for Emmanuel and his grandmother.

Per the risk of harm protocol, Emmanuel's case triggered several red flags—suicidality, urgent medical concerns—and barriers to accessing services. With Emmanuel's permission to break confidentiality, and permission from his grandmother, the study team immediately contacted the health centre social worker and nurse at the health centre's infectious disease clinic. The social worker helped the family enroll in *mutuelle de santé* and immediately referred Emmanuel to Kirehe District Hospital for mental health services. A community health worker from a neighbouring village also agreed to watch over Emmanuel due to conflicts with the *accompagnateur* in his village and his adherence to his medications improved. He is no longer suicidal. His grandmother was also provided with psychoeducation to monitor his mental health needs and received follow-up visits from the social work team.

Emmanuel's case highlights the need to act quickly through all the possible intervention channels. As a result of the field team's preparedness, Emmanuel was kept safe and linked to ongoing care; several members of the health system acted quickly to ensure he received help for both his physical and mental health concerns.

Anticipating referral networks

Case study: Sierra Leone

In Sierra Leone, 11 years of civil war destroyed the country's infrastructure as well as its health and social services. At the end of the war, these public sectors were still not functioning (53). While a few such services were reinvigorated on a small scale, their funding usually came from foreign NGOs, and few of these programmes were able to be integrated and sustained within the country's health system after the surge of funding that had been available at the war's end dried up. When our research team began work in Sierra Leone in 2002 to conduct a longitudinal study of war-affected youth (LSWAY), many NGOs were still operating in the region to serve war-affected youth. However, over time, as the country transitioned from a crisis situation to fragile state, many of these programmes discontinued their operations. As a result, our research-related outreach was some of the only follow-up that many of the war-affected youths in our sample had received.

Outreach was conducted as part of our longitudinal study, which examines risk and protective factors shaping social reintegration and psychosocial adjustment in war-affected youth in Sierra Leone over time. Interviews were conducted in three phases in 2002, 2003–4, and 2008 (51, 54). Before we began the phase III interviews in 2008 (55–57), we spent 7 months preparing mechanisms and identifying formal and non-formal supports to help anticipate and prepare to address risk of harm cases. We did this by phoning and visiting with youth and family service providers in each of the six districts where the study would be active. Upon meeting providers at each agency, we inquired about the nature of the services provided and associated costs, fee waivers for impoverished groups, how to make a referral, and whom at the agency to contact. In order to do so, we emphasized organizations that could provide mental health and social services without 'labels,' such as services specific to only one gender or to children with a narrow eligibility criteria (e.g. only HIV-positive children) and those providing free or low-cost care. As a result, in follow-up research conducted in 2008, the research team was able to successfully respond to nine risk of harm cases identified as comprising a range of risk situations, from untreated medical needs and hunger to young people who had a history of suicide attempts and active suicidal ideation. A larger group of participants demonstrating less severe risk of harm cases was also provided with information about resources in their community given their specific needs.

Using mixed methods to understand local perceptions of mental health problems

Conducting mental health services research in cross-cultural settings with vulnerable populations requires an understanding of local perceptions of and terminology used to describe mental health problems. Involvement of the community of interest in the research process is essential to understand mental health in the local context and for developing and testing locally relevant and culturally sensitive informed interventions. Utilizing a mixed-methods research approach can inform intervention development and assessment techniques by aiding in understanding local terms and symptoms for describing mental health problems and also protective processes that are associated with resilient mental health outcomes. Figure 7.1 describes an iterative mixed methods approach used in Rwanda to understand the mental health problems and resilience among children affected by HIV and AIDS (58).

A variety of qualitative research techniques may be used in such mixed-methods research. In Rwanda, for example, key informant interviews, free-listing exercises, and focus groups were conducted with a variety of community members, such as parents

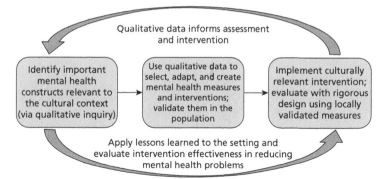

Fig. 7.1 A model for designing and evaluating mental health services in diverse cultural settings.

Table 7.1 Problems of HIV/AIDS-affected children and adolescents in Rwanda. (From Betancourt, et al. (2011) (59))

Local syndrome	Meaning	Example indicators
agahinda kenshi	persistent sorrow	is lonely (arigunga) is unhappy (ntiyishimye) cries (ararira)
kwiheba	severe hopelessness	wishes to die (yifuza gupfa) feels life is meaningless (yumva ubuzima ntacyo buvuze) has no hope for life (yumva nta)
guhangayika	anxiety/depression	is never at ease (sinjya ntuza) does not play with others (ntakina n'abandi) overthinks about life (atekereza cyane ku buzima)
ihahamuka	trauma/anxiety	thinking a lot (aratekereza cyane) is always afraid (ahorana ubwoba) feels like he/she has lost his/her mind (yumva ameze nk'uwataye umutwe) is lonely (numva ndi jyenyine)
uburara	bad/delinquent behaviour	being unruly (ni ikigenge) roaming around (arabungera) taking drugs (gufata ibiyobyabwenge) playing dangerously (akinanana ubugome)
umushiha	persistent irritability/anger	talks badly (avuga nabi) becomes annoyed (ararakara) becomes grouchy (azinga umunya) quarrels (aratongana)

and children, and with local clinicians to identify local terms for mental health problems and protective processes (see Tables 7.1 and 7.2). The qualitative research formed the foundation for the development of a Family Strengthening Intervention for Rwanda (FSI-R) to bolster naturally occurring protective processes as well as assessment tools that have been validated for use with Rwandan children and families (59, 60).

Table 7.2 Protective processes in Rwandan children and families affected by HIV/AIDS. (From Betancourt, et al. (2011) (60))

Local protective factors	Meaning	Example indicators
kwihangana	patience/ perseverance	interacts with peers (*asabana n'abandi bagenzi be*) does not lose hope (*ntajya yiheba*) plays with others (*akina n'abandi*) is well behaved (*yitwara neza*)
kwigirira ikizere	self-esteem	thinks of his/her future (*atekereza ku buzima bwe bw'ejo hazaza*) feels he/she will live (*yumva akamaro ko kubaho*) feels strong (*yumva akomeye*)
kwizerana	family unity/trust	they talk to reach agreement (*baraganira bagahuza*) they cooperate (*barafatanya*) they live together well (*babana neza*)
kurera neza	good parenting	teach good discipline (*kugira ikinyabufura*) training a child (*gutoza umwana kujijuka*) provide resources (*kubaha ibikenewe*) speak with love (*bavugana urukundo*)
ubufasha abaturage batanga	communal/social support	they don't discriminate (*ntibabaha akato*) provide comfort (*barabihanganisha*) visit (*barabasura*) provide help when able (*babafasha uko bashoboye*)

Addressing power differentials: CBPR with vulnerable populations

Another important issue when conducting research with vulnerable populations is the power differential that exists between researchers and the very vulnerable populations they may be studying. A less hierarchical stance as a researcher that can contribute to even greater research insights and positive and engaged involvement of the community is that of community based participatory research or CBPR. At its core, CBPR work relies on a collaborative partnership that equitably and actively involves community partners in all aspects of the research process (61–64). Israel and colleagues present a cogent framework for CBPR. A participatory stance in mental health services research through CBPR may often involve an exploration and enhancement of inherent strengths and resources within the community in addition to preventing or treating mental health problems.

Another important feature of CBPR within vulnerable communities is co-learning between stakeholders, who can include academic teams and populations for which services are being developed. For instance, research leadership may share and engage in capacity building among community partners on methodological issues, such as techniques for qualitative or quantitative data analysis, while partners' knowledgeable about the community of focus may provide historical and cultural knowledge, thus ensuring two-way learning. Data collection using CBPR methods often means the involvement of both community and academic partners in designing and implementing data collection. Once collected, such data can be analysed in a collaborative process and iteratively applied to the design, implementation, and evaluation of intervention models that are a good fit to the culture and context (61, 65–68).

A CBPR approach not only can help to illuminate critical issues related to mental health and resilience in a community, but also is a means of ensuring the buy-in of all key stakeholders. Such commitment to a shared vision can have effects far beyond the narrow scope of a clinical trial. For instance, in work with CABs in Sierra Leone on the issue of intervention components, our research team was able to learn about several Sierra Leonean proverbs that captured the essence of key messages the intervention team was looking to impart to affected youth. Some examples include the proverb *Yu need for paddle yu one canoe*, which means, 'One has to set one's own direction in life'. This proverb and related terms in the local language were then integrated into the manual for the Youth Readiness Intervention, making it easy for participants to connect to the core intentions of the intervention.

Using CABs

CABs are a common feature of many CBPR approaches, but certainly not the only technique. Nonetheless, CABs provide a rich resource to help guide investigators working within communities and can be an excellent method for deepening research questions, ensuring the relevance and applicability of research, designing interventions that are a good fit, as well as reviewing and analysing data in a more collective fashion. Figure 7.2 describes the process of using CABs in Rwanda to adapt an evidence-based intervention, the Family-Based Preventive Intervention (FBPI) for the prevention of depression in children with depressed caregivers, for use with families affected by HIV and AIDS in Rwanda. In order to understand the context of HIV and the multiple challenges facing HIV-affected families, we convened CABs comprised of caregivers, youths, clinicians, and the broader community.

We used CAB input to review intervention materials for cultural appropriateness and acceptability and to recommend thematic content to complement and reinforce the modules for the Family Strengthening Intervention in Rwanda (FSI-R). We reviewed qualitative study findings with the CABs and their feedback reinforced the salience of our findings and helped us identify Rwandan stories, proverbs, songs, and parenting practices useful in fostering such protective processes in children.

CABs can play a critical role in raising community awareness about mental health, particularly when such issues are frequently misunderstood and stigmatized. In a collaborative project in Rwanda between the Harvard School of Public Health and PIH to develop and evaluate FSIs, CABs have played a critical role. In this project, CABs have provided insight into local understandings of mental health problems in children and adolescents, as well as community responses to children struggling with mental health problems.

In 2011, one of our CAB members, Therese Mukukamari, inspired by training and ongoing discussions in the CAB meetings, took action in her own community

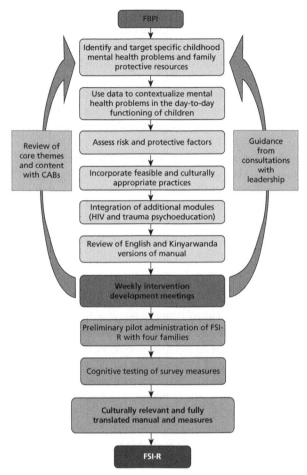

Fig. 7.2 Process of using CABs for intervention adaptation and assessment tool development in Rwanda.

to help a boy, Uwimana, who had suffered years of neglect and abuse which contributed to a pattern of conduct problems, or *uburara*. She was interviewed by study staff in 2011:

'When we first met Uwimana he was 10 or 11. Because he was an orphan living in [a] refugee camp, we still aren't quite sure how old he is,' recalls Therese. He had been living in Kageyo, a region home to Rwandan refugees—families repatriating to Rwanda from Tanzania after fleeing during the Rwandan Genocide. Some of his time had been spent living on and off with a woman from the camp. 'Instead of providing good parenting, of being motherly, [this woman] beat the child, leaving him to feel like no one ever loved him,' said Therese. In fact, like many orphans living in refugee camps, he had been abused and mistreated for much of his life. When he came to her village, she recalled, 'He was a delinquent who would roam up and down the streets. [He] would seek shelter for a night from someone, and the following morning he would leave without telling anyone. He would sleep under trees, or next to the home of people in the neighborhood who would offer some food in the morning. I would ask why he was sleeping outside; I learned that he was hungry and alone.' Knowing that Uwimana had slept outside of her home one night, Therese got up early the next morning to ensure that he would not run away. She convinced him to come inside and eat breakfast. She invited him to stay; however, her act of generosity quickly took a dangerous turn for the worse. When he began to have conflicts with her children, 'Uwimana fought with my daughter . . . beating her until she became unconscious,' says Therese. 'We rushed her to the hospital.' Having worked for 2 years on PIH's FSI CAB, a project that trains people to recognize and deal with mental illness and depression, Therese recognized Uwimana was sick and needed care. Most people would have given up on a boy after such an act of violence, but Therese did not.

At CAB meetings, members had extensive conversations and training about mental health and mental illness. They had reviewed both western criteria and local data on how people think about what causes mental health problems and how they manifest, specifically in children. This included talking about illnesses caused by violence, maltreatment, and neglect. The CAB had discussed what family-based mental health interventions might look like and what families and other helpers in the community, such as community health workers, might do to help children with problems. Therese would later learn that Uwimana had no memory of his parents. He had never lived with a family, and even worse he had never felt loved. Therese was more determined than ever to take Uwimana in. 'If I had not been trained, I probably would have just shown him pity and provided him with some food,' explains Therese. 'Instead, I took the responsibility to accept the child into my home and to become his caregiver.' This new journey required patience, but Therese knew what she had to do. 'I stayed with him, showed him love, and he started calling me "mother". I talked with him and I showed him how people live together in harmony. He would show me the scars on his hands; they used to tie his hands. He was so quiet.' As time passed, so too did Uwimana's anger. 'He began to trust me,' says Therese. 'If someone beat him in the community during the day he would resist fighting, Uwimana would come and tell me. He realized that I loved him, and whatever I would give to my own children, I would give him so as to be convinced that someone loves him . . . Now', Therese says, 'Uwimana is a part of our family and works around our home, he takes care of the cows and even builds fires for them at night,' Therese remarks proudly: 'He used to sleep with goats, now he knows I love him and he lives with us. I treat Uwimana the same way I did my own children.' When asked what Therese sees in his future, the answer comes quickly and with confidence: 'He is striving and I plan to take him to school this next year. If Uwimana grows older and is able to look after himself, I would be incredibly pleased . . . I am grateful for the training I received from the Family Strengthening Intervention Project,' says an empowered Therese. 'Not only has the training helped change the life of this boy, but it has allowed me to help many people in my village through my work as a community health worker . . . The training opened my mind about mental illness and helped me better understand what children like this experience—as a result I am educating other adults in my village on how harmful physical abuse is.'

Therese and Uwimana's story underscores the importance of raising awareness of mental health problems in vulnerable communities. Through her involvement in the CAB, she became knowledgeable about mental health issues that are often misunderstood and not discussed. Therese is now in a position to be an advocate for mental health in her local community. This story also captures the essence of the CBPR element of capacity building. Therese would not have learned what she had about child mental health had our CAB—many of them illiterate—not offered training and routine discussions on child vulnerability and mental health.

Attending to the needs of vulnerable populations while trials are underway

In addition to using more participatory methods, learning about local terminology, and developing rich and intact referral networks to support the conduct of a clinical trial, issues may arise during the course of a mental health clinical trial which require certain adjustments or accommodations to meet the needs of vulnerable groups. The Applied Mental Health Research group of Johns Hopkins University has a new manual for design, implementation, monitoring, and evaluation of clinical trials that provides some excellent examples from field trials (69).

For instance, they describe encountering logistical and security complications while treating torture survivors in southern Iraq, some of whom had to travel several hours and cross multiple check points in order to meet with their therapist in a trial of cognitive behavioral therapy for traumatic stress reactions and depression. In order to address concerns about this burden on participants, the team adjusted the treatment schedule so that individuals could extend the length of their treatment sessions to 1.5 hours rather than 1 hour, allowing them to thus complete all of the CBT modules in more rapid sequences, which reduced the amount of time needed for travelling to the treatment site.

In another example from the Democratic Republic of Congo using cognitive processing therapy (CPT) for the treatment of depression and PTSD among survivors of sexual violence (70), the research team utilized a version of the therapy that does not include the trauma narrative because of the greater ease to utilize in a group format (71, 72). This version of the therapy has equal efficacy as the version that does include a trauma narrative and limits the chances of exposing group members to the details of others' traumatic events. The structure of CPT and its core treatment elements were retained, although aspects of the treatment were simplified. For example, the manual was adapted to remove technical jargon and simplify its language, reducing theory-heavy content on PTSD, and providing greater emphasis on the basics of group therapy and skills for managing group interactions. Clinical case examples of relevance to sexual violence survivors in the Democratic Republic of Congo were also added. Since many of the participants were illiterate, homework typically assigned in CPT to recognize and change problematic beliefs that maintain PTSD and depression was modified to be short and simple so that it could be done from memory without additional materials. Pictures were also used on worksheets to provide a visual reminder of each step of the skill being practised while doing the homework. These modifications underscore the need to continually monitor issues of fit to the context and culture as well as the safety of participants during a clinical trial and to be open to making adjustments as research with vulnerable groups is planned and implemented.

Conclusion

This chapter has presented several key sensitivities necessary for carrying out trials/mental health services research in vulnerable populations. The discussion has presented both field-based examples and promising approaches to moving beyond short-term, crisis-focused responses to longer-term advocacy. With such practices at the forefront, clinical trials and other mental health services research can inform and strengthen sustainable service models for children, youths, families, and other vulnerable populations in situations of adversity, such as those due to armed conflict or HIV/AIDS. In closing, the following points emphasize the importance of new directions for advancing the research agenda on children, youths, and families in situations of compounded adversity.

Clinical trials focused on children and families facing adversity, such as those affected by HIV/AIDS or armed conflict (73–75), must be sensitive to the unique needs of vulnerable populations in research. If not done with great care, research among vulnerable populations may endanger subjects, their families, and research staff, especially in communities where the research may invoke taboo or legal issues. In the case of stigmatized populations, such as former child soldiers or individuals living with HIV, research and intervention also run the risk of exposing individuals who have veiled their status or wish to remain anonymous (75). All research on youths in vulnerable populations should receive approval from local and international ethical review committees, but community input and oversight is additionally needed. CABs have been used with success in research with vulnerable populations and can help to ensure implementation of clinical trials and other mental health services research that is sensitive and responsive to the local culture and context (76), and to ensure ethical implementation and appropriate dissemination of findings (58). In programming, an additional and critical part of upholding best practices when working with vulnerable groups is to ensure that participants can access additional supports and services as needed in order to be safe and mentally healthy and that treatment protocols can be adjusted to meet their unique needs.

Our work in Rwanda highlights different kinds of ethical concerns. Was it possible that discussions about HIV/AIDS in families could cause harm to participants? Through extensive work with our advisory boards in both developing core constructs of resilience and difficulty and devising the intervention, this proved not to be the case, but it does emphasize that assessing the possible harmfulness of interventions is a crucial part of research with vulnerable populations. Finally, as mentioned, anticipation of and planning in response to risk of harm cases before beginning a study proved essential both in Sierra Leone and Rwanda and are an essential part of the conduct of research with vulnerable groups worldwide. Examples from others, such as the Applied Mental Health Research Group of Johns Hopkins, also underscore the need to be flexible in how clinical trials are implemented for vulnerable groups.

In conclusion, the benefits of culturally sensitive and contextually collaborative mental health research within vulnerable communities cannot be underestimated. Provision of untested interventions is unethical and wasteful, but the implementation of high-quality research must be balanced against sensitive practices and participatory research approaches within vulnerable communities. Such efforts are critical to advancing informed decision-making and the development and evaluation of optimal interventions to assist vulnerable populations and for promoting their resilience and strength. Implementation of high-quality, ethical, and evidence-based mental health services research—including clinical trials—is possible in LAMIC. Greater attention to the vulnerabilities facing populations and mechanisms for illuminating their strengths are critical to advancing approaches such as those described in this chapter. Anticipating and implementing risk of harm protocols and application of CBPR principles, including the use of CABs and flexible approaches to the implementation of trials, can all deepen and enrich research processes and findings. Likewise, participation methods can promote greater community buy-in, creating a context in which recommendations and intervention models derived from the research are more likely to be implemented and sustained in vulnerable communities.

Appendix—risk of harm protocol

We have discussed the role of confidentiality in making the research process respectful of our participants. However, as an organization serving the health and wellbeing of children and families, there are some very specific circumstances in which we cannot keep information a secret and may need to break confidentiality. These are explained to our participants in the informed consent form.

From the informed consent form

What you tell us will not be shared with anyone besides the study team. We will not let anyone else find out who gave a certain answer unless we think that you or someone else might be in danger. In that case, we cannot keep what you say a secret and we will take steps to make sure that all people in this study are kept safe. For example, if you say that you want to hurt yourself, we will do everything we can to keep that from happening, and we will make sure that you see a doctor and/or social worker right away.

Throughout the research, study staff should also consistently ask participants open-ended questions to assess anxiety or stress (e.g. *'Do you have any concerns or questions about our conversation today? Do you feel you need any additional care or services due to your experiences today? Are there any questions or concerns that you would like to discuss with a mental health provider or other health professional?'*)

Instances where we must intervene to ensure safety

Risk of suicide (thoughts about or actual actions taken to harm self)

Risk of physical or sexual abuse

Risk of committing a serious crime against another person (i.e. murder, rape)

Risk of being victimized by a serious crime (i.e. murder, rape)

During the course of this study, it is possible that situations involving study participants in immediate risk of harm (e.g. physical or sexual abuse) may arise. These situations are to be triaged by the research staff member present at the time of interview with support from study supervisors. When one or more of the risk of harm criteria are met, the staff member present must follow the safety plan, reporting and documenting each step.

All risk of harm cases must be discussed with the research coordinator and the project manager, in addition to being reported to the study principal investigator. All Safety Plan Activation notes will be kept on file at the research offices during data collection and then transferred securely to the university research offices, where they will be stored securely.

Any participant deemed to be in immediate risk of harm will be referred to appropriate local mental health providers and emergency facilities as needed. In addition, mental health worker staff at the regional hospital and local health centres can provide additional individual support, assessment of individuals for additional mental health services, as well as clinical supervision and support to the study staff.

When to activate the safety plan

The following situations will initiate activation of the safety plan:

1 *Flagged questions.* Some survey items are designed to assess participants' risk behaviours and welfare, including critical issues such as suicidal ideation, physical abuse, and sexual abuse. Specific questions related to these problems are 'flagged' (see 'Flagged questions'). A positive response to a flagged question will mandate activation of the risk of harm protocol. These flagged items are coded in your Android phones and will issue prompts for further follow-up.

2 *Concerning or excessive punishment/intimate partner violence (IPV).* If you are concerned that a child or adult participant is the victim (or perpetrator) of physical or sexual abuse, activate the risk of harm protocol.

3 *Distress during intervention or at the time of interview.* Participants may exhibit distress during interviews. In these cases, the research assistant/interventionist present at the time of distress should follow the risk of harm protocol as appropriate.

In situations where you are not sure

Sometimes young people won't directly state that they are thinking of harming themselves or are at risk of being harmed. However, your instincts are very important and are not to be ignored. If you have an interaction that leads you to believe that a participant is possibly 'at risk' of harm to self or others, please express concern to the young person and/or their family. If they admit further information, then you can follow the protocol as described. If ever you feel any sort of significant concern for the wellbeing of a participant that you have interacted with, be sure to express this concern and get their permission for follow-up. In any such instance, the first line of defence should be to make contact with the research coordinators and project manager, and have a social worker conduct a follow-up visit.

Flagged responses

Ag23/Ag23P: *Mu cyumweru gishize natekereje kwiyahura.* Over the last week, I thought about suicide.

Ag27/Ag27P: *Mu cyumweru gishize nashakaga gupfa kuko numvaga ubuzima ntacyo buvuze.* Over the last week, I wanted to die because I felt life is meaningless.

Gu3/Gu3P: *Ubu cyangwa mu mezi atandatu ashize nagerageje kwigirira nabi cyangwa kwiyica ku bushake.* Now or during the last 6 months, I deliberately tried to hurt or kill myself.

Gu14/Gu14P: *Ubu cyangwa mu mezi atandatu ashize natekerezaga kwiyahura.* Now or during the last 6 months, I thought about killing myself.

HSCL20: *Ibitekerezo byo kwiyahura (utarabigerageje, kubitekereza gusa).* I have thoughts of ending my life.

Other questions that may indicate harm

HP11/HP11P: *Baraguhondaguye cyane?* Have you been severely beaten?

ORB15: *Mu minsi 30 ishize, wigeze witwaza icyuma kugira ngo ugikoreshe nk'intwaro?* In the last 30 days, have you ever carried around a knife with intentions to use it as a weapon?

What to do if you encounter indications of risk

1 Express concern
   - Express your concern to your participant. Help them to understand that you see this as a very serious situation that must be addressed to make sure that they are safe.
   - You may use language such as, '*You mentioned having thoughts of hurting yourself or wishing you were dead. I am concerned about you and want to make sure that you are safe. As we mentioned in the consent, if we are concerned that someone is at serious risk of harm we cannot keep that information private.*'

2 **Assess severity**
   - Get information. Talk with the participant to find out the nature of the problem.
   - As appropriate, talk with caregivers and other people important to the participant.
   - Find out when the thoughts or behaviours started.

- In the case of suicidal ideation, find out if the participant has ever made a previous suicide attempt.
- Find out what triggered the thoughts or behaviours now and in the past.
- Find out how serious the problem is RIGHT NOW. Does the participant have immediate thoughts of ending their life? Do they have a plan to act on these thoughts? How lethal is the action being considered?
- **If a participant is having thoughts of ending his/her life, ask:**
  - How long have you been having these thoughts?
  - How often do you have these thoughts?
  - Have you ever done anything to harm yourself in the past?
    - § Can you tell me about what you tried?
  - Do you currently have a plan for harming yourself?
  - *Observe the behaviour of the participant. Look for signs of distress.*
- **If a participant reports a situation involving other people, find out:**
  - Who are the people involved and how are they related to the participant?
  - How often does the participant see them?
  - Is there an immediate risk of someone being harmed (such as murdered or raped)?
  - Have the authorities ever been notified about this situation?
  - *If there is a risk of murder or rape, the police or other legal authority must be notified right away. As appropriate, you may want to consult with the relevant village leadership and NGO staff.*

3   **Identify supports**

- If the participant is a child, ask him/her to identify an adult or guardian whom they are close to and feel they could discuss this problem with to keep them safe. Sometimes this may be the caregiver; at other times it may be a relative, neighbour, village leader, teacher, etc.
- If the participant is an adult, ask him/her to identify a trusted adult whom they are close to and feel they could discuss this problem with to keep them safe. This might be a spouse, friend, or village leader.
- Help the participant to identify his/her strengths, as well as activities that he/she finds enjoyable or relaxing.

4   **Contract for safety**

- *Do not leave the situation until you have ensured that some other person has been notified who can help keep the participant safe.*
- Inform the participant (and caregiver if a child) that you will be taking additional steps to ensure their safety (e.g. *'Based on your responses to some of these questions, I have concerns about your safety and would like to have someone on our team touch base with you.'*).

- If it seems helpful, you can write out an agreement and have all parties sign it. We call this a 'contract for safety'. For example, you can write a contract that states something like:

I (participant's name) agree to the following contract:

If I have thoughts of ending my life, I promise not to do this and to keep myself safe. Instead, I will do the following things to keep myself safe: (for example: talk to my auntie, tell my mother, talk to the village chief)

Signed:

Participant's name
Research Assistant or social worker's name
Guardian or other adult

5 Get backup

- In all risk cases, both the supervising research coordinator and project manager must be phoned immediately so that they can help trouble shoot.
- The supervising research coordinator and project manager will help facilitate referrals to mental health/social work services:
  - *If suicidality/self-harm is reported*, a study social worker or psychologist may conduct a follow-up diagnostic interview to assess severity. The participant will subsequently be referred to mental health services if appropriate.
  - *If ongoing physical or sexual abuse is reported*, a local social worker and local authority will be contacted. The study team member should inform the village head/leader and tell him/her to contact the police. The study team member should also tell the village head/leader to request medical expertise from the nearest health centre. The local social worker will work to substantiate indications of abuse. If the abuse relates to a child under 18 years of age, a report will be submitted to the appropriate authorities, as required by national law. In abuse cases involving participants aged over 18 years, the safety plan recommends informing the participants' primary care or mental health providers. Additionally, individuals/couples/families may be referred for mental health services.
  - *If high levels of IPV are reported*, referrals for appropriate care will be made through the health centre to the social work department. If the situation is an emergency, local health programme staff will provide immediate services and will refer the subject to appropriate services.
- Research staff, the research coordinator, and the project manager should work with the mental health/social work teams to track progress about what services are provided for the participant(s) in each case.
- Emergency services may be contacted if suicidal ideation is ongoing and the participant cannot be kept safe with social work and family-level interventions.

Risk of harm action flowchart

RISK OF HARM ACTION FLOWCHART

	Suicidality	Harming others	Being harmed by others
	Did the participant endorse any of the following:	Did the participant endorse any of the following:	Did the participant endorse any of the following:
Flag	• Thought about suicide • Wanted to die because I felt life is meaningless • Deliberately tried to hurt or kill myself • Thought about killing myself	• Ever carried around a knife with intentions to use it as weapon • Expression of intent to harm	• Excessive punishment • Excessive Intimate Partner Violence (IPV)
	If YES	*If YES*	*If YES*
Urgency	*IMMEDIATE* *Assess whether participant can be kept safe*	*IMMEDIATE* *Assess whether participant is at immediate risk of harming others*	*IMMEDIATE* *Assess whether participant is at immediate risk of being harmed by others*
	Ask:	*Find out:*	*Find out:*
Assess severity	• When did thoughts of killing yourself start? • How often do you have these thoughts? • Now and in the past, what triggered the thoughts? • Have you ever done anything to harm yourself in the past? • Do you currently have a plan for harming yourself?	• Who are the people involved and how are they related to the participant? • How often does the participant see them? • Is there an immediate risk of someone being harmed (such as murdered or raped)? • Have the authorities ever been notified?	• Who are the people involved and how are they related to the participant? • How often does the participant see them? • Is there an immediate risk of physical or sexual abuse? • Have the authorities ever been notified about this situation?
	Is the participant actively suicidal? *If YES*	*Is there immediate risk of harm to others?* *If YES*	*Is there immediate risk of physical or sexual abuse?* *If YES*
Contact supports	• Ask participant to identify an adult, guardian, or important person whom they are close to • Contact the identified person and express your concern to them	*The police or other legal authority must be notified right away. As appropriate you may want to consult with the relevant village leadership and IMB staff*	*If abuse relates to a child under 18 years of age:* • Inform the umudugudu (village) head/leader • Tell him/her to inform the police • Make sure that he/she tells the police to request medical expertise from the interventionist *If abuse relates to a participant aged over 18 years:* • Research coordinator and Project Manager will inform the correct authorities
Contract for safety	*Do not leave until you have ensured that a responsible adult can keep the participant safe* • Create a signed contract for safety	• Create a signed contract for safety	
Make the referral	Fill out referral form	Fill out referral form	Fill out referral form
	Alert Health Centre to case	Alert Health Centre to case	Alert Health Centre to case
	Give form to caregiver/ guardian; inform them of next steps	Give form to caregiver/ guardian; inform them of next steps	Give form to caregiver/ guardian; inform them of next steps
Backup	• Contact research coordinator and Project Manager immediately	• Contact research coordinator and Project Manager immediately	• Contact research coordinator and Project Manager immediately

References

1 US Department of Health and Human Services (2013) Regulations. <http://www.hhs.gov/regulations/>.

2 Mello M, Wolf L (2010) The Havasupai Indian Tribe case—lessons for research involving stored biological samples. N Engl J Med, **363**(3):204–7.

3 Heimlich H, Chen X, Xiao B, Liu S, Lu Y, Spletzer E, et al. (1997) Malariotherapy for HIV patients. Mech Age Dev, **93**(1–3):79–85.

4 Brandt A (1978) Racism and research: the case of the Tuskegee syphilis study. Hastings Center Rep, **8**(6):21–9.

5 Angell M (1997) The ethics of clinical research in the third world. N Engl J Med, **337**(12):847–9.

6 UNAIDS (2008) Report on the global AIDS epidemic. Geneva: WHO.

7 Otunnu OA (2002) 'Special comment' on children and security, disarmament forum No. 3. Geneva: United Nations Institute for Disarmament Research.

8 Mason E (2006) Positioning paediatric HIV in the child survival agenda. Presentation to UNICEF–WHO consultation, 11–13 January, New York. New York: UNICEF.

9 UNAIDS (2012) Core epidemiology slides. Geneva: WHO.

10 UNICEF (2010) Children and AIDS: fifth stocktaking report. New York: UNICEF, UN-AIDS, WHO, UNFPA, UNESCO.

11 Mellins CA, Ehrhardt AA (1995) Families affected by pediatric acquired immunodeficiency syndrome: sources of stress and coping. J Dev Behav Pediatrics, **15**(3):S61.

12 Mellins CA, Kang E, Leu C-S, Havens JF, Chesney MA (2003) Longitudinal study of mental health and psychosocial predictors of medical treatment adherence in mothers living with HIV disease. AIDS Patient Care STDs, **17**(8):407–16.

13 Cluver L (2011) Children of the AIDS pandemic. Nature, **474**(7349):27–9.

14 Rotheram-Borus MJ, Flannery D, Rice E, Lester P (2005) Families living with HIV. AIDS Care, **17**(8):978–87.

15 Forehand R, Biggar H, Kotchick BA (1998) Cumulative risk across family stressors: short- and long-term effects for adolescents. J Abnorm Child Psychol, **26**(2):119–28.

16 Garcia-Moreno C, Watts C (2000) Violence against women: its importance for HIV/AIDS. AIDS, **14**(3):S253–65.

17 Gielen AC, Ghandour RM, Burke JG, Mahoney P, McDonnell KA, O'Campo P (2007) HIV/AIDS and intimate partner violence. Trauma Violence Abuse, **8**(2):178–98.

18 Lipsitz JD, Williams JB, Rabkin JG (1994) Psychopathology in male and female intravenous drug users with and without HIV infection. Am J Psychiatry, **151**:1662–8.

19 Cluver L, Gardner F (2007) Risk and protective factors for psychological well-being of children orphaned by AIDS in Cape Town: a qualitative study of children and caregivers' perspectives. AIDS Care, **19**(3):318–25.

20 Betancourt TS, Meyers-Ohki SE, Charrow A, Hansen N (2013) Annual research review: mental health and resilience in HIV/AIDS-affected children—a review of the literature and recommendations for future research. J Child Psychol Psychiatry, **54**(4):423–44.

21 Bachmann MO, Booysen FL (2003) Health and economic impact of HIV/AIDS on South African households: a cohort study. BMC Public Health, **3**:14.

22 Nampanya-Serpell N (ed.) (2000) Social and economic risk factors for HIV/AIDS-affected families in Zambia. AIDS and Economics Symposium, 7–8 July, Durban.

23 Brouwer CN, Lok CL, Wolffers I, Sebagalls S (2000) Psychosocial and economic aspects of HIV/AIDS and counselling of caretakers of HIV-infected children in Uganda. AIDS Care, **12**(5):535–40.

24 Seeley J, Russell S (2010) Social rebirth and social transformation? Rebuilding social lives after ART in rural Uganda. AIDS Care, **12**:1–7.

25 Denison JA, McCauley AP, Dunnett-Dagg WA, Lungu N, Sweat MD (2009) HIV testing among adolescents in Ndola, Zambia: how individual, relational, and environmental factors relate to demand. AIDS Educ Prev, **21**(4):314–24.

26 Biddlecom A, Awusabo-Asare K, Bankole A (2009) Role of parents in adolescent sexual activity and contraceptive use in four African countries. Int Perspect Sex Reprod Health, **35**(2):72–81.

27 Messam T, McKay MM, Kalogerogiannis K, Alicea S (2010) HOPE committee champ collaborative board MHHC. Adapting a family-based HIV prevention program for homeless youth and their families: the HOPE (HIV prevention Outreach for Parents and Early adolescents) family program. J Hum Behav Soc Environ, **20**(2):303–18.

28 Bell CC, Bhana A, Petersen I, McKay MM, Gibbons R, Bannon W, et al. (2008) Building protective factors to offset sexually risky behaviors among black youths: a randomized control trial. J Natl Med Assoc, **100**(8):936–44.

29 Coates T, Richter L, Caceres C (2008) Behavioural strategies to reduce HIV transmission: how to make them better. Lancet, **372**(9639):669–84.

30 Li L, Liang L, Lee S, Iamsirithawron S, Wan D, Rotherham-Borus MJ (2012) Efficacy of an intervention for families living with HIV in Thailand: a randomized controlled trial. AIDS Behav, **16**:1276–85.

31 Rochat T, Mkwanazi N, Bland R (2013) Maternal HIV disclosure to HIV-uninfected children in rural South Africa: a pilot study of a family-based intervention. BMC Public Health, **13**(1):147.

32 Visser M, Finestone M, Sikkema K, Boeving-Allen A, Ferreira R, Eloff I, et al. (2012) Development and piloting of a mother and child intervention to promote resilience in young children of HIV-infected mothers in South Africa. Eval Program Plan, **35**:491–500.

33 Rochat TJ, Bland T, Coovadia H, Stein A, Newell ML (2011) Towards a family-centered approach to HIV treatment and care for HIV-exposed children, their mothers and their families in poorly resourced settings. Future Virol, **6**(6):687–96.

34 UNICEF (2009) Machel study 10-year strategic review: children and conflict in a changing world. New York: UNICEF.

35 UNICEF (2008) State of the world's children 2008. New York: UNICEF.

36 United Nations High Commissioner for Refugees (2012) A framework for the protection of children. Geneva: UNHCR.

37 Guha-Sapir D, van Panhuis WG, Degomme O, Teran V (2005) Civil conflicts in four African countries: a five-year review of trends in nutrition and mortality. Epidemiol Rev, **27**(1):67–77.

38 Child Soldiers International (2012) Louder than words: an agenda for action to end state use of child soldiers. London: Child Soldiers International.

39 Otunnu OA (2005) 'Era of application: instituting a compliance and enforcement regime for CAAC'. Statement before the Security Council. New York: United Nations.

40 UNICEF (2013) Child protection from violence, exploitation and abuse: child recruitment by armed forces or armed groups. <http://www.unicef.org/protection/57929_58007.html>.

41 UNICEF (2009) Progress for children: a report card on child protection. New York: UNICEF.

42 Betancourt TS, Borisova I, Williams TP, Meyers-Ohki SE, Rubin-Smith JE, Annan J, et al. (2013) Research review: psychosocial adjustment and mental health in former child soldiers—a systematic review of the literature and recommendations for future research. J Child Psychol Psychiatry, **54**(1):17–36.

43 Derluyn I, Broekaert E, Schuyten G, De Temmerman E (2004) Post-traumatic stress in former Ugandan child soldiers. Lancet, **363**(9412):861–3.

44 Bayer CP, Klasen F, Adam H (2007) Association of trauma and PTSD symptoms with openness to reconciliation and feelings of revenge among former Ugandan and Congolese child soldiers. JAMA, **298**(5):555–9.

45 Kohrt BA, Jordans MJ, Tol WA, Speckman RA, Maharjan SM, Worthman CM, et al. (2008) Comparison of mental health between former child soldiers and children never conscripted by armed groups in Nepal. JAMA, **300**(6):691–702.

46 Betancourt TS, Agnew-Blais J, Gilman SE, Williams DR, Ellis BH (2010) Past horrors, present struggles: the role of stigma in the association between war experiences and psychosocial adjustment among former child soldiers in Sierra Leone. Social Sci Med, **70**(1): 17–26.

47 Fontes L (2004) Ethics in violence against women research: the sensitive, the dangerous, and the overlooked. Ethics Behav, **14**(2):141–74.

48 Gorin S, Hooper C, Dyson C, Cabral C (2008) Ethical challenges in conducting research with hard to reach families. Child Abuse Rev, **17**:275–87.

49 Draucker C, Martsolf D, Poole C (2009) Developing distress protocols for research on sensitive topics. Arch Psychiatr Nurs, **23**(5):343–50.

50 Fisher C, Higgins-D'Allessandro A, Rau J, Kuther T, Belanger S (2008) Referring and reporting research participants at risk: views from urban adolescents. Child Dev, **67**(5):2086–100.

51 Betancourt TS, Borisova II, Brennan RB, Williams TP, Whitfield TH, de la Soudiere M, et al. (2010) Sierra Leone's former child soldiers: a follow-up study of psychosocial adjustment and community reintegration. Child Dev, **81**(4):1077–95.

52 Betancourt T, Scorza P, Meyers-Ohki S, Mushashi C, Kayiteshonga Y, Binagwaho A, et al. (2012) Validating the center for epidemiological studies depression scale for children in Rwanda. J Am Acad Child Adolesc Psychiatry, **51**(12):1284–92.

53 Donnelly J (2011) How did Sierra Leone provide free health care? Lancet, **377**(9775):1393–6.

54 Betancourt TS, Brennan RT, Rubin-Smith J, Fitzmaurice GM, Gilman SE (2010) Sierra Leone's former child soldiers: a longitudinal study of risk, protective factors, and mental health. J Am Acad Child Adolesc Psychiatry, **49**(6):606–15.

55 Betancourt TS, Simmons S, Borisova I, Brewer SE, Iweala U, de la Soudiere M (2008) High hopes, grim reality: reintegration and the education of former child soldiers in Sierra Leone. Comp Educ Rev, **52**(4):565–87.

56 Betancourt TS, Khan KT (2008) The mental health of children affected by armed conflict: protective processes and pathways to resilience. Int Rev Psychiatry, **20**(3):317–28.

57 Betancourt TS, Ettien A (2010) Transitional justice and youth formerly associated with armed forces and groups in Sierra Leone: acceptance, marginalization and psychosocial adjustment. Innocenti Working Paper. Florence: UNICEF Innocenti Research Centre.

58 Betancourt TS, Meyers-Ohki S, Stevenson A, Ingabire C, Kanyanganzi F, Munyana M MC, et al. (2011) Using mixed-methods research to adapt and evaluate a Family Strengthening Intervention in Rwanda. Afr J Traum Stress, 2(1):32–45.

59 Betancourt TS, Rubin-Smith J, Beardslee WR, Stulac SN, Fayida I, Safren SA (2011) Understanding locally, culturally, and contextually relevant mental health problems among Rwandan children and adolescents affected by HIV/AIDS. AIDS Care, 23(4):401–12.

60 Betancourt TS, Meyers-Ohki S, Stulac SN, Elizabeth Barrera A, Mushashi C, Beardslee WR (2011) Nothing can defeat combined hands (Abashize hamwe ntakibananira): protective processes and resilience in Rwandan children and families affected by HIV/AIDS. Social Sci Med, 73(5):693–701.

61 Israel BA, Schultz AJ, Parker EA, Becker AB (1998) Review of community based research: assessing partnership approaches to improve public health. Annu Rev Public Health, 19:173–202.

62 Laverack G, Wallerstein N (2001) Measuring community empowerment: a fresh look at organizational domains. Health Promot Int, 16(2):179–85.

63 Krieger J, Allen C, Cheadle A, Ciske S, Schier JK, Senturia K, et al. (2002) Using community-based participatory research to address social determinants of health: lessons learned from Seattle Partners for Healthy Communities. Health Educ Behav, 29(3):361–82.

64 Cornwall A, Jewkes R (1995) What is participatory research? Social Sci Med, 41(12):1667–76.

65 Israel BA, Schurman SJ, House JS (1989) Action research on occupational stress: involving workers as researchers. Int J Health Serv, 19(1):135–55.

66 Hall B (1992) From margins to center? The development and purpose of participatory research. Am Sociologist, 23(4):15–28.

67 Macaulay A, Commanda L, Freeman W, Gibson N, McCabe M, Robbins C, et al. (1999) Participatory research maximises community and lay involvement. BMJ, 319(7212):774–8.

68 Schulz AJ, Parker EA, Israel BA, Becker AB, Maciak BJ, Hollis R (1998) Conducting a participatory community-based survey for a community health intervention on Detroit's East Side. J Public Health Manage Practice, 4(2):10–24.

69 Johns Hopkins University, Bloomberg School of Public Health, Applied Mental Health Research Group, Center for Refugee and Disaster Response (2013) Design, implementation, monitoring, and evaluation of cross-cultural mental health and psychosocial assistance programs for trauma survivors in low resource countries: a user's manual for researchers and program implementers (adult version). Module 5: intervention selection, adaptation, and implementation. <http://www.jhsph.edu/research/centers-and-institutes/center-for-refugee-and-disaster-response/response_service/AMHR/dime/VOT_DIME_MODULE5_FINAL.pdf>.

70 Bass JK, Annan J, McIvor Murray S, Kaysen D, Griffiths S, Cetinoglu T, et al. (2013) Controlled trial of psychotherapy for Congolese survivors of sexual violence. N Engl J Med, 368(23):2182–91.

71 Chard KM, Resick PA, Monson CM, Kattar KA (2008) Cognitive processing therapy group manual: veteran/military version. Washington, DC: Department of Veterans Affairs.

72 Resick PA, Galovski TE, Uhlmansiek MOB, Scher CD, Clum GA, Young-Xu Y (2008) A randomized clinical trial to dismantle components of cognitive processing therapy for posttraumatic stress disorder in female victims of interpersonal violence. J Consult Clin Psychol, 76(2):243–58.

73 **Allden K, Jones L, Weissbecker I, Wessells M, Bolton P, Betancourt TS, et al.** (2009) Mental health and psychosocial support in crisis and conflict: report of the Mental Health Working Group. Prehosp Disaster Med, **24**(2):s217–27.

74 **Betancourt TS** (2011) Attending to the mental health of war-affected children: the need for longitudinal and developmental research perspectives. J Am Acad Child Adolesc Psychiatry, **50**(4):323–5.

75 **Kohrt BA, Jordans MJ, Morley CA** (2010) Four principles of mental health research and psychosocial intervention for child soldiers: lessons learned from Nepal. Int Psychiatry, **7**(3):58–60.

76 **Betancourt TS, McBain R, Newnham EA, Brennan RT** (2013) Trajectories of internalizing problems in war-affected Sierra Leonean youth: examining conflict and postconflict factors. Child Dev, **84**(2):455–70.

Chapter 8

Ethical issues in global mental health trials

Athula Sumathipala and Buddhika Fernando

Introduction

The aim of this chapter is to examine crucial ethical issues related to conducting RCTs that evaluate innovative packages of care and delivery systems for mental disorders in low-resource settings as well as to offer a framework to address relevant ethical issues. However, we attempt to not limit the discussion solely to factual information and technical skills but to link ethics to the overall research endeavour. We also aim to achieve the attitude change required to perceive ethics as an essential component of high-quality research similar to methodology including trial designs and sample sizes. Scientists who believe in high-impact research should have a sound understanding of basic ethical principles and the skill to integrate ethics into the design, execution, and dissemination of research: in summary, to recognize that ethics and research are two sides of the same coin and not as competing or opposing elements.

The objective of clinical research is to develop generalizable knowledge to improve health and/or increase scientific knowledge, i.e. 'to do good', but it also has the potential to inflict harm and treat participants as mere 'subjects' and means to an end. The role of ethics is to ensure that participants are treated with dignity and respect while they contribute to the social good and to find the 'least harmful' ways to do research. Ethics aims to protect participants from harm caused by science and experimentation and to promote their welfare. However, ethics can and should also promote and protect good science.

Broader context of ethics in relation to global mental health

As the strength of the link between resource availability and health becomes clearer, bioethics is finding it hard to remain within the glass walls separating it from the philosophical issues of justice and fair distribution of resources. We view the global 90:10 divide in health, research, and publications as the focal point of the ethical issues surrounding global mental health trials; no one with an interest in global health research can now remain oblivious to this primary issue.

There is enormous inequity existing in global health as well as research (1). Less than 10% of research funds are spent on the diseases that account for 90% of the global disease burden. Though 93% of the world's burden of preventable mortality occurs in LAMIC, too little research funding is dedicated to health problems in these countries (2). There is also a publication divide in medical and mental health research, with less than 6% of mental health research and 8% of other medical disciplines research publications originating in LAMIC (3, 4). In a similar vein, even though LAMIC bear the brunt of the burden of risk factors for mental disorders, underrepresentation of the most at-risk populations for mental disorders and underproduction of relevant knowledge remain an insurmountable impediment in reducing the disease burden (1). We believe strengthening health research capacity and a greater focus on the health issues of LAMIC are critical elements for achieving health equity, and the need to carry out clinical research (and mental health research) in LAMIC if these dual aims are to be achieved is therefore evident.

The issue, however, lies in the process. Though the need for health and mental health research in LAMIC is enormous, and it is currently *en vogue* as it is considered a 'popular need of the hour', the attempt to strengthen research capacity in LAMIC should not result in a repetition of the historical injustice of exploitation of resource-poor settings for easy and cheap research. The *New England Journal of Medicine* poignantly expressed the reason for this necessity:

> One reason ethical codes are unequivocal about investigator's primary obligation to care for the human subjects of their research is the strong temptation to subordinate the subjects' welfare to the objectives of the study. That is particularly likely when the research question is extremely important and the answer would probably improve the care of future patients substantially. In those circumstances it is sometimes argued explicitly that obtaining a rapid, unambiguous answer to the research question is the primary ethical obligation. With the most altruistic of motives, then researchers may find themselves slipping across a line that prohibits treating human subjects as means to an end. When that line is crossed, there is very little left to protect patients from a callous disregard of their welfare for the sake of research goals (5).

In the light of this bitter truth one extreme view based on precautionary principles may be to advocate against conducting RCTs in LAMIC. We reject this approach of not carrying out RCTs that evaluate innovative care and delivery system packages in LAMIC as unethical, because it neglects the social responsibility of research by not contributing to resolving the complex, onerous, and challenging task of addressing the issue of the 90:10 divide. Our strategic approach lies in encouraging and empowering those across the divide to form a mutually respectful and beneficial partnership to carry out suitable RCTs in LAMIC using robust scientific methods and incorporating the highest ethical standards. We have no doubt that such collaborations will result in benefits to the local host community as well as wider benefits globally.

In the next section, we cite three case studies to support our argument that research that is both scientifically rigorous and of high ethical standards can be carried out in LAMIC. Furthermore, these case studies yielded results that were of global benefit. We also emphasize that research here referred relates not only to pharmaceutical intervention research but also to psychological and psychosocial interventions of public health importance.

The role of intervention trials in LAMIC— justification for conducting robust, locally relevant, and ethical interventions in the context of the 90:10 divide

Can RCTs (including mental health trials) carried out in LAMIC contribute to global knowledge, or are they limited to providing local benefit alone? We wish to refer to three high-quality collaborative research projects conducted in LAMIC that generated evidence of relevance and value to both LAMIC and the developed world. The first case is exclusively related to physical illness and pharmaceutical treatment research: the use of anticonvulsants in the management of eclampsia. This had been a controversial subject for over 70 years, until a large clinical trial (1687 patients) conducted in South America, Africa, and India, coordinated by the Oxford Eclampsia Trial Collaborative Group (ETCG), conclusively demonstrated that magnesium sulphate was the drug of choice (6). The trial results were widely accepted, resulting in recognized institutions such as the Royal College of Obstetricians and Gynaecologists incorporating this evidence into its practice guidelines.

A second good example relevant to mixed physical and psychological morbidity is the large population-based cohort study carried out in Goa, India, investigating the aetiology of vaginal discharge, one of the most common and disabling reproductive and sexual symptoms affecting women in developing countries (7, 8). Previous WHO treatment guidelines recommended syndromic management, treating women for all or several of the five common reproductive tract infections—Chlamydia, gonorrhoea, and trichomoniasis, which are sexually transmitted infections (STI)—as well as for bacterial vaginosis and candidiasis, due to disturbance in normal bacterial flora. This approach had significant marital and social implications on women and their families due to the implied connotation of a woman having contracted a sexually transmitted disease (STD). This study revealed that the condition had strong associations with bacterial vaginosis, psychosocial stressors, and common mental disorders, but significantly not with STIs. These findings resulted in the syndromic approach no longer being considered fool-proof and diagnostic tests for STI are now recommended before antibiotics. Although the mental health issues were not adequately addressed, it did result in a policy shift initiation.

The third project, which resulted in benefits for both the developing and developed countries, was carried out in Pakistan to test an exclusively psychological intervention: a community-based complex intervention for maternal depression and child development delivered by community health workers (9). This provided conclusive evidence that suitably modified CBT can be effectively given by community health workers who had not completed high school, when sufficiently trained and supervised (10). These examples amply demonstrate that intervention research can be undertaken successfully in LAMIC and yield global benefits. The challenge, however, lies in conducting such research while observing the highest ethical standards.

Brief introduction to fundamental ethical principles and issues in human subject research

The strong focus of contemporary biomedical ethics on the individual patient appears to have resulted in marginalizing other important ethical concepts such as global justice and fair distribution of resources (11). Popular reference to ethical research is often limited to carrying out research with the 'informed consent' of the participants (12). This is partly due to the widespread adoption of the 'four principles' approach, which is based on the fundamental tenets of autonomy, non-maleficence, beneficence, and justice (13). While these principles provide the buttress for an ethical framework for research, there are other equally or more important considerations that need to be factored in when carrying out research with human subjects.

Starting from the Nuremberg Code in 1947, there have been numerous codes and guidelines on the conduct of ethical research (12). The Declaration of Helsinki (DoH) (14) was formulated to fulfil the gaps in the Nuremberg Code, and the Council for International Organizations of Medical Sciences (CIOMS) guidelines (15) extended the applicability of the DoH to developing countries. In an attempt to broaden the ethical considerations to be undertaken in clinical research, the Nuffield Council of Bioethics, UK, supplemented the four principles approach by introducing a duty to (16):

1 alleviate suffering;

2 show respect for persons;

3 be sensitive to cultural differences; and

4 not to exploit the vulnerable when conducting research in LAMIC.

Given the ambiguity in the guidelines and the wide scope for interpretation, there have been several attempts to build a simplified but comprehensive practical framework for ethical evaluation of clinical research involving human subjects. A good example is the seven principle framework proposed by Emanuel and colleagues (12) for multinational research, where they suggest social/scientific value, scientific validity, fair subject selection, favourable risk-benefit ratio, independent review, informed consent, and respect for potential and enrolled subjects as the criteria essential for clinical research to be ethical. Later on, collaborative partnership between researchers, policy makers, and the community was added as an eighth criterion (17).

Given the almost universal familiarity with the four principles approach, we do not discuss this here in detail but refer the reader to Beauchamp and Childress's *Principles of Biomedical Ethics* (13). Following a brief look at these ethical principles, we will consider their application in mental health and in resource-poor settings.

Autonomy in the four principles approach to clinical research ethics refers to the right of a person to be self-determining. Often enough, in practice, this translates to informed consent—giving the relevant information to the patient/research subject and obtaining his or her voluntary consent for research. Non-maleficence dates from the time of Hippocrates, where the doctor is required to 'first—do no harm'. Beneficence is the other side of the same coin—affirmative action to generate wellbeing. Justice encompasses a broader ethical requirement, most simply described as fairness.

The requirement for a study to increase scientific knowledge or human wellbeing arises from the finite nature of available resources. Similarly, research must be scientifically valid; the CIOMS guidelines explain this as 'Scientifically unsound research on human subjects is ipso facto unethical in that it may expose subjects to risks or inconvenience to no purpose'. Fair subject selection refers to the need to select participants based on the scientific needs of research, and not on cost or convenience. This also encompasses a need to ensure that vulnerable populations are not exploited. As the Belmont report states, 'efficiency cannot override fairness in recruiting subjects'.

The risk-benefit ratio assessment requires that a proposed research project fulfils three conditions: risk to the participants must be minimized, potential benefits to the participant must be enhanced, and benefits to the participant and society must be proportionate or outweigh the risks (17). Respect for study participants encompasses the requirement to protect the participants from harm; including protection of their privacy, planning for interventions in case of study-related damage to meet at least the local standards, and providing all relevant information regarding their conditions to the study participants. Approval from an independent review board for the proposed research is required to ensure transparency and public accountability, as well as to ensure that the requirements discussed in this section are met in the study design.

Collaborative partnership is a concept that arose as the prevalence of research carried out in countries and communities different from that of the researchers increased. In this model, representatives of the country or the community where the research is taking place are involved in the project from the very early stages, from feasibility and risk-benefit assessment to carrying out the research and disseminating results. It is expected that this will give a voice to the research participants and help avoid exploitation of vulnerable persons. The partnership model for collaboration can produce high-quality research with greater influence on national policy and practice (18).

Ethicists are in general agreement that the broader ethical context should be similar wherever any human subject research is carried out, irrespective of the level of resources. However, as Macklin points out, there are certain areas in which there is 'stark disagreement' on what constitutes ethical behaviour in a modern setting (19). Though the basic principles are universal, ethics deal with moral rights and wrongs, which are not universal, and therefore it is essential to consider the sociocultural norms of the research milieu.

Exploitation is the key concern in conducting trials in resource-poor settings

Simply put, the concerns relating to conducting research in resource-poor settings arise around the issue of exploitation. Exploitation exists at two extremes: unfair burden of risks and unfair level of benefits. A exploits B when B receives an unfair level of benefits or unfair burden of risks as a result of interacting with A (17). Participants receiving 'unfair level of benefits' may be considered as being exploited due to 'undue inducement for participation' (20).

Entire volumes have been written about why exploitation is not exploitation if it is voluntary, how being exploited may not be harmful, and why exploitation should not necessarily be prevented (21, 22). In the context of clinical research in LAMIC, we see certain fundamental problems with such an approach. The highest level of ethical standards should be the norm in carrying out research in LAMIC due to the extreme powerlessness of the study participant in such cases. One can always mention legal redress. The practicalities of financial costs, logistical issues, cultural issues, and risk, combined with the lack of publicly available evidence and the complicated legal issues of liability and obligation of the primary company/sponsor, make it virtually impossible for a LAMIC research participant to seek redress through courts. The EU and the US have both recognized this disparity and have published draft proposals to address these issues by measures such as extending the jurisdiction of the US/EU courts where the parent companies sponsoring research are domiciled outside the US/EU, shifting the burden of proof from the purported victim, and seeking collective means of redress (23, 24).

Is there a need for special considerations in mental health research?

There should be no presumption of lack of capacity on the mere grounds of mental illness, although certain persons with mental disorders may not have the capacity to give informed consent to research. Where participant capacity is impaired, there is a greater obligation on the part of the researcher to protect such participants, but there are further unique challenges in mental health research that necessitate special protection for participants in such studies. Dubois undertakes a detailed discussion of why both the EU and US have considered legislating for special protection for people with mental health disorders (though it is yet to happen) and concludes that even if legislative protection does not materialize, educating researchers about this need should be mandatory (25):

> Research involving individuals with a mental illness poses unique ethical challenges due to the cognitive impairment, debilitation and stigma associated with many psychiatric diagnoses. These ethical challenges can arise at many points throughout the research process, including the trial design phase, the recruitment and inclusion stages, the process of gaining informed consent and the treatment washout period (26).

One concern is the heightened level of risk a participant may be subjected to in certain types of mental health research. For example, the use of placebos in an RCT could, under most circumstances, lead to an aggravation of the disease condition: greater risk of self-harm or suicide. Another concern is protection of confidentiality, which is imperative.

Controversies in conducting research in resource-poor settings

In general, the controversies in conducting research in resource-poor settings have centred on three issues (17):

1 the standard of care that should be used in research in LAMIC;

2 the 'reasonable availability' of interventions proven to be useful during the trials;

3 the quality of informed consent.

Even though the financial conflict of interests will not be a crucial issue in non-pharmaceutical research, most of the other issues will be similar. We believe vulnerability is another controversial issue in conducting research in LAMIC that cannot be ignored (27, 28).

Vulnerability

Conventional definitions of vulnerable populations included prisoners, disaster-affected populations, the mentally ill, and children (28). Vulnerability here is defined somewhat restrictively as 'those who have to bear unequal burden in research' because 'they are readily available in settings where research is conducted' (29).

However, taking a broader outlook at the concept, in certain societies women should be considered a vulnerable group. Also, students can be placed in a vulnerable position in respect to their superiors. Therefore, it is our argument that vulnerability is a relative and fluid concept that should be understood in the context of power issues. Through this view, we believe researchers as a group could be considered vulnerable in certain situations. Particularly, junior researchers could be vulnerable due to the power their senior counterparts, such as supervisors, hold. Vulnerability issues could also crop up between resource-poor and resource-rich partners in research conduct. As ethics is about moral rights and wrong, there is an intimate link between ethics and power/authority (30).

Trials with vulnerable and displaced populations

This issue needs special attention due to the large number of mental health research trials that take place in the wake of natural disasters. The fundamental philosophical approach to disaster research ethics is that the research undertaken should be particularly relevant to the disaster situation and limited to essential research that is not possible in non-disaster situations (27). The objectives of all research in disasters should be weighed very carefully for their potential contribution to the survivors and their communities, as well as their value in future disaster situations. All phases of research must be culturally sensitive and should involve experts familiar with the community.

Therapeutic misconception

When research is combined with humanitarian aid or clinical care there can be lack of clarity whether this is research or routine care. If information provided to potential participants does not explicitly mention research as well as therapeutic intent there is a likelihood of participants mistaking research for clinical services. This scenario is termed 'therapeutic misconception' (31). Therefore, it is vital that presence/absence of therapeutic intent is made clear to potential participants, and informed consent procedures should reduce the likelihood of participants mistaking research for clinical services.

Philanthropic misconception

Similar misconceptions are likely to exist among beneficiaries of philanthropy or humanitarian aid when these agencies conduct or sponsor research projects. The participants may start believing that the aim of such researchers is primarily human welfare and the best interests of individuals, instead of research. Ahmed and colleagues have termed this misconception 'philanthropic misconception' (32).

Ethics of conducting research in LAMIC

We now consider the three main concerns surrounding the ethics of conducting research in LAMIC.

Standard of care, clinical equipoise, and the ethics of study design

What constitutes clinical equipoise and is standard of care universal? The Helsinki Declaration stated that, 'In any medical study, every patient, including those of a control group, if any, should be assured of the best proven diagnostic and therapeutic method' (14). The DoH provision is based on the principle that an RCT comparing two substances is carried out because there is no evidence that one of the substances is more effective than the other in treating a condition. This state of clinical equipoise is necessary simply because if it were known that there was a more effective substance, the research would be redundant and the trial participants would be exposed to harm for no valid scientific reason. Clinical equipoise is an essential condition to be fulfilled for ethical approval of a study to be carried out in the West. As a result, placebo-controlled trials are carried out in the West only in situations where there is no known effective treatment. Active-controlled trials are indicated for situations where a known effective treatment exists, except under specific circumstances (see Box 8.1).

Box 8.1 DoH guidelines on the standard of care required in RCTs

Section 33 of the 2013 revised version

The benefits, risks, burdens, and effectiveness of a new intervention must be tested against those of the best, proven intervention(s), except in the following circumstances:

- ◆ Where no proven intervention exists, the use of placebo, or no intervention, is acceptable; or
- ◆ where for compelling and scientifically sound methodological reasons the use of any intervention less effective than the best proven one, the use of placebo, or no intervention is necessary to determine the efficacy or safety of an intervention, and the patients who receive any intervention less effective than the best proven one, placebo or no intervention will not be subject to additional risks of serious or irreversible harm as a result of not receiving the best proven intervention. Extreme care must be taken to avoid abuse of this option (14).

The controversy arises when the research is conducted in a location where the known effective treatment is not available. In the well-known case of azidothymidine (AZT) trials in Africa, a placebo-controlled trial was carried out to test the efficacy of a less intense treatment regimen for controlling the perinatal transmission of HIV (33). As an effective treatment regimen had already been established in the West as the standard of care, a placebo-controlled trial was not ethically permissible in the West, but the investigators in the AZT trials held that ethical norms only required that a control group in an RCT be given the current standard of care for the condition researched *in the country where the trial is conducted*. In both the AZT trials and the similarly well-known Surfaxin trials (where a placebo-controlled trial was carried out with premature neonates, although at least four other established treatments were available in the West), the argument was that as the usual standard of care for these women and babies was no treatment at all, they never had the opportunity of receiving treatment to begin with, and therefore the placebo group patients were not made 'worse off' by the lack of treatment. As such, the researchers argued that they were mere observers of what would happen to the participant women and babies, and that there was no ethical transgression. Furthermore, they argued that a placebo-controlled study provided the most reliable response to the research question at hand. Whilst recognizing that some participants would not benefit, defenders of the trials 'felt that this was morally acceptable as long as using placebo controls was necessary to gain the knowledge sought and no participant was made "worse off" than before the trial' (33). Defenders also commented on the issue of consent, citing *volenti non fit injuria*—to those consenting, no injury is done (34).

Is this double standard of less stringent ethical standards being good enough for developing countries acceptable? Macklin rejects this double standard for the simple reason of being the 'lowest common denominator that determines the minimal ethical obligations' (35). She argues that the principle of beneficence requires clinicians and researchers to maximize benefits as well as to minimize the harm suffered, and that a higher standard of care during the research is ethically preferable to providing the bare minimum. We believe that despite the guidelines at the time being open to interpretation, the morality of the action of knowingly allowing an infant to die, so that its path from respiratory distress/HIV to death can be recorded, is deplorable. Pogge points out that benefit to part of the group does not justify abandoning universal standards of care (36). The researcher is in a position to avoid the control group being harmed but fails to do so and compounds the moral wrong by extracting benefit to himself from the resulting harm. Even the justification of benefit to society through gaining scientific knowledge fails when the tested compound is merely a competitor drug. On a broader level, justice requires a researcher to be responsive to the health needs of his subjects, particularly if they are vulnerable subjects. Given that the majority of drugs that are tested in LAMIC are not for diseases unique to the country they are tested in, the commonest reasons for carrying out placebo-controlled trials in these locations are cheapness and lax ethical controls. Therefore, it is critical to assess if a placebo control is essential to the scientific needs or if it is simply due to economic and time convenience, before enabling such trials in LAMIC. After much deliberation and argument following the AZT and Surfaxin trials, the DoH was twice amended, and the standard of care required in medical research was finally restated in 2008.

What has changed in this version is the insistence that a placebo must not be used in cases where the subject is likely to suffer serious or irreversible harm. The use of placebo is permissible 'where no current proven intervention exists'. We interpret 'exists' as 'existing anywhere in the world' but are pessimistic about universal adoption of this interpretation, given the wriggling room still available to interpret it as 'existing in the country where the research is carried out'. The clause was revised again in October 2013 to further relax the requirements and now the use of placebo/less effective intervention/ no intervention is permissible as long as it does not lead to the patient being subjected to "additional" risks of serious harm.

Ironically, almost all these guidelines are centred on pharmaceutical research. Therefore, the challenge for those who will embark on conducting non-pharmaceutical RCTs and evaluating innovative packages of care and delivery systems for mental disorders in LAMIC lies in adapting the intention of these guidelines to such research. In most cases, the comparable in such interventions is 'treatment as usual', which may be neither evidence based nor the best treatment. The situation will be worse if there is no existing treatment or 'care', leading to the ethical and methodological challenge in establishing the existing intervention/care protocol.

> In order to support health research in developing countries that is both relevant and meaningful, the focus must be on developing health research that promotes equity and on developing local capacity in bioethics (37).

The considerations relating to the standard of care argument can be summarized as shown in Fig. 8.1.

Responsiveness of research to health priorities and reasonable availability

There is an inherent probability of exploitation in most research. If the trial is conducted in a resource-rich country, this concern is limited as there is also a reasonable probability of the participant and the community benefitting from the outcomes when

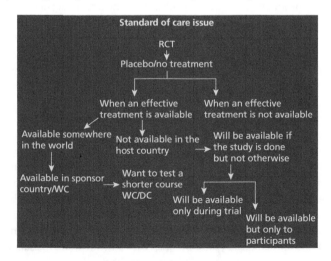

Fig. 8.1 The issue of standard of care at a glance.

Box 8.2 CIOMS guidelines on responsiveness to research

- ◆ The research is responsive to the health needs and priorities of the community in which it is to be carried out.
- ◆ Any intervention or product developed or knowledge generated will be made reasonably available for the benefit of that population or community.

these are integrated into the health care system. In contrast, in a LAMIC, the host country and the participants may not receive benefits that are fairly proportionate to the risk assumed during the trials. If, as the CIOMS guidelines state (see Box 8.2), the results of the research primarily benefit the people of rich countries, then such research can be rightly characterized as exploitative. Therefore, there exists a moral imperative to ensure that the host community/country is in a position to benefit from the results of the research, be it a product or knowledge gained (16).

In practice, the concept involves two distinct parts: (1) what is owed to the trial participants when the trial is over; and (2) what is owed to the community/country where the trial is conducted. Regarding what is owed to the participants, the CIOMS guidelines specifically require the sponsor to continue to provide successful treatment to the participants after the conclusion of the trials, while it is pending approval from the regulatory authorities. Regarding the host community/country, the highest ethical standards, as specified in the CIOMS guidelines, require that prior to undertaking the research, the investigators, including the sponsor, negotiate the requirements for safe and rational use of the interventions in the host country, should the research trial prove to be beneficial. In making the treatments 'reasonably' available, it is necessary to consider the duration for which the treatment will be provided in relation to the risk undertaken, the effect of withdrawal of the treatment, as well as the costs involved in such an undertaking. The CIOMS guidelines specifically mention that this applies primarily to research where a commercial product is the outcome. When the outcome is scientific knowledge, the requirement is only that this knowledge be used for the benefit of the population.

The best possible approach during non-pharmaceutical intervention research to ensure benefit for the community where research is conducted is local capacity building through proper planning in advance by networking with local colleagues via collaborative partnerships. Encouragingly, the major funding agencies for LAMIC research, such as the Wellcome Trust, Medical Research Council (MRC, UK), and National Institute of Health (NIH) (US), strongly encourage policy impact and involvement of local policy planners right from the start of research. They also encourage local capacity building and allocate 100% indirect costs to LAMIC partners.

Informed consent

Looking at the ethics of health research from the perspective of the four principles, where autonomy is a paramount requirement, neither the issue of a universal standard of care nor that of reasonable availability would arise. As long as the research participant was given all relevant information about the trial and steps were taken to ensure that this information was given in a form understandable to the participant, and if the participant freely agreed to assume the risks of the trial, such a trial would fulfil the ethical requirements of clinical research.

The DoH states: 'when obtaining informed consent for a research project, the physician should be particularly cautious if the subject is in a dependent relationship to him or her or may consent under duress. In that case a physician who is not engaged in the investigation and who is completely independent of this official relationship should obtain the informed consent' (14).

Consent is taken to be 'informed' when it is given by a person who understands the purpose and the nature of the research, what participating in the study requires the person to do and to risk, and what benefits are intended to result from the study (15, 38) (see Box 8.3).

Informed consent and information leaflets are mandatory requirements in today's research environment. Without using these words, no research is likely to be approved by an ethics review committee. As such, anyone with the remotest interest in ethics would be aware of what constitutes informed consent and the basic requirements of competency, full disclosure of all relevant information, comprehension, and the voluntary nature of the consent. Force, coercion, and undue inducement would undermine the validity of informed consent. The issue of informed versus understood consent results from concerns regarding information overload and presenting information in a format understood by participants (39).

Our discussion here therefore focuses on why informed consent alone may not be sufficient for assessing the ethicality of mental health trials in LAMIC, as autonomy has unfortunately served to subjugate other equally critical ethical aspects of research, particularly in settings of vulnerability or disadvantage. In mental health research, these disadvantages are further heightened as the participants may lack the capacity to understand or consent for research. There is also a strong probability of therapeutic misconception. When consent is given when there is no other favourable alternative, such consent may not be a valid consent. Pogge states that such a situation is rendered morally questionable even more in cases where those who benefit from the research have

Box 8.3 Factors affecting consent

◆ Consent/compliance
◆ Role of authority
◆ Obedience
◆ Conformity
◆ Duress
◆ Vulnerability
◆ Competence

colluded/participated in creating the circumstances that have placed the subject at a disadvantage: for example, in the case of lack of affordability of a high-priced drug in a LAMIC, the pharmaceutical company that is complicit in pricing the LAMIC patient out of the market may then benefit by that patient having to choose trial participation as a result of being priced out of the market (36).

In developed countries, informed consent is based on the autonomy of the individual, but in some LAMIC settings the initial decision-making for informed consent is typically vested in the community rather than the individual (40). However, such collective community agreement or the consent of the community leader or other authority or advocate substitute for an individual's informed consent (27).

A comprehensive publication entitled *Ethical challenges in study design and informed consent for health research in resource-poor settings* by Patricia A. Marshall is excellent further reading on the subject (41).

Ethics review and the role of the Ethics Review Committee

It is in this context of extreme powerlessness often faced by a trial participant in a LAMIC that there is a crucial need for independent ethics review of research projects. The role of the Ethics Review Committee (ERC) is primarily to ensure participant protection; most guidelines are now unequivocal that this is the paramount requirement.

Ethical responsibility beyond ethical clearance

Ethical clearance is a stamp that is given by an ERC to say that the work proposed has been planned and will be conducted ethically. However, there are many issues with this one-off certification:

- ◆ whether the proposed and approved work will be carried out in the same spirit and scientific rigor;
- ◆ whether the ethical clearance given or refused is valid and ethical in the first place.

The integrity of the committee members, and their capacity and experience determine the quality of the ethical clearance granted or rejected. As the quantum of research in LAMIC grow, there is, on the one hand, a significant growing demand for ethical review, and universities and other research-driven institutions are pressed to set up ethics committees. On the other hand, these committees may be formed without adequate capacity. Mushrooming of such ethics committees without adequate capacity is similar to having heads without brains! Major grant-awarding bodies encourage local capacity building in ethics review in LAMIC and some also have dedicated schemes supporting this endeavour.

Ethical responsibilities of those sitting on ERCs

ERCs exist to serve the specific purpose of providing peer reviews for research proposals submitted. When reviewing a research proposal there are certain fundamental principles that cannot be ignored by anyone who reviews research (see Box 8.4).

Box 8.4 Indicators: how to evaluate ethical conduct of an intervention

- Choice of the population and specific participants; not for easy and cheap research but for wider public good.
- Engaging locals—the process before starting the trial, managing unreasonable resistance from local professionals.
- Sensitivities in relation to the society and its culture.
- Informed and understood consent, making it work.
- Ethics review process—proactively identifying the ethical issues inherent in the proposal and clarifying how you will address them to suit the local context.

As bioethics is a relatively new area of study but is growing fast, those who review research need to keep up with the expanding knowledge base, because ignorance will result in injustice. Considering that ERCs review research in many different disciplines, they may not necessarily have expertise in the specific area of inquiry reviewed. It is therefore the duty and responsibility of the researcher to assist ethicist(s), by identifying specific ethical issues in their area of research interest and to propose proactive measures to deal with them.

Conclusion

Despite the myriad issues that could arise during the conduct of RCTs in low-resource settings, we believe there is a critical need for such research and that the challenges can be overcome effectively, provided certain prerequisites are achieved and there is goodwill from both sides of the 90:10 divide. It is therefore our objective to reshape the minds of researchers, to view ethics as an essential component and a friend of research, rather than one that is antagonistic to its aims. This can be achieved by empowering researchers to understand that addressing inherent ethical issues is not merely for the purposes of ethical review but to ensure a high quality of research, which will in turn strengthen their own research proposals. This model will be a mutual catalyst for both research and ethics. We hope this book not only provides factual information concerning ethics, but also instils an attitude change amongst researchers, especially those new and budding researchers in LAMIC as well as in the West.

References

1 Razzouk D, Sharan P, Gallo C, Gureje O, Lamberte EE, Mari JJ, et al. (2010) Scarcity and inequity of mental health research resources in low- and-middle income countries: a global survey. Health Policy, **94**:211–20.

2 Global Forum for Health Research (2000) The 10/90 report on health research. Geneva: WHO.

3 Sumathipala A, Siribaddana A, Patel V (2004) Under-representation of developing countries in the research literature: ethical issues arising from a survey of five leading medical journals. BMC Med Ethics, 5:5.

4 Patel V, Sumathipala A (2001) International representation in psychiatric literature: survey of six leading journals. Br J Psychiatry, 178:406–9.

5 Angell M (1997) The ethics of clinical research in the third world. N Engl J Med, 337(12):847–9.

6 Mari JJ (1997) Erasing the global divide in health research: collaborations provide answers to developing and developed countries. BMJ, 314:390.

7 Patel V, Pednekar S, Weiss H, Rodrigues M, Barros P, Nayak B, et al. (2005) Why do women complain of vaginal discharge? A population survey of infectious and pyschosocial risk factors in a South Asian community. Int J Epidemiol, 34:853–62.

8 Patel V, Weiss HA, Kirkwood BR, Pednekar S, Nevrekar P, Gupte S, et al. (2006) Common genital complaints in women: the contribution of psychosocial and infectious factors in a population-based cohort study in Goa, India. Int J Epidemiol, 35(6):1478–85.

9 Rahman A, Malik A, Sikander S, Roberts C, Creed F (2008) Cognitive behaviour therapy-based intervention by community health workers for mothers with depression and their infants in rural Pakistan: a cluster-randomised controlled trial. Lancet, 372(9642):902–9.

10 Patel V, Kirkwood B (2008) Perinatal depression treated by community health workers. Lancet, 372(9642):868–9.

11 O'Neill O (2002) Autonomy and trust in bioethics. Cambridge: Cambridge University Press.

12 Emanuel EJ, Wendler D, Grady C (2000) What makes clinical research ethical? JAMA, 283(20):2701–11.

13 Beauchamp T, Childress F (2001) Principles of biomedical ethics, 5th edn. Oxford: Oxford University Press.

14 World Medical Association (2013) WMA Declaration of Helsinki—ethical principles for medical research involving human subjects. 1964 and latest revision 2013. <http://www.wma.net/en/30publications/10policies/b3/>.

15 Council for International Organizations of Medical Sciences (1993) International ethical guidelines for biomedical research involving human subjects. Geneva: CIOMS.

16 Nuffield Council on Bioethics (2013) Exploring ethical issues in biology and medicine. <http://www.nuffieldbioethics.org/research-developing-countries>.

17 Emanuel EJ, Wendler D, Killen J, Grady C (2004) What makes clinical research in developing countries ethical? The benchmarks of ethical research. J Infect Dis, 189:930–7.

18 Costello A, Zumla A (2000) Moving to research partnership in developing countries. BMJ, 321:827.

19 Macklin R (2001) After Helsinki: unresolved issues in international research. Kennedy Inst Ethics J, 11:17–36.

20 Martin R (2005) Undue inducement in clinical research. Lancet, 366:275–6.

21 Hawkins J, Emanuel EJ (2008) Exploitation and developing countries: the ethics of clinical research. Princeton: Princeton University Press.

22 Feinberg J (1990) Harmless wrongdoing. Oxford: Oxford University Press.

23 Schipper I (2009) Clinical trials in developing countries: how to protect people against unethical practices? Brussels: Directorate-General for External Policies of the Union, European Parliament.

24 **Presidential Commission for the Study of Bioethical Issues** (2011) Research across borders. Proceedings of the International Research Panel of the Presidential Commission for the Study of Bioethical Issues. <http://www.bioethics.gov, http://www.mariestopes.org/sites/default/files/PCSBI-IRP_Research-Across-Borders_0_0.pdf>.

25 **Dubois J** (2007) Ethics in mental health research, Chapter 6. Oxford: Oxford University Press.

26 **Anderson KK, Mukherjee SD** (2007) The need for additional safeguards in the informed consent process in schizophrenia research. J Med Ethics, **33**:647–50.

27 **Sumathipala A, Jafarey A, De Castro L, Ahmed A, Marcer D, Srinivasan S, et al.** (2010) Ethical issues in post-disaster clinical interventions and research: a developing world perspective. Key findings from a drafting and consensus generation meeting of the Working Group on Disaster Research and Ethics (WGDRE) 2007. Asian Bioethics Rev, **2**(2):124–42.

28 **Sumathipala A, Siribaddana S** (2005) Research and clinical ethics after the tsunami: Sri Lanka. Lancet, **366**:1418–20.

29 **National Commission for the Protection of Human Subjects of Biomedical and Behavioral Research** (1979) The Belmont report. <http://www.hhs.gov/ohrp/humansubjects/guidance/belmont.html>.

30 **Benatar S** (2001) Justice and medical research. A global perspective. Bioethics, **15**(4):335–40.

31 **Henderson GE, Churchill LR, Davis AM Easter ME, Grady C, Joffe S, et al.** (2007) Clinical trials and medical care: defining the therapeutic misconception. PLoS Med, **4**(11).

32 **Ahmad A, Mahmud SM** (2010) Philanthropic misconception. Asian Bioethics Rev, **2**:154–61.

33 **Gu SM, Sayle A** (2006) The ethics of placebo-controlled studies on perinatal HIV transmission and its treatment in the developing world. Penn Bioethics J, **2**:21–4.

34 **Hawkins J, Emanuel EJ** (2000) Exploitation and developing countries: the ethics of clinical research. Princeton: Princeton University Press.

35 **Macklin R** (2004) Double standards in medical research in developing countries. Cambridge: Cambridge University Press.

36 **Pogge T** (2008) Testing our drugs on the poor abroad. Exploitation and developing countries: the ethics of clinical research. Princeton: Princeton University Press, p. 106.

37 **Bhutta ZA** (2002) Ethics in international health research: a perspective from the developing world. Bull World Health Organ, **80**:114–20.

38 **Alderson P, Goodey C** (1998) Theories of consent. BMJ, **317**:1313–15.

39 **Bhutta ZA** (2004) Beyond informed consent. Bull World Health Organ, **82**:771–7.

40 **Krogstad DJ, Diop S, Diallo A, Mzayek F, Keating J, Koita OA, et al.** (2010) Informed consent in international research: the rationale for different approaches. Am J Trop Med Hygiene, **83**(4):743–7.

41 **Marshall OA** (2007) Ethical challenges in study design and informed consent for health research in resource-poor settings. Geneva: WHO.

Part 2

Case studies of global mental health trials

Chapter 9

Trials of interventions for people with psychosis

Sudipto Chatterjee, Smita Naik,
Hamid Dabholkar, R. Padmavati, Sujit John,
Mirja Koschorke, and Rangaswamy Thara

Introduction

Schizophrenia is a severe mental disorder with a median lifetime prevalence of 4 per 1000 persons (1) that usually has an onset in early adulthood and then frequently takes a chronic or episodic course. According to the most recent estimates, mental and substance use disorders contribute to 7.4% of the global disability burden; within this category, schizophrenia accounts for 7.4% of the total DALYs (2). The psychotic, cognitive, and behavioural symptoms associated with the disorder contribute to serious disabilities in many domains of functioning. People with schizophrenia are further disadvantaged by a number of associated difficulties that contribute to their poor health and social outcomes. These include higher rates of suicide, premature mortality due to co- existing physical health problems (3), social exclusion due to widespread stigma and discrimination, and poverty due to the costs of treatment and the lack of economically viable work options (4–6). This combination of serious impairments, disabilities, and social disadvantages makes people with schizophrenia a highly vulnerable group. In addition, people with schizophrenia are often subjected to serious human rights violations across the world. Responding to their health and social needs is, therefore, a public health and ethical imperative for all countries.

In recognition of the complex needs of people with schizophrenia, a range of clinical and social services for people with schizophrenia coordinated by specialist community-based multidisciplinary teams within a well-defined health system, policy, and legal framework is the norm in many HIC. However, the situation for people with schizophrenia and their families in LAMIC is very different where similar community-based services, delivered by a specialist mental health workforce, do not exist in most countries. The reasons for this situation are a set of well-known and formidable challenges—the serious shortage of trained human resources, the lack of a clear mental health policy, the inadequate budgetary allocation for service development, and the inefficient and inequitable use of limited resources (7). Thus, the vast majority of people with schizophrenia in LAMIC cannot access community-based services, contributing to a very substantial treatment gap (8).

Schizophrenia is a priority mental health disorder in the WHO mhGAP that seeks to reduce the treatment gap for selected mental and neurological disorders in LAMIC through 'task-sharing'. (9). In the context of service provision for persons with schizophrenia, task-sharing generally involves the training and supervision of lay or non-specialist CHWs to deliver interventions such as psychoeducation, ensuring timely follow-up, rehabilitation, adherence management, improving access to employment opportunities, and networking with community agencies for social and social inclusion (Box 9.1). CHWs are most effective when they are part of a team and work closely with and under the supervision of specialist mental health professionals. CHWs have been successfully trained to identify and refer persons for specialist assessments, deliver accessible, need-based interventions in collaboration with the specialists, help develop mechanisms for initiating collective action through organizing self-help groups (SHGs), and engage with the community to enhance social inclusion and developmental opportunities (10, 11) (see Box 9.1).

Thus, there is now a small but growing and consistent observational evidence base from a number of community-based programmes that 'task-sharing' with lay or non-specialist health workers is a feasible and effective option in LAMIC. Involving lay or non-specialist CHWs can increase equitable access to services and has been shown to improve disability and social outcomes for people with schizophrenia and other severe mental disorders. In this chapter, we present a brief overview of intervention trials that have evaluated the effectiveness of psychosocial interventions for schizophrenia from LAMIC and then briefly describe the community care for people with schizophrenia in India (COPSI), using a case study to highlight the challenges involved in conducting

Box 9.1 mhGAP recommendations for psychoses (such as schizophrenia)

1 Pharmacological treatment using older antipsychotic medications (oral and injectable preparations) for both acute and maintenance phases of the treatment.

2 Psychosocial intervention comprising of:

- providing information to persons with psychosis and carers about the nature of illness, need for adherence, lifestyle modifications, and promotion of human rights;

- specific psychological treatments such as family therapy, social skills therapy, and CBT after specific training and under specialist supervision;

- facilitating rehabilitation in the community by coordinating health and social needs through appropriate networking with community agencies, by actively encouraging the person to resume social, educational, and vocational activities, by addressing stigma and discrimination, and by provision of supported community residential facilities, if necessary;

- regular follow-up to support adherence, assess needs, and provide ongoing support.

RCTs of complex interventions. Finally, we highlight the key learning experiences that may be of value to other researchers in this area.

Intervention studies for schizophrenia conducted in LAMIC

Similar to for other mental disorders, there is little evidence about the clinical and cost-effectiveness of community-based interventions in schizophrenia from RCTs conducted in LAMIC settings. This has been the most common observation of a number of recent systematic reviews evaluating psychosocial interventions for people with schizophrenia in LAMIC (12, 13). The bulk of the limited RCTs have been from China where various psychoeducational interventions with participants and family members have been shown to improve functioning for people with schizophrenia (12). More recently, two well-conducted RCTs from Pakistan (14), Iran (15), and Thailand (16) have demonstrated the effectiveness of structured adherence management and psychoeducational interventions across a range of outcomes. Thus, the available evidence, however limited, suggests that various psychosocial treatments can improve outcomes for people with schizophrenia in these settings.

However, two main issues with these studies limit their applicability when considering scaling up these interventions in LAMIC. First, these trials have been conducted in specialist hospital settings which makes their generalizability to community settings uncertain. Second, in these studies the psychosocial interventions were delivered by specialist mental health workers, making it unclear whether the reported benefits would be seen for similar interventions when delivered by lay or non-specialist CHWs.

The dearth of RCTs that can have a direct translational value for developing affordable and evidence-based services in LAMIC has been consistently identified as a serious research gap in a number of recent influential publications (13, 17). All of these have indicated that there is an urgent need to conduct RCTs that evaluate the effectiveness and costs of community-based interventions from LAMIC settings. However, as yet, there is no available RCT evaluating a community-based, multicomponent intervention delivered by CHWs from LAMIC settings. The trial described as a case study in the next section was specifically designed to address this research gap.

Case study: COPSI

The COPSI study is a multicentre effectiveness RCT (ISRCTN 56877013) designed to compare the clinical and cost-effectiveness of two service delivery methods for people with schizophrenia and their caregivers in India (18).

Study design

The COPSI study is a parallel group RCT to test the hypothesis that over 12 months, a combination of usual, facility-based care (FBC) plus a systematically developed collaborative community-based care (CCBC) intervention will be superior to FBC alone for people with moderate to severe schizophrenia. The primary outcomes were changes in overall symptoms and disability over 12 months. In addition, a number of secondary outcomes were assessed for persons with schizophrenia and their caregivers over 12 months.

In *persons with schizophrenia*, the *secondary objectives* were to determine whether FBC + CCBC will be more effective than FBC alone, in:

+ improving adherence to antipsychotic treatment;
+ reducing experiences of stigma and discrimination.

For *caregivers of people with schizophrenia*, the *secondary objectives* were to determine whether FBC + CCBC will be superior to FBC alone, in:

+ improving their knowledge and attitudes about the illness;
+ reducing their burden of caring;
+ reducing experiences of stigma and discrimination.

The *health economic objective* is to compare the costs and assess the cost-effectiveness and cost-utility of the FBC + CCBC intervention compared to FBC alone. In addition, the COPSI trial included a nested qualitative study to explore experiences of stigma and discrimination, the impact of the illness across key areas of life, and experiences of treatment at the point of entry into the trial and after 1 year.

Settings

The trial was conducted at three sites in India: in four blocks or sub-districts of the Kancheepuram district of the southern state of Tamil Nadu; across the state of Goa; and in the district of Satara in the western state of Maharashtra. The Tamil Nadu site was exclusively rural with no locally accessible mental health services available in the area. Both Satara and Goa had a mixed urban and rural population who had relatively easier access to specialist care in public and private care facilities. These three sites were chosen to reflect a diversity of health system contexts, to strengthen the generalizability of the study findings, and to meet trial recruitment targets within the allocated time frame.

Sample size and description

Since the COPSI trial was an effectiveness RCT, broad inclusion criteria were employed to identify potential participants. These were:

+ age between 16 and 60 years;
+ a primary International Classification of Diseases Diagnostic Criteria for Research (ICD-10 RCD) diagnosis of schizophrenia;
+ an illness duration of at least 12 months of at least overall moderate severity;
+ continued residence in the study catchment areas for the next 12 months.

In the rural Tamil Nadu site, a key-informant-based community survey was conducted to identify participants who met the inclusion criteria, while in Goa and Satara participants were recruited from the clinical practices of the collaborating psychiatrists. Based on data from the only available relevant study in India (10), it was assumed that a difference of 20% reduction on the mean PANSS total score would be clinically significant. The intra-class correlation between sites in the FBC arm was estimated at

0.05; for the FBC + CCBC arm (which also includes between-CHW clustering), this was assumed to be 0.1. An allocation ratio of 2:1 was used to allow for the between-CHW clustering effect in the FBC + CCBC arm. The estimated total sample size of 241 was increased to 282 to allow for 15% attrition during the course of the study. Using alpha = 0.05, this sample size had 80% power to detect an effect size of 0.8 (difference in PANSS score of 7.2 units, standard deviation (SD) = 9 units) and 90% power to detect an effect size of 1 (difference in PANSS score of 9 units, SD = 9 units).

Randomization and masking

Once baseline assessments were completed, randomization was stratified by site, and conducted using random block sizes chosen from 3, 6, and 9 using the '*ralloc*' routine in Stata (StataCorp, College Station, US), with individual participants being randomly allocated to receive either the FBC + CCBC intervention or FBC alone, respectively. For each site, a randomization list was generated independently by the trial statistician in London and transferred to the site data manager prior to the commencement of recruitment. The data manager had no part in recruiting participants and held the passwords for the randomization lists, while those recruiting participants did not have access to the randomization lists. The site data manager was responsible for assigning the unique trial ID for each participant. If the participant was assigned to the CCBC arm, the data manager notified the site intervention coordinator to communicate the required contact information to the intervention team. Treating psychiatrists were then provided with the allocation details to help record treatment information for the next 12 months for participants in both arms.

To maintain masking, all outcome measures were administered by researchers blind to the allocation status of individual participants and caregivers. However, neither participants nor the family caregivers were blind to their allocation status, making unmasking during the outcome assessments possible. To minimize this possibility, a number of measures were employed a priori:

◆ the intervention and research teams did not have any interactions during the trial and were located separate locations;

◆ prior to the assessment, CHWs were asked to specifically remind them about the need for blinding in data collection and, therefore, not to mention if they received any visits from CHWs;

◆ researchers were asked to complete the primary outcome measures- the Positive and Negative Syndrome Scale (PANSS) and the Indian Disability Evaluation and Assessment Scale (IDEAS) first.

All instances of unmasking were recorded and reported by the researchers. If this occurred at the time of the 6-month assessment, a separate researcher was allocated to undertake the 12-month assessments.

Trial intervention: CCBC

The CCBC intervention was systematically developed in iterative phases, in line with the recommendations of the MRC guidelines for developing and evaluating complex interventions (see Chapters 2 and 3). First, the individual components of the intervention were selected on the basis of a systematic review of the available scientific literature. For the selection of the CCBC components, two previous observational studies from a rural site in India were particularly important. The first study compared the effectiveness of a community-based rehabilitation (CBR) service, with routine facility-based outpatient (OP) services for people with chronic schizophrenia. The results indicated that the CBR service was more effective in retaining people in treatment and in improving symptoms, disability, and adherence (10). The second paper described the longer term outcomes of a CBR service for people with psychotic disorders in a defined catchment area. The CBR service, again provided by a specialist and CHWs, was associated with improved disability and a range of improved social and economic outcomes (11).

Second, to help improve the acceptability of the intervention, outcomes that mattered to people with schizophrenia and their caregivers were identified in Goa and in rural Tamil Nadu (19). Persons with schizophrenia and their caregivers identified 11 broad domains as being important outcomes of services. These were: symptom control; employment/education; social functioning; activities of daily living; fulfilment of duties and responsibilities; independent functioning; cognitive ability; management without medication; reduced side-effects; self-care; and self-determination. Across participants and caregivers, improvements in social functioning, employment/education, and activities of daily living were the most important desired outcomes of interest. When comparing the groups, symptom control and cognitive ability were more important to persons with schizophrenia, while independent functioning and fulfilment of duties were more important to caregivers. This information was useful to develop a more detailed understanding of the complex relationships between the components and the domains that were important for potential participants and their caregivers.

Third, pilot studies were carried out in two sites to identify the operational challenges involved in delivering the planned CCBC intervention (20). This process led to several changes to help improve the operational aspects of the intervention, such as developing more detailed methods of recording contact, specific strategies to address the issue of scheduling home-based sessions when caregivers were working, the development of a range of intervention material such as the information hand-outs about managing schizophrenia for participants and caregivers in relevant local languages, and a flip-chart to help CHWs communicate the contents of the psychoeducation sessions in a more interactive manner. Fourth, the experiences of the piloting exercise were collated and deliberated upon by the collaborators in order to finalize the CCBC intervention for the main trial.

The final CCBC intervention was designed to deliver a flexible, individualized, and needs-based intervention through an active collaboration between the person with schizophrenia, their caregivers, and the treatment team, including the CHWs. To standardize the intervention across the sites, a manual (<http://sangath.com/details.php?nav_id=60>) was developed, while allowing for flexibility in tailoring components to the individual needs of participants. The intervention was delivered in three phases: the initial, intensive engagement phase (0–3 months), the subsequent stabilization phase (4–7 months), and the maintenance phase (8–12 months). The sessions were delivered by the CHWs through home visits, or by delivering the session in the treatment facility or in any other location nominated by the participants; each session lasted between 45 and 60 minutes.

To meet the quality assurance and fidelity standards of the intervention across the sites, CHWs were supervised by intervention coordinators who were trained and mentored in the necessary supervision and monitoring skills. The treating psychiatrists supervised the overall intervention delivery through ongoing supervision sessions with the concerned CHWs and through a quarterly review and update of the individualized care plan. In addition, a set of predetermined process, fidelity, and quality assurance indicators were collected and collated from across the three sites on a monthly basis; this allowed a real-time monitoring of the progress of the trial.

The individual components of the final CCBC intervention are as follows:

- *Structured needs assessments* at enrolment and every 3 months thereafter, to develop personalized treatment plans.
- *Structured clinical reviews by treating team and supervision for CHWs.*
- *Psychoeducational information* for both participants and caregivers.
- *Adherence management strategies.*
- *Health promotion strategies* to address physical health problems in participants.
- Personalized *rehabilitation strategies* to improve the personal, social, and work functioning of participants.
- Specific efforts with participants and caregivers to deal with experiences of *stigma and discrimination.*
- Linkage to *self-help groups* and other methods of user-led support.
- *Networks with community agencies* to address social problems and facilitate social inclusion, access to legal benefits, and employment opportunities.

Control intervention: FBC

The comparison arm was designated FBC to reflect the usual care provided by specialist mental health practitioners for persons with schizophrenia and their families in India. However, there were differences between the operational aspects of the care facilities across the trial sites. In Goa and Satara, the recruiting facilities were the private clinics of the collaborating psychiatrists, backed up by separate inpatient facilities. In contrast, in rural Tamil Nadu, participants were identified through a population-based key informant survey and care services were provided through outreach camps at a designated community facility once every 2 weeks by a clinical team comprising the treating psychiatrists and trained assistants.

Across the sites, the FBC intervention was delivered by the psychiatrists through consultations lasting between 10 and 30 minutes. All persons with schizophrenia were prescribed antipsychotic medication by their treating psychiatrists. In addition to the medical treatments, psychiatrists provided information about the illness, encouraged medication adherence, and discussed other specific concerns that the person with schizophrenia or their family members mentioned, as and when felt to be necessary.

The FBC was available to participants in both study arms; thus, the treating psychiatrists were aware of the allocation status of the participant.

Outcomes

While a number of outcome measures were used to compare the interventions, in this chapter we discuss the primary outcomes—changes in symptom and disability scores in participants at baseline and at 12 months. The symptoms of schizophrenia were assessed by using the PANSS, a widely used measure of psychopathology in schizophrenia. The PANSS comprises 30 items measuring three broad domains of symptoms: positive, negative, and general psychopathology. Each item is rated on a 1–7 point scale, with increasing scores reflecting a greater severity of symptoms. Since this is a highly structured assessment that requires a suitable degree of clinical expertise, the scale was administered by mental health professionals who were trained, certified, and supervised by external experts.

To assess disability, the IDEAS was used at baseline and at 12 months. The IDEAS is used to assess four domains of disability related to schizophrenia: self-care; interpersonal activities; communication and understanding; and work. Each item is rated on a 1–4 scale to generate a total disability score; similar to the PANSS, a higher score is indicative of greater disability levels. The information related to the IDEAS was collected by generic researchers through interviewing both the participant and the primary caregiver.

Ethical procedures

Formal ethical approval for conducting the trial was obtained from the ethics committees of all the organizations involved in the study—the Kings' College, London, the London School of Hygiene and Tropical Medicine, and the institutional review boards at the Schizophrenia Research Foundation Centre (SCARF) and Sangath. The trial was also registered with the International Society for the Registration of Clinical Trials (RCT: ISRCTN 56877013).

Apart from this, the trial was regulated by an independent trial monitoring committee (TMC) which comprised mental health experts and a service user who reviewed and approved the protocol independently before commencement of subject recruitment. The TMC was provided with periodic updates describing the trial progress. The reports included information on four specific serious adverse events—death, suicide attempt, hospitalization (from any cause), and serious medication side-effects.

GCP guidelines related to data management and protecting the confidentiality of study participants were incorporated, and this was principally achieved by separating study data from participant-identifiable data by replacing the latter with unique trial IDs. The original data were kept in a restricted password-protected file that could be accessed by the data manager alone.

Consent procedure

People with schizophrenia constitute a vulnerable group who pose unique challenges in relation to their informed participation in clinical trials. One of the key assumptions underlying the informed consent procedure is that the person has adequate decision-making capacity to make an informed choice. Although most people with schizophrenia have adequate decisional capacity to provide meaningful consent, decision-making ability is sometimes compromised during the course of the illness. The most common or 'universal' challenge, therefore, is to ensure that the person with schizophrenia has adequate decision-making ability when making the choice to participate in a trial or not.

In countries like India, there are additional, contextual challenges that significantly influence consent procedures for clinical trials. First, in comparison to HIC, the construct of informed consent is not as uniformly embedded in the local culture. Second, there is a highly skewed power differential between doctors and participants which can adversely influence the achievement of a truly free informed consent process. Third, information related to the purpose, procedures, risks, and potential benefits of trials is often presented in a technical and unfriendly manner, which is a particular problem because many participants are of limited literacy and are unable to read or understand the contents of the information sheets. Fourth, the close involvement of caregivers in all aspects of decision-making related to accessing treatments in India makes it difficult to ensure autonomous decision-making, as envisaged in the existing ethical guidelines.

The COPSI informed consent procedure was systematically designed to address these important challenges. First, to understand the challenges involved in conducting informed consent procedures with people with schizophrenia and their caregivers, a pilot study was conducted in Goa. A set of information sheets were developed for this purpose, and trained researchers conducted the informed consent procedure in a standardized manner with persons separately with schizophrenia and their caregivers. A number of dimensions related to the consent procedure, such as the adequacy and ease of understanding of the information and the involvement of the caregivers in making an informed choice, and perceived levels of privacy were explored through in-depth interviews.

Most persons with schizophrenia and their caregivers felt that they could make an independent decision to participate and, if needed, could also have the option of discussing any issues with their caregivers. The recall of the essential sections of the information sheet varied widely between participants, suggesting the need for the information to be provided in a more interactive manner. Both primary caregivers and persons also identified the need for improvements in making the information sheets and consent forms simpler. Another specific suggestion was to use visual prompts to supplement the procedure, especially for people who could not read or understand the written material clearly.

Based on this feedback, a number of adaptations were made to the procedure. First, the language used in the information sheets was simplified and systematically translated into the five relevant regional languages across the sites. A flipchart (<http://sangath.com/details.php?nav_id=60>) containing simple a set of diagrams to explain the key elements of the study was developed to promote a more interactive method of information provision during the consent procedure for the main trial.

Second, to ensure that only persons with schizophrenia having the capacity to make an informed choice were approached for participation, specific screening for capacity was conducted by the treating psychiatrist prior to consent procedure being carried out and by the consent interviewer at the time of the consent interview.

Third, to promote autonomous decision-making by participants, the consent interview was delinked from the treating psychiatrist. Separate consent interviews were independently carried out for participants and caregivers by highly trained researchers; as an additional requirement, both persons with schizophrenia and their caregivers had to independently consent to participate in the study.

Fourth, other specific steps taken to reduce possible attrition during the procedure included having the capacity to conduct the consent interviews in a flexible location of convenience for the participants and caregivers. For example, participants could nominate an alternative place of interview other than at home, to negate worries about public disclosure due to the home visit by the researcher. All of these measures led to a high acceptability of the procedure as well as overall satisfaction from the perspective of the participants and caregivers across the sites.

Results

Across the three sites, a total of 1021 people with schizophrenia were screened for eligibility. Of these, 587 (57%) did not meet one or more of the inclusion criteria. Of the 434 eligible persons with schizophrenia, the consent procedure could be conducted for 332 (76%) of them. Of these 332 persons, a total of 282 (85%) persons with schizophrenia and their primary caregivers were enrolled in the trial. One hundred and eighty seven of the participants were randomly allocated to the FBC + CBCC arm, while 95 were randomly assigned to the FBC arm, as per protocol and without any instance of unmasking. The overwhelming majority of participants in both arms (91% in the FBC + CBCC arm; 90% in the FBC arm) were available for the 12-month endpoint assessments.

The intervention was monitored on an ongoing basis across the sites by collecting key process indicators that described essential aspects of the interventions. For example, the mean number of sessions with CHW received by participants in the CCBC intervention arm was 18, and 169 (90.3%) received the predefined 'minimally effective' 12 sessions. The mean number of contacts with a treating psychiatrist was 10 (95% CI 9.53–10.89) in the CBCC arm and 8 (95% CI 6.98–9.11) in the FBC arm. In addition, a number of supervision mechanisms, such as onsite supervision of live sessions by the intervention facilitator/coordinator, team reviews, and interactions with the treating psychiatrist, were conducted as per protocol. The process and supervision data indicate that the intervention was delivered according to predefined fidelity and quality assurance standards across the sites.

The baseline sociodemographic and clinical characteristics of participants were very similar across arms, indicating that randomization was successful in achieving balance between the two arms. The mean age of participants was 36 years (SD 10.2); approximately half (47%) were female and about 20% had no formal education, while the median duration of illness was 7 years in the FBC + CCBC arm and 6.25 years in the FBC arm. Though many were on treatment for some time prior to the baseline assessments, only a small number of participants (20% in the CCBC arm; 25% in the FBC arm) were engaged in some income-generating work at the time of recruitment and fewer than half were married. This profile of being both unmarried and not working is unusual in India for the age of the participants and is indicative of the severity of their social disabilities.

At 12 months, there was a greater reduction in overall symptoms and disabilities in the FBC + CCBC arm participants. After adjusting for baseline PANSS scores and site, the total PANSS score was lower at 12 months in the FBC + CCBC arm than in the FBC arm, (adjusted mean difference: –3.75; 95% CI –7.92 to 0.42; p = 0.08).

The FBC + CCBC intervention was more effective in reducing disabilities than symptoms. Participants in this arm had both a statistically (adjusted mean difference in IDEAS score: –0.95; 95% CI –1.68 to –0.23; p = 0.01) and a clinically significant reduction in total disability scores, as indicated by the analysis of the odds of improving by 20% or more on the IDEAS total score (46.6% vs 34.2%, respectively) (adjusted odds ratio: 1.78; 95% CI 0.95–3.33; p = 0.07).

Overall, these results indicate that the FBC + CCBC intervention appears to be more effective than FBC alone in improving symptoms and disabilities in people with moderate to severe schizophrenia in India. The overall benefits of the intervention are modest at 12 months and most evident in reducing the disabilities associated with schizophrenia. There was also a trend for improvement in the severity of symptoms with the intervention; however, this was not statistically or clinically significantly different in comparison to FBC at 12 months.

Strengths and limitations

The COPSI trial was a multisite effectiveness study to examine whether augmenting usual, FBC with an additional, CCBC intervention would improve symptoms and disabilities in people with moderate to severe schizophrenia. The strengths of the COPSI trial include the large sample size and allocation method that specifically accounts for the effects of clustering between sites and CHWs, the successful masking of allocation, the delivery of the CCBC intervention according to protocol across the sites, and the low attrition rates. The broad inclusion criteria and the fact that participants were recruited from real-world clinical settings across three diverse sites and practice arrangements in India suggest that the findings of the trial are generalizable to similar settings in other parts of India and, possibly, other LAMIC.

The modest improvements seen with a more resource-intensive CCBC intervention is surprising, given the large benefits of these measures reported from a number of previous observational studies. This could be due to the nature of the trial sample, the quality of the FBC intervention, or the duration of follow-up involved in the study. For example, participants in the trial had a median duration of about 7 years of the illness, at least a moderate severity of symptoms and disabilities, as well as elevated rates of social adversity such as being single and unemployed. In addition, the majority of participants, though adherent with ongoing treatment, continued to cross the threshold of severity that enabled their inclusion in the trial. For this group of people with long-term and severely disabling symptoms and with multiple social problems, these modest improvements in disability and symptoms may reflect the limits of effectiveness of the CCBC intervention.

In addition, another reason for the limited effectiveness of the FBC + CCBC intervention could be in the choice of the trial recruiting facilities and the quality of the FBC intervention delivered in the trial sites. Recruitment for the trial was from purposively chosen sites selected on the basis of their motivation to participate in such a trial and their ability to manage the fairly complex technical requirements of the trial; this non-random selection of the trial facilities makes selection bias possible. Thus, another likely reason for the modest additional effectiveness of the CCBC intervention was the high quality of the FBC intervention delivered at the sites by the highly trained and experienced psychiatrists participating in the trial.

Clinical improvement in people with more severe schizophrenia is often a gradual process and, in that context, the relatively short follow-up duration of 12 months is a limitation. The longitudinal analysis of the disability data shows that significant improvements in the CCBC arm occurred between the 6- and 12-month period, suggesting that a longer duration of follow-up is necessary to demonstrate the additional benefits of non-pharmacological interventions.

Lessons learned

The COPSI trial is one of the largest RCTs conducted for people with schizophrenia in a LAMIC setting. There were obviously many complexities and challenges involved in conducting this multicentre trial in a successful manner. Some of the important challenges included recruiting subjects in a timely manner across the sites and in ensuring their continued participation in the trial, maintaining the fidelity and quality assurance standards of a psychosocial intervention delivered by CHWs across three diverse sites, and effectively coordinating the various dimensions of the trial administration between the many teams and individuals. The success in implementing the COPSI trial as per protocol can be attributed to the closely coordinated and effective process that was employed to address challenges proactively. Some of these are challenges and the solutions tried in the study may be relevant to other researchers conducting RCTs in LAMIC settings; hence they are briefly summarized in Table 9.1.

Undertaking and successfully managing clinical trials involving the evaluation of complex psychosocial interventions is an inherently complicated exercise, as even the best planned clinical trials can be adversely influenced by completely unanticipated developments. For example, the COPSI trial was seriously threatened by the sudden and unilateral exit of one of the two original sites (a government mental hospital) just 6 months before the initiation of the main trial. In response to the crisis, a unanimous decision was made by the trial collaborators to invite suitable psychiatrists working in the private sector to participate in the trial. In retrospect, this crisis was an opportunity to demonstrate that it was very much possible to work with specialists in the private sector while conducting rigorous RCTs of complex mental health interventions. This is of particular relevance in countries like India where a large proportion of services are provided by the private sector and are yet not included conventionally in research studies. On the other hand, our 'usual care' arm no longer represented the typical care received in the government sector and could have, as mentioned earlier, contributed to the smaller effects observed in favour of the intervention.

Table 9.1 Summary of the challenges and solutions in the COPSI trial

Challenge	Solutions
Working with multiple partners across sites and countries	Developed memoranda of understanding (MoUs) between collaborating institutions and individual psychiatrists with clear outlines of roles and responsibilities
	Developed clear trial administrative structure and reporting requirements
	Developed clear financial management guidelines with all institutional partners
	Maintained commitment to adhere to plans and protocols through regular updates on trial progress and problems
Recruitment and retention of key study staff	Recruited highly committed and effective senior management team across the sites
	Continued capacity building to sustain interest and competence of the management, research, and intervention teams
	Retained staff through adopting clear human resource policies, building in adequate support and supervision resources, fostering a sense of common purpose and morale, managing interpersonal problems proactively in a transparent manner, building team rituals, and assistance in career advancement pathways
	Planned for staff turnover during the period of the study, and ensured systems are in place for ongoing training
Recruitment and retention of participants over 12 months	Developed a process for highly informed participation and by involving caregivers
	Offered encouragement by treating psychiatrist to continue in the study during follow-up visits
	Developed an online tracking system using Google apps which was used to generate timely alerts for impending assessments
	Had well-trained research and intervention teams interacting with participants and caregivers in a competent and professional manner
Trial management and coordination across multiple sites	Developed a detailed protocol with timelines for the conduct of the trial across the various phases
	Ensured close oversight of trial progress by trial coordinator and regular consultations with teams at each site as well as with the study collaborators
	Used three key qualities to characterize the successful onsite study teams: (1) organizational commitment; (2) effective leadership by onsite study coordinators; and (3) effective lines of communication between the onsite study coordinators and study staff
	Ensured effective operational implementation of study procedures, subject recruitment timelines, data management, and funds management (which includes planning, spending, and reconciling budgets)
	Developed clear standard operating procedures (SOP) governing recruitment procedures, flow of participants, timing and content of research assessments, intervention delivery as per protocol, AE monitoring, and reporting across the sites
	Had a clear reporting structure and clear accountability of various personnel for monitoring the progress of the trial
	Used key process, fidelity, and quality assurance indicators to monitor trial progress in real time

Table 9.1 (continued) Summary of the challenges and solutions in the COPSI trial

Challenge	Solutions
Managing the requirements for independent oversight	Ensured timely completion of trial registration update and closure reports Had well-developed protocol for communication with the TMC, including planned meetings Provided periodic updates of the trial progress to the TMC as per agreed protocol
Managing the nested qualitative study	Had dedicated human and financial resources for conducting the qualitative study across the sites Offered ongoing training and close supervision to build high level of competencies in the study researchers Ensured close and ongoing communication between the main trial and the nested study teams Managed the considerable logistical challenges involved in conducting the nested study such as the transcription, translation, and coding of the interviews in a time-bound and quality-assured manner
Closing the trial to comply with all financial and regulatory standards	Managed and supported the exit of study staff across sites Ensured continuity of care for trial participants by handing over care to treating psychiatrists in a structured manner Provided necessary trial closure report to collaborating institutions and funders

A very important and optimistic lesson from the COPSI trial is that high-quality psychosocial RCTs that have a direct bearing on the issue of providing services to people with schizophrenia can be successfully implemented in LAMIC settings with limited resources. At the heart of a successful trial is having a highly committed and stable trial senior management team who have the leadership and shared vision to achieve a high benchmark of quality. Similar lessons emerge from other RCTS of interventions for people with schizophrenia, as shown in Table 9.2. In our experience, the quality of the trial will only be as good as the quality of the staff involved in conducting the trial. The success of meticulous planning and close monitoring of trials is more likely in situations where all personnel involved in the trial are highly trained, competent, and motivated.

Another key lesson from the COPSI trial is the importance of conducting relevant formative research and piloting of the intervention before initiating the main trial. Adopting a systematic and sequential approach in developing and refining a psychosocial intervention is well worth the trouble. As mentioned in earlier sections of the chapter, the quality of the final COPSI trial was significantly improved by following this iterative and phased approach, and this approach is highly recommended for similar future trials.

Table 9.2 Overview of RCTs of interventions for people with schizophrenia in LAMIC

Country	Setting	Study design	Human resource used	Target sample	Type of intervention	Comparison group	Outcomes selected	Main findings
China, 2005 (21)	Psychiatric hospital	RCT, 3 and 9 months follow-up	An experienced nurse provided the intervention, with the aid of research assistants who had worked in psychiatric nursing for at least 10 years. The research assistants were provided with direct supervision and 12 hours of training in the intervention. To ensure consistency, they were observed in a pilot scenario before the main study	101 patients with schizophrenia and their families	Psychoeducation programmes for patients and families (8 hours with the patient and 36 hours with the family in hospital, and then 2 hours per month for 3 months after discharge for patient and family together)	Routine care provided in the clinic	Knowledge about schizophrenia, psychopathology, functioning, relapse rates, and medication compliance	Significant improvement in knowledge about schizophrenia, reduction in symptoms, and improvement in functioning in the intervention group at 9 months after discharge. Intervention did not have an impact on readmission rates and medication adherence
Pakistan, 2011 (15)	Psychiatry department of general hospital	RCT, 3, 6, and 12 months follow-up	Two consultant psychiatrists, 3 postgraduate trainees with a minimum of 2 years training in psychiatry, 2 qualified psychiatric nurses, and a master's degree level social worker	110 patients with schizophrenia or schizoaffective disorder and their respective caregivers	Psychoeducation programme for caregiver along with training in techniques for administering and supervising the medication	Routine care provided in the clinic	Medication adherence, symptoms, and functioning	Participants in the intervention group had better adherence (complete adherence 67.3% vs 45.5%) and significant improvement in symptoms and functioning

Table 9.2 (continued) Overview of RCTs of interventions for people with schizophrenia in LAMIC

Country	Setting	Study design	Human resource used	Target sample	Type of intervention	Comparison group	Outcomes selected	Main findings
Iran, 2012 (16)	Three psychiatric centres	RCT, immediately after intervention and 1 month follow-up	One psychiatrist/psychiatric nurse, 1 recovered patient	70 patients with schizophrenia and their respective caregivers	Psychoeducation programme for caregiver (10 sessions comprising 2 sessions per week of 90 minutes for 5 weeks)	Routine care provided in the clinic	Symptoms and family burden	The intervention group showed significantly reduced symptom severity and caregiver burden both immediately after intervention and 1 month later
Malaysia, 2010 (17)	Six community psychiatric clinics	Controlled trial, cluster allocation, 3 and 6 months follow-up	Psychiatrists and psychoeducation team comprising staff nurses and medical assessments	109 patients and their respective caregivers	Psychoeducation programme for caregivers (5 sessions of 1 hour each over 2 weeks)	Routine care provided in the clinic	Knowledge, burden, relapse, and clinic follow-up rates	The intervention group showed significant improvement in knowledge, and reduction in burden in assistance in daily living (severity), and a reduced defaulter rate was seen in the patients' follow-up

The final important lesson learned from the COPSI trial was the benefit of investing time and effort in developing a detailed dissemination strategy and a consensus publication plan well before the scheduled completion of the trial duration. Effectiveness trials like COPSI have a relevance to a range of stakeholders, including participants and their families, the scientific community, agencies in national governments in LAMIC that deal with public health policy and financing, as well as a number of global agencies involved in this sector. While publication of the trial results in high-impact scientific journals is an obvious dissemination strategy, our experience suggests the need to go beyond this conventional approach to effectively appeal to a larger audience. In the context of the COPSI trial, a range of dissemination materials were produced and combined as a multipurpose resource kit. The dissemination kit contained the manual for the CHWs, a set of information hand-outs for persons with schizophrenia and their caregivers, the flipchart used by the CHWs to communicate the individual treatments of the CCBC intervention, a booklet describing the real life stories of recovery of trial participants and their caregivers in the course of the study, and two documentary films of the experiences of participants and caregivers at the rural Tamil Nadu and the Satara sites. All these resources are free to access from the You Tube Satara video- http://youtu.be/HYGkgh4lXio; Chennai video http://www.youtube.com/watch?v=VBFeStQJtJo-Part1 http://www.youtube.com/watch?annotation_id=annotation_447286&feature=iv&src_vid=VBFeStQJtJo&v=U7Xu_-gNtvY- Part 2) the website of Sangath (<http://www.sangath.com>) and the Centre for Global Mental Health. A multimodal approach to disseminating trial results that have translational value to a wide range of stakeholders in LAMIC is a necessary requirement and needs to be planned for carefully from the very beginning of the trial.

Conclusion

The COPSI trial results demonstrate that the strategy of involving trained and well-supervised CHWs to deliver a community-based intervention for people with schizophrenia is modestly more effective in comparison to the high-quality specialist care provided from facilities. These results strengthen the evidence base for the use of CHWs in enhancing access to services for people with schizophrenia in LAMIC settings where specialist resources are scarce. The COPSI findings are an important addition to the ongoing policy and advocacy efforts for making evidence-based services available for many more people with schizophrenia in LAMIC in the near future.

References

1 Saha S, Chant D, Welham J, McGrath J (2005) A systematic review of the prevalence of schizophrenia. PLoS Med, 2(5):e141.

2 Whiteford HA, Degenhardt L, Rehm J, Baxter AJ, Ferrari AJ, Erskine HE, et al. (2010) Global burden of disease attributable to mental and substance use disorders: findings from the Global Burden of Disease Study 2010. Lancet, 382(9984):1575–86.

3 Brown S, Kim M, Mitchell C, Inskip H (2010) Twenty-five year mortality of a community cohort with schizophrenia. Br J Psychiatry, 196:116–21.

4 Thornicroft G, Brohan E, Rose D, Sartorius N, Leese M, INDIGO Study Group (2009) Global pattern of experienced and anticipated discrimination against people with schizophrenia: a cross-sectional survey. Lancet, 373:408–15.

5 Lund C, De Silva M, Plagerson S, Cooper S, Chisholm D, Das J, et al. (2011) Poverty and mental disorders: breaking the cycle in low-income and middle-income countries. Lancet, 378:1502–14.

6 Drew N, Funk M, Tang S, Lamichhane J, Chávez E, Katontoka S, et al. (2011) Human rights violations of people with mental and psychosocial disabilities: an unresolved global crisis. Lancet, 378(9803):1664–75.

7 Saxena S, Thornicroft G, Knapp M, Whiteford H (2007) Resources for mental health: scarcity, inequity, and inefficiency. Lancet, 370(9590):878–89.

8 Kohn R, Saxena S, Levav I, Saraceno B (2004) The treatment gap in mental health care. Bull World Health Organ, 82:858–66.

9 Dua T, Barbui C, Clark N, Fleischmann A, Poznyak V, van Ommeren M, et al. (2011) Evidence-based guidelines for mental, neurological, and substance use disorders in low- and middle-income countries: summary of WHO recommendations. PLoS Med, 8(11):e1001122.

10 Chatterjee S, Patel V, Chatterjee A, Weiss HA (2003) Evaluation of a community-based rehabilitation model for chronic schizophrenia in rural India. Br J Psychiatry, 182:57–62.

11 Chatterjee S, Pillai A, Jain S, Cohen A, Patel V (2009) Outcomes of people with psychotic disorders in a community-based rehabilitation programme in rural India. Br J Psychiatry, 195:433–9.

12 De Silva MJ, Cooper S, Li HL, Lund C, Patel V (2013) Effect of psychosocial interventions on social functioning in depression and schizophrenia: meta-analysis. Br J Psychiatry, 202:253–60.

13 Eaton J, McCay L, Semrau M, Chatterjee S, Baingana F, Araya R, et al. (2011) Scale up of services for mental health in low-income and middle-income countries. Lancet, 378(9802):1592–603.

14 Farooq S, Nazar Z, Irfan M, Akhter J, Gul E, Irfan U, et al. (2011) Schizophrenia medication adherence in a resource poor setting: randomised controlled trial of supervised treatments for out-patients for schizophrenia (STOPS). Br J Psychiatry, 199:467–72.

15 Sharif F, Sheygan M, Mani A (2012) Effect of a psycho-educational intervention for family members on caregiver burdens and psychiatric symptoms in patients with schizophrenia in Shiraz, Iran. BMC Psychiatry, 12:48.

16 Parantahaman V, Kaur S, Lim J-L, Amar-Singh HS, Sararaks S, Nafiza MN, et al. (2010) Effective implementation of a structured psychoeducation programme among caregivers of patients with schizophrenia in the community. Asian J Psychiatry, 3:206–12.

17 Lancet Global Mental Health Group, Chisholm D, Flisher AJ, Lund C, Patel V, Saxena S, et al. (2007) Scale up services for mental disorders: a call for action. Lancet, 370:1241–52.

18 Chatterjee S, Leese M, Koschorke M, McCrone P, Naik S, John S, et al. (2011) Collaborative community based care for people and their families living with schizophrenia in India: protocol for a randomised controlled trial. Trials, 12:12.

19 Balaji M, Chatterjee S, Brennan B, Rangaswamy T, Thornicroft G, Patel V (2012) Outcomes that matter: a qualitative study with persons with schizophrenia and their primary caregivers in India. Asian J Psychiatry, 5:258–65.

20 **Balaji M, Chatterjee S, Koschorke M, Rangaswamy T, Chavan A, Dabholkar H, et al.** (2012) The development of a lay health worker delivered collaborative community based intervention for people with schizophrenia in India. BMC Health Serv Res, **12**:42.

21 **Li Z, Arthur D** (2005) Family education for people with schizophrenia in Beijing, China. Randomised controlled trial. Br J Psychiatry, **187**:339–45.

Chapter 10

Trials of interventions for people with depression

Neerja Chowdhary, Atif Rahman,
Helena Verdeli, and Vikram Patel

Introduction

Common mental disorders (CMD) are the heterogeneous ICD-10 categories of mood-, anxiety-, and stress-related disorders. Since they often co-occur, and share similar risk factors and interventions, they are frequently clubbed together for public health purposes. Depression is by far the most recognized CMD and is estimated to affect 350 million people worldwide (1). Its cardinal features are low mood, loss of interest in daily life, and fatigue; other common complaints include sleep and appetite disturbances, aches and pains, poor concentration, rumination, irritability, and suicidal thoughts. The WHO World Mental Health Survey initiative collected data on the prevalence and determinants of depression from ten HIC and eight LAMIC (1). The findings reveal that the average lifetime and 12-month prevalence estimates of depression were 14.6% and 5.5% in HIC and 11.1% and 5.9% in LAMIC respectively. Depression is projected to be, overall, the second leading cause of burden of disease by 2020 (2, 3). The average age of onset ascertained retrospectively was 25.7 years in HIC and 24.0 years in LAMIC. The female:male ratio is approximately 2:1. There is consistent, cross-cultural evidence showing a strong, bidirectional association between depression and social disadvantage (4).

Depression is often co-morbid with other chronic diseases and contributes significantly to the disability associated with them (5). The relationships between physical health and depression are complex. Depression is a risk factor for a number of communicable and non-communicable diseases, and many physical health conditions increase the risk for depression (6). Co-morbidity complicates help-seeking, diagnosis, and treatment, and affects the outcomes of treatment for physical conditions, including disease-related mortality. For example, depression is an independent risk factor for cardiovascular diseases (CVD) including angina, myocardial infarction, and stroke (7, 8). Furthermore, depression predicts reinfarction and death after myocardial infarction. Depression also increases the risk for onset of type II diabetes, and there is extensive co-morbidity between diabetes and mood disorders (9).

There may be a particular salience of depression for women, given its higher prevalence in women and significant associations with reproductive, maternal, and child health. Depression has been associated with dysmenorrhea, dyspareunia, and pelvic pain (10). Maternal depression may also have important implications for infant growth and survival. A meta-analysis of 17 studies from 11 LAMIC reported that the children of mothers with depression or depressive symptoms were more likely to be underweight (odds ratio (OR) 1.5; 95% CI 1.2–1.8) or stunted (OR 1.4; 95% CI 1.2–1.7) (11). Maternal depression reduces adherence to child-health promotion and disease-prevention interventions, for example immunization, and there is evidence that suggests that maternal depression is associated with sub-optimal breast-feeding (12, 13).

Apart from worsening the outcomes of co-morbid physical health problems, depression is associated with increased mortality through suicide. Each year at least 800,000 people commit suicide, 86% in LAMIC (6). Mental disorder is overwhelmingly the most important preventable factor for suicide, and depression is by far the most important mental disorder that predicts suicide (14). A systematic review of psychological autopsy studies identified depression (along with other mental disorders) as the important proximal risk factor for suicide, with a median prevalence of mental disorder of 91% in suicide completers and a population-attributable fraction of 47–74% (15).

Thus, depression is a global health priority because of its frequency, early onset, and strong association with premature mortality, poor physical health, functional impairment, and social adversity. The WHO mhGAP provides evidence-based recommendations for the treatment of depression (16). These are:

♦ Antidepressants, i.e. serotonin reuptake inhibitors (SSRIs), e.g. fluoxetine, and tricyclic antidepressants, e.g. amitriptyline, which are effective for adults with moderate to severe depressive disorder. When initial antidepressant treatment is beneficial, it should not be stopped before 9–12 months after recovery and should be regularly monitored, with special attention to treatment adherence.

♦ Brief structured psychological treatments, i.e. CBT, problem-solving therapy (PST), interpersonal psychotherapy (IPT), and behaviour activation (BA), are effective treatments for depression but require substantial dedicated time and more intensive use of human resources.

♦ Relaxation training and physical activity may be considered as treatment of adults with depressive episode/disorder in addition to antidepressants and brief structured psychological treatments.

Despite the evidence on burden and effective treatments, the vast majority of individuals affected by depression do not receive these treatments. In an attempt to understand and improve treatment for CMD, the WHO World Mental Health Survey initiative described worldwide use of mental health services for anxiety, mood, and substance disorders (17). The results reveal very high levels of unmet need for mental health treatment worldwide, even among cases with the most serious disorders. The situation appears to be most dire in less-developed countries, with only small fractions of even severe cases receiving any form of care in the prior year; however, even in more developed countries, roughly half of severe cases received no services. Among the minority of cases receiving some services, even fewer were likely to have been *effectively* treated. In many countries, nearly one-quarter of those initiating treatments failed to receive any follow-up care. Finally, a minority of treatments were observed to meet minimal standards for adequacy and quality.

Major challenges exist for implementation of evidence-based treatments, especially in LAMIC (18–20). These include the inadequate number of mental health specialists, the low recognition rate of depression in primary care where these individuals usually seek treatment, the inadequate or inappropriate use of antidepressant drugs or psychosocial treatments in these settings, and low adherence to treatments. The situation is compounded by lack of research in contextualized interventions and services in LAMIC.

This chapter aims to analyse opportunities and barriers to conducting trials of interventions for depression in LAMIC. An overview of the recent literature on large randomized trials for treatment of depression in low-resource contexts is presented, followed by a case study of a trial conducted in India that evaluated the effectiveness of a lay counsellor-delivered intervention for CMD in primary care and highlights the logistics and methodological considerations in undertaking such a study.

Intervention studies for depression in low-resource contexts

Over the past decade, a number of clinical trials have shown the effectiveness of treatment for depression across a range of low-resource settings (Table 10.1). Most of these trials have evaluated the effectiveness of structured psychological treatments or collaborative care programmes, compared to usual care or no-treatment control conditions (21).

An RCT carried out in rural Uganda, for example, showed that group IPT conducted in communities substantially reduced the symptoms and prevalence of depression among 341 men and women meeting criteria for major or sub-syndromal depression (22). After intervention, 6.5% of the intervention group met the criteria for major depression compared to 54.7% in the control group. A trial in Chile was conducted with 240 low-income women suffering from major depression in order to examine the effectiveness of a multicomponent intervention that included psychoeducational group intervention, structured and systematic follow-up, and drug treatment for those with severe depression. The trial found that there was a substantial difference in favour of the stepped-care programme as compared to standard treatment in primary care. A depression measure (the HDRS) administered at the 6-month follow-up point showed that 70% of the stepped-care group had recovered, as compared with 30% of the usual-care group (23). A cluster RCT of perinatally depressed women in rural Pakistan reported a 78% reduction in prevalence of depression at 6 months and 77% reduction at 12 months in the intervention arm compared to 47% and 41% in the control arm respectively (24). The intervention consisted of psychological treatment incorporating cognitive and behavioural techniques delivered at home over 16 sessions starting from the last month of pregnancy until 10 months post-partum. An RCT compared the effectiveness of a multicomponent intervention with usual care to treat postnatal depression in low-income mothers in primary care clinics in Santiago, (25). The intervention involved a psychoeducational group, treatment adherence support, and pharmacotherapy if needed. The mean depression score on the HDRS was lower for the multicomponent intervention group than for the usual-care group at 3 months: 8.5 (95% CI 7.2–9.7) vs 12.8 (95% CI 11.3–14.1). Although these differences between

Table 10.1 Characteristics of trials of psychological treatments in LAMIC. (Adapted with permission (26))

Trial	Country	Design	Target population and sample size	Psychological treatment and other active intervention	Comparison group	Primary outcome effects
MANAS	India	Cluster RCT in 12 PHCs and 12 GP facilities	Adults over 17 years attending primary care facilities and screening positive for CMD. 2796 patients enrolled	Psychoeducation, IPT, antidepressants, and specialist referral delivered in a collaborative stepped-care framework	Enhanced usual care—screening and antidepressant treatment guidelines for doctors	24% reduction in prevalence of depressive or anxiety disorder in participants with depression over 12 months in intervention arm in public facilities: RR = 0.76 (95% CI 0.59–0.98; $p = 0.04$). No effect in private facilities
Thinking Healthy Programme (THP)	Pakistan	Cluster RCT of women living in 40 Union Councils in two sub-districts	Married women aged 16–45 years, in the third trimester of pregnancy, meeting SCID criteria for DSM-IV major depressive episode. 903 mothers enrolled	Psychological treatment incorporating cognitive and behavioural techniques delivered at home over 16 sessions, starting from the last month of pregnancy until 10 months post-partum	Enhanced routine care, including a similar number of sessions	78% reduction in prevalence of depression at 6 months in intervention arm (adjusted odds ratio (AOR) 0.22; 95% CI 0.14–0.36; $p < 0.0001$); 77% reduction at 12 months (AOR 0.23; 95% CI 0.15–0.36; $p < 0.0001$)
Uganda IPT (IPT-GU)	Uganda	Cluster RCT in 30 villages	Adults ≥ 18 years who: (1) were identified by others or self-identified with local syndromes equating to DSM-IV depression, and (2) screened positive for DSM-IV major depression or a dissociative disorder not otherwise specified (DD-NOS). 248 participants enrolled	IPT adapted for local population; delivered in 2 individual and 16 weekly group sessions	Information about using other locally available resources (e.g. local healers, NGO services)	In the intervention arm: 79.5% reduction in prevalence of depression at termination (4 months), using adjusted difference in mean depression score change (AOR 13.91, 95% CI 10.99–16.84; $p < 0.0001$); 74.3% reduction in prevalence of depression at 6 months following termination (AOR 13.98, 95% CI 12.17–15.79; $p < 0.0001$)

Table 10.1 (continued) Characteristics of trials of psychological treatments in LAMIC. (Adapted with permission (26))

Trial	Country	Design	Target population and sample size	Psychological treatment and other active intervention	Comparison group	Primary outcome effects
Multicomponent stepped-care programme	Chile	RCT in three primary care clinics	240 adult female patients with DSM-IV major depression	Stepped care was a 3-month, multicomponent intervention which included a psychoeducational group intervention, structured and systematic follow-up, and drug treatment for patients with severe depression	Usual care consisted of all services normally available in the primary care clinic, including antidepressant medication or referral for specialty treatment	The adjusted difference in mean depression score between the groups was –8.89 (95% CI –11.15 to –6.76; $p < 0.0001$). At 6 months follow-up, 70% (95% CI 60–79) of the stepped-care group compared with 30% (95% CI –21–40) of the usual-care group had recovered
Postnatal depression trial	Chile	RCT in three postnatal clinics	208 women with DSM-IV major depression detected within 12 months post delivery	The multicomponent intervention involved a psychoeducational group, treatment adherence support, and pharmacotherapy if needed	Usual care included all services normally available in the clinics, including antidepressant drugs, brief psychotherapeutic interventions, medical consultations, and external referral for specialty treatment	The depression score remained better in the multicomponent intervention group than in the usual-care group: 10.9 (95% CI 9.6–12.2) vs 12.5 (95% CI –11.1–13.8)). The adjusted difference in mean scores between the two groups at 3 months was –4.5 (95% CI –6.3 to –2.7; $p < 0.0001$)

groups decreased by 6 months, the depression score remained better in the multicomponent intervention group than in the usual-care group: 10.9 (95% CI 9.6–12.2) vs 12.5 (95% CI 11.1–13.8).

The MANAS trial in India was conducted to test the effectiveness of a collaborative care intervention led by lay health counsellors in primary care settings to improve outcomes for people with CMD. The intervention consisted of case management; psychosocial treatment led by a trained lay health counsellor supervised by a mental health specialist; and medication from a primary care physician. The trial found that patients in the intervention group had reduced prevalence of CMD, suicidal behaviour, psychological morbidity, and disability days at 12 months than patients in the control group (26). This trial is described in more detail in the section titled 'Case study' in this chapter.

The common threads running through many of these trials were (27):

◆ lay or community health workers were trained to deliver the psychological treatments and/or play the role of case managers;

◆ the psychological treatments were systematically adapted to contextual factors;

◆ mental health care was integrated with routine health care or community delivery systems.

While the collaborative care trials reported (Chile and India) included antidepressant medication as part of a stepped-care package, there are also a few trials that specifically evaluate the efficacy of antidepressant pharmacotherapy for primary care patients in LAMIC. For example, a randomized trial in India found fluoxetine superior to placebo (specifically at 2-month follow-up) among primary care patients with raised levels of psychological distress (28). Such trials are frequently carried out for pharmaceutical licencing purposes rather than to evaluate interventions aimed at improving access to evidence-based interventions.

In the section 'Case study', we describe the MANAS study in detail to illustrate the important considerations in carrying out trials of the effectiveness of a comprehensive package of interventions for depression in LAMIC and the challenges that are encountered in carrying out such research.

Case study: a collaborative stepped-care intervention for CMD in primary care in India—the MANAS trial

The MANAS (MANashanti Sudhar Shodh, which means 'project to promote mental health' in Konkani) trial aimed to evaluate the effectiveness and cost-effectiveness of a lay counsellor-led collaborative care intervention for CMD in primary care. MANAS was implemented in Goa, India, from April 2007 to September 2009 in two sequential phases: phase 1 was conducted in government-run primary health care clinics (PHCs) and phase 2 was conducted in private GP clinics.

Study design

The study design comprised a cluster RCT, with the facility as the unit of randomization. Outcomes were evaluated at the level of individual participants.

Study setting

The trial was carried out in the state of Goa, in western India, with a population of 1.4 million. It is estimated that at least 50% of primary care in India (and in Goa) is delivered in the private sector and about half the population lives in rural areas. The trial comprised two consecutive phases: an evaluation of the intervention in 12 public centres for primary health care that were operated by the government of Goa (phase 1), and an evaluation of the same intervention in 12 private GP clinics (phase 2). In each phase, health care facilities were randomized to the intervention arm (i.e. collaborative and stepped care) or the control arm (i.e. enhanced usual care). In phase 1, facility consent was obtained from the Government of Goa's Directorate of Health Services (DHS). In phase 2, facility consent was obtained from each GP. The participation of GPs was sought through letters to over 400 registered practitioners; however, as the response rate was poor, the research team then visited a sub-sample of practitioners who had not responded. Through this process, 22 eligible facilities were identified, of which 12 were randomly selected for inclusion in the trial.

Participants

Participants who met the initial eligibility criteria (e.g. aged > 17 years and spoke one of the four study languages) were screened for depression and/or anxiety by means of a pretested GHQ (29). Subjects found positive for either of these CMD were invited to participate. If the individual gave written or verbal consent, a structured clinical diagnostic interview—the Revised Clinical Interview Schedule (CIS-R) (30)—was administered to provide a baseline assessment of severity and ICD-10 diagnostic categorization. Based on these assessments, trial participants were categorized into four a priori groups for analyses: all participants (screen-positive group); the sub-group of those who screened positive who had ICD-10 diagnoses of CMD (ICD-10 diagnosis group); the sub-group of those with ICD-10 CMD diagnoses with the specific diagnosis of depression (depression sub-group); and the sub-group of those who screened positive who did not meet ICD-10 criteria for CMD (sub-threshold sub-group).

Intervention

The original intervention plan was based on two principles: first, the treatments selected were based on evidence from published trials in LAMIC and, thus, included psychoeducation (31, 32), antidepressants (22, 23), and group IPT (22, 33); and, second, the intervention would address the challenges highlighted earlier and be based on the best global evidence available. The intervention was intended to be a lay counsellor-led collaborative stepped-care intervention that emphasizes the efficient use of scarce resources and tailors the intervention to the needs of patients. This delivery model has strong evidence in support of its effectiveness from a number of trials in HIC (34).

Development of the intervention

Before initiating the trial, extensive preparatory work over a period of 15 months was conducted, to examine the feasibility and acceptability of the planned intervention (35). The preparatory stage had three distinct phases: (1) consultation with stakeholders; (2)

formative research to evaluate key components of the intervention; and (3) piloting of the entire intervention. Although the final intervention protocol continued to use the same specific treatments that were originally envisaged, there were a number of key modifications to improve their feasibility and acceptability.

Some examples are considered in this discussion. First, IPT was initially planned as a group intervention with eight to twelve sessions; however, it became clear during the pilot that formation of groups was not feasible in the clinics. Thus, IPT was modified to be delivered in an individual format over six to eight sessions. Furthermore, the role of IPT was modified and instead of being provided as an alternative to antidepressants initially, it was reserved for patients not improving with antidepressants. This was an important adaptation that was deemed necessary, since the doctors were more comfortable with prescribing medicines than offering a 'talking treatment' and the patients' expectations of receiving 'medicines' for their problems (as was the prior treatment offered in the PHC) was met. Second, adherence management moved from being a peripheral component of the intervention to becoming a central feature, running across the intervention from the first psychoeducation session onwards, with a proactive set of strategies. Third, it was originally anticipated that the health counsellor would carry out both screening and delivery of the intervention. This proved to be unfeasible, and an additional, low-cost, human resource (the health assistant) was used to administer the screening instrument. Fourth, the scope of the health counsellors' role expanded to include a range of additional activities, such as managing adherence and being a link between the health centre and existing resources (e.g. social welfare agencies) in the community. Fifth, yoga, though not a part of the intervention package, was retained as a means to both promote mental health and reduce the stigma associated with a mental health intervention. Sixth, the process indicators allowed for setting of realistic and appropriate targets for the delivery and monitoring of the intervention.

The content of IPT was adapted in a number of ways during the formative research phase in order to suit the local context. These adaptations were in the following areas:

◆ Language: the sessions were structured in greater detail with simplified scripts in the local language.

◆ Concepts: explaining depression as a stress-related illness rather than using the term 'depression', 'mental' illness, or any other psychiatric label.

◆ Use of metaphors: mood ratings were elicited from patients by showing a picture of a mood ladder, with each rung depicting a higher or lower level of mood intensity.

◆ Use of handouts: with simplified explanation of the psychological treatment for patients and family members.

◆ Exploration of the use of religious practices as a coping method.

The final intervention

The specific components of the intervention were psychoeducation, antidepressant drug therapy, IPT, proactive monitoring and adherence support, and referral to specialists, delivered in stepped-care fashion (see Fig. 10.1). The collaborative approach

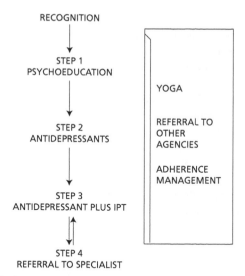

RECOGNITION

STEP 1
PSYCHOEDUCATION

YOGA

STEP 2
ANTIDEPRESSANTS

REFERRAL TO
OTHER
AGENCIES

ADHERENCE
MANAGEMENT

STEP 3
ANTIDEPRESSANT PLUS IPT

STEP 4
REFERRAL TO SPECIALIST

Fig. 10.1 Steps of the MANAS intervention.

involved three key team members: the lay health counsellor, the primary care physician, and a visiting psychiatrist (the clinical specialist). The lay health counsellors were recruited from the local community, did not have any prior health training or experience, and underwent a structured 2-month training course followed by supervision by mental health specialists with clinical experience in the psychological treatment (IPT). Supervision was conducted individually, initially once in 2 weeks, reduced to once every month, as well as group supervision once a month. The lay health counsellor acted as a case-manager for all patients who screened positive for CMD, and took overall responsibility for delivering all the non-drug treatments in close collaboration with the primary care physician and the clinical specialist, with the ultimate goal of a planned discharge on recovery.

Psychoeducation was offered to all patients who screened positive for CMD and focused on educating the person about their symptoms, the association of CMD with interpersonal difficulties, the importance of discussing mood-related symptoms with the doctor, and the importance of sharing personal difficulties with family members or significant others in their social network (this component was based on the initial phase of IPT). Psychoeducation also taught patients strategies to alleviate symptoms, such as breathing exercises for anxiety symptoms and scheduling pleasurable activities for symptoms of depression. Encouraging adherence to antidepressant drug treatment (if prescribed by the primary care physician) and providing information about social and welfare organizations when needed were other key strategies of psychoeducation. Psychoeducation was provided for one to three sessions delivered at weekly/fortnightly intervals, each session lasting for 45–60 minutes.

Antidepressant drugs were recommended only for moderate or severe CMD (i.e. with a GHQ score > 7) and for those who did not respond to psychoeducation alone on the basis of routine clinical assessments by the lay health counsellor. In phase 1, the antidepressant drug offered was fluoxetine, which was provided by the project to integrate with the existing model of free drugs prescribed by the PHC doctor. In the GP clinics, doctors could prescribe antidepressant drugs of their choice, from recommendations in a manual. Once initiated, antidepressant drugs were recommended for a minimum of 90 days at an adequate dose (at least 20 mg per day of fluoxetine or the equivalent, which could be titrated up to 40 mg if clinical response was inadequate). The recommended duration of the drug therapy was a minimum of 6 months. Physicians were given training for half a day and a manual. The other key roles of the physicians were to encourage patients to meet the lay health counsellor, to avoid the use of unnecessary medication, and to provide usual care for any coexisting physical health problems.

IPT, delivered by the lay health counsellor, was the structured psychological treatment. This was chosen because of its documented feasibility and effectiveness in another low-resource setting (22), and because of its focus on interpersonal problems such as grief, disputes, and role transitions, which were common in the adverse life experiences of patients with depression in previous research in Goa (36, 37). A minimum of six sessions, with an optimum of eight and a maximum of 12, were offered. IPT was reserved only for patients who had moderate or severe CMD, and was offered as an alternative to or in addition to antidepressant drugs for those who did not respond to antidepressant treatment.

Referral to the clinical specialist was reserved for patients who were assessed as having a high suicide risk at any stage, were unresponsive to the earlier treatments, posed diagnostic dilemmas (e.g. an elderly patient who has notable memory problems along with depressive symptoms, or a patient who has hallucinations in addition to depressive symptoms), had co-morbidity with alcohol dependence, had other associated substantial medical problems (e.g. a patient who has uncontrolled diabetes or hypertension in addition to depression), or for whom the primary care physician requested a consultation. Every facility team was supported by a clinical mental health specialist who visited once or twice a month and was also available for consultation on the telephone to discuss cases. Patients' discharge was either planned (e.g. if they were deemed to have recovered) or unplanned (e.g. if they did not return for reviews despite adherence management procedures).

The control arm

In order to assemble comparable samples of patients in the intervention and control practices, it was necessary to conduct systematic screening in both groups. It would have been unethical to conceal these screening results from treating physicians. Consequently, physicians in usual care practices received screening results. This enhancement to usual care in the control practices ran the risk of reducing the difference in outcomes between intervention and control arms, but this risk was deemed to be minimal given that screening or the provision of evidence-based guidelines are not, by themselves, sufficient to lead to clinical improvements (38, 39). Thus, the control intervention was 'enhanced usual care' (EUC) where usual care was enhanced in two key ways: physicians and patients received screening results and physicians were given the treatment manual prepared for primary care. Physicians were free to initiate treatments of their choice.

Outcomes

The mental health outcomes were prevalence of CMD, psychiatric symptom scores, and suicidal behaviour (plans, attempts, completed suicide). These were assessed using the CIS-R, a structured interview for use by trained lay interviewers which generates both CMD case and depression case outcomes based on ICD-10 criteria. The CIS-R is one of the most widely used measures of CMD globally, with extensive prior use in the study setting (10, 28, 30).

Disability outcomes were assessed using the 12-item WHODAS II, a brief questionnaire that has been used in Goa previously (40). The questionnaire generates two types of outcomes: a score that summates Likert scale responses on ten items assessing a range of six domains of functional impairment; and two items assessing the number of days in the previous month that the patient was unable to work in the previous 30 days.

Economic outcomes were measured using the Costs of Illness Schedule, developed for economic analyses of mental disorders in India and used in an earlier efficacy trial in Goa (28, 41). Two key categories of costs were estimated: health-system costs (including those related to the intervention itself, comprising the costs of inpatient and outpatient care, medications, and clinical investigations) and the 'time costs' for the subjects and their families (i.e. the opportunity costs of time spent travelling to, waiting for, or receiving care, plus the wages from any days of work lost). The additional human resource use associated with the lay health workers employed in the intervention was evaluated using the clinical process indicator records. Some of the costs of the intervention were estimated by multiplying the total number of minutes a subject in the intervention arm had contact with a lay health worker by the per-minute cost of the health worker.

The outcomes were assessed through home visits at three time points: 2, 6, and 12 months after randomization. Assessments were carried out by a team of researchers independent of the intervention team and blind to the allocation status of the patient. Six months was chosen as the primary endpoint because it marks the maximum duration of the drug and psychological treatments. The 2- and 12-month endpoints assessed the rate and persistence of clinical recovery.

Ethical issues

In cluster RCTs, consent for participation in a trial is needed both from the clusters and, depending on the type of intervention being delivered and outcomes assessed, from individual participants. In the MANAS trial, cluster level consent was obtained for phase 1 in two steps: first, from the Government of Goa's DHS; and second, after the final 12 PHCs were identified and randomized, specific written consent was obtained from the DHS for the participation of these 12 PHCs. In phase 2, individual facility-level consent from each GP was implicit, since only those who had expressed an interest to participate were included in the sampling frame. Individual participant consent was obtained in two stages: consent for screening and subsequently after the screening, those who were screen-positives were invited to participate in the trial.

The MANAS trial addressed whether a lay counsellor-led collaborative stepped-care intervention enables these treatments to be provided effectively in primary care and, if so, what are the marginal benefits and costs. There is genuine clinical equipoise concerning this research question in the context of developing countries where the intervention presents additional costs and where there are several other public health priorities. Underpowered trials are unethical for patients; the sample size calculations were therefore based on conservative estimates and high power. No participant was deprived of any treatment they would ordinarily receive. Participants in the enhanced usual care control facilities could have benefitted as a consequence of the screening and, in the PHCs, the provision of antidepressants to the pharmacy. They were provided with the results of the screening questionnaire, and those who remained ill at 12 months were offered psychiatric consultation by the clinical specialist. In addition, if any trial participant (in either arm) was found to have attempted suicide (assessed during outcome evaluation), the fieldwork team reported this through an administrator to the intervention team who made arrangements to provide psychiatric care for the participant. Explicit referral guidelines were provided to doctors in the enhanced usual care control arm for patients who were suicidal or needed specialist advice.

Formal ethical approval was obtained from the Institutional Review Boards (IRBs) of the lead Goan organization (Sangath), the London School of Hygiene and Tropical Medicine, and the Indian Council for Medical Research. A Trial Steering Committee and a Data Monitoring and Ethics Committee monitored the progress of the trial through quarterly reports and annual meetings.

Delivery of the intervention

Process data, both quantitative and qualitative, was collected to identify key challenges during the course of the trial as well as to help explain the outcome findings. Process indicators were obtained from four sources: the separate clinical records maintained by the lay health counsellor and the clinical specialist, antidepressant use from the clinic records, and quality assessments done for every component of the intervention.

Overall, there was little variation between clinics in the two phases in most of the key process indicators. In summary:

- A high proportion (96%) of screen-positive patients received the first session of psychoeducation.
- The majority of patients with moderate/severe depression received antidepressant medication (85%) as first line of treatment in addition to psychoeducation, in keeping with the stepped-care protocol.
- Over half of all patients (53%) on antidepressant medication completed the minimum of 3 months of treatment. This was made possible by proactive monitoring of follow-up appointments and institution of adherence management strategies especially for those who had missed their appointments.
- In phase 1, only a small proportion of patients with moderate to severe depression received IPT (3%) and a very small proportion of these completed the minimum of six IPT sessions (33%).
- More than half of all patients (57%) had a planned discharge from the programme. This included reasons such as completion of the treatment course, referral to

previously treating psychiatrist, and referral out of the programme by the clinical specialist.

♦ A very small number of patients needed a clinical specialist's consultation—seven in the PHC phase and four in the GP phase of the programme.

Key findings

1 The effectiveness of the intervention: a total of 2796 participants were recruited in both phases. The proportions completing the outcome assessment were 89% at month two, 87% at month six, and 85% at month 12. Overall, 2181 (78%) of all screen-positive participants were seen at all three follow-up visits. In public facilities, the intervention was consistently associated with strong beneficial effects over the 12 months on all outcomes. There was a 30% decrease in the prevalence of CMD among those with baseline ICD-10 diagnoses (risk ratio (RR) = 0.70; 95% CI 0.53–0.92), and a similar effect among the sub-group of participants with depression (RR = 0.76; 95% CI 0.59–0.98). Suicide attempts/plans showed a 36% reduction over 12 months (RR = 0.64; 95% CI 0.42–0.98) among baseline ICD-10 cases. Strong effects were observed on days out of work and psychological morbidity, and modest effects on overall disability. In contrast, there was little evidence of impact of the intervention on any outcome among participants attending private facilities. Thus, participants in both arms of phase 2 had comparable outcomes, and these were similar to those of the intervention arm of phase 1 participants.

2 The cost-effectiveness of the intervention: despite the additional resources required for the intervention led by lay health workers, the health system costs incurred over the 12 months of follow-up were similar across the two arms. In the public facilities investigated, time costs were lower and health outcomes were significantly better in the intervention arm than in the control arm. In these facilities, therefore, the intervention appeared to be not only cost-effective but also cost-saving; the subjects in the intervention arm used and/or lost less cash and showed greater improvement in their mental state than the control subjects. As mentioned, there were no statistically significant between-arm differences in any of the health outcomes investigated in private facilities. In these facilities, however, the care of the subjects with depression and/or anxiety was cheaper in the intervention arm than in the control arm and therefore the intervention still appeared advantageous from a cost-minimization perspective.

3 The intervention suggested some preventive effect in reducing the prevalence of CMD in sub-threshold cases, though this was of weak statistical significance (RR at 6 months for all facility types 0.52; 95% CI 0.29–0.96; $p = 0.04$).

4 High specificity of the screening procedure was observed—2242 participants who screened positive with the GHQ met ICD-10 criteria for CMD at baseline (about 80%).

In addition to the quantitative evaluations, we carried out nested qualitative studies with the MANAS and PHC workers and a sub-group of trial participants.

♦ Semi-structured interviews were conducted with participants of both arms
($n = 115$): the first interview within 2 months of recruitment and the second
6–8 months after recruitment (42). More participants in the intervention than
control arm reported relief from symptoms and an improvement in social functioning and positive impact on work and activities of daily life. The intervention
arm participants attributed their improvement both to medication received from
the doctors and the strategies suggested by the lay counsellor. However, two key
differences were observed in the results for the two types of facilities. First, the
intervention arm participants in the public sector clinics were more likely to consider the counsellors to be an important component of providing care who served
as a link between patient and doctor, provided them with skills in stress management, and helped in adherence to medication. Second, in the private sector, doctors performed roles similar to those of the counsellors, and participants in both
arms placed much faith in the doctor, who acted as a confidante and was perceived
to understand the participant's health and context intimately.

♦ Qualitative semi-structured interviews were conducted with key members ($n = 119$)
of the primary health care teams upon completion of the trial and additional interviews with control arm GPs ($n = 6$) upon completion of the outcome analyses,
which revealed non-inferiority of this arm (43). The analyses were carried out separately for each of the two types of facilities in order to understand better the reasons for the differential quantitative findings. Data from health providers revealed
that several components of the MANAS intervention were seen to be critically
important for facilitating integration: notably screening and the categorization of
the severity of CMD; provision of psychosocial treatments and adherence management; and the support of the visiting psychiatrist. Non-adherence was common,
often because symptoms had been controlled or because of doubt that 'talking
treatment' could 'solve' real-life problems. IPT was intended to be provided face
to face by the counsellor; however, it could not be delivered for most eligible patients due to the cost implications related to travel to the clinic and the time lost
from work. The counsellors had particular difficulty in working with patients with
extreme social difficulties or alcohol-related problems, and elderly patients, as the
intervention seemed unable to address their specific needs. The control arm GPs
adopted practices similar to the principles of the MANAS intervention; GPs routinely diagnosed CMD and provided psychoeducation, advice on lifestyle changes
and problem-solving, prescribed antidepressants, and referred to specialists as
appropriate. This may partly explain the findings that they were as effective as the
MANAS intervention arm GPs in enabling recovery.

Strengths and limitations of the trial

The strengths of the MANAS trial include: large samples from rural and urban populations with inclusion of both public and private facilities (the latter being a decision
taken to enhance the generalizability of the findings in the study context where at least
half of all primary care takes place in the private sector); high follow-up rates; high
levels of fidelity and quality of the intervention; excellent uptake of the low-intensity

psychoeducation component and moderate uptake of the antidepressant component; and consistent documentation of effect in PHCs for each diagnostic group apart from depression. Additionally, MANAS was able to confirm the high specificity of the screening procedure in a real-world context. About 13% of patients were not seen at the 6-month outcome, and these patients were more likely to be younger and male. However, separate models by age-group and sex were fitted, and showed no evidence of differential recovery rates by sex or age. Missing data are thus unlikely to affect the results.

We also experienced a number of limitations. Among patients receiving IPT, the proportion who completed at least six sessions was lower than expected. A major barrier was the indirect and direct costs associated with the need for patients to return to the facility for regular sessions. While it is notable that our intervention was able to lead to favourable outcomes in public facility participants that were at least as good as those observed in private facility participants, no additional impact was observed on any outcome, apart from a non-significant reduction in the risk of suicidal behaviours, for any diagnostic group in participants attending the intervention arm private facilities. This finding could be, at least in part, attributed to the difficulties encountered in recruiting a representative group of private facilities in the trial, leading to a highly motivated group of practitioners with a strong interest in mental health ultimately participating.

Conclusion

The lessons learned from MANAS can be summarized under three broad headings: future research, clinical practice, and policy.

- *Future research:* several lessons can be drawn from MANAS to inform future trials. First, integrating mixed methods process evaluation into the design of trials of complex mental health care interventions is essential to provide greater understanding of the generalizability of the findings and provide explanatory data for unpacking the primary outcome analyses results. Second, estimating the cost-effectiveness of interventions is important to inform the wider adoption and scale-up of the intervention. Third, MANAS illustrates how ensuring relevant contextual adaptations enhances the acceptability, feasibility, and effectiveness of evidence-based interventions. Fourth, the effect modification by facility type illustrates both the need to recruit representative samples of facilities and the limits to generalizability of findings of implementation trials from one health service context to another.

- *Clinical practice:* lay health counsellors such as the ones in MANAS could undertake several healthcare roles, from case management to the delivery of specific psychological treatments, are fairly low cost to recruit, and are readily available in most developing countries. They can thus play an important role in reducing the treatment gap for CMD in these settings. The importance of ongoing supervision and support for the counsellors emphasizes that they must always be part of a collaborative care team, including a mental health specialist. MANAS also demonstrates that screening is feasible because of the high prevalence of CMD in primary care attenders, the brevity of screening instruments, and a relatively high specificity of diagnosis of these disorders by ICD-10 criteria. Also, increasing literacy rates in many countries may make self-completion feasible, for example while patients are waiting to see the doctor. Screening might have been a crucially important component accounting for the good outcomes in the control private facilities in the MANAS study. However, the fact that the intervention had no effect on the sub-group of patients with depression also indicates the need for more effective treatments—for example, psychological treatments that are more specific to the needs of the patient or more aggressive pharmacotherapy. MANAS demonstrates the importance of adherence management for patients receiving treatment for CMD much in the same way as for any chronic disease management. Furthermore, technological and practical flexibility is essential for the delivery of psychological treatments. Thus strategies such as conducting sessions on the telephone, broadening the settings for psychological treatment delivery to include homes and community settings, and tapping into family and community resources enhance opportunities for non-medical interventions to facilitate recovery.

Policy: the MANAS trial has provided evidence that trained lay counsellors working within a collaborative care model can reduce prevalence of CMD, suicidal behaviour, psychological morbidity, and disability days among those attending public primary care facilities. The main implication from this research is the demonstration that the addition of a lay counsellor in public primary care facilities greatly improves the outcomes of patients with CMD and that these are comparable to the outcomes achieved by private physicians. The findings demonstrate that the additional investments needed to scale up the MANAS intervention via task-sharing with lay health counsellors would be offset by reduced overall health care costs. Such evidence, particularly in the context of the findings from other trials of the treatment of depression in community and primary care settings in LAMIC outlined in the chapter, needs to be scaled up into routine health programmes. Indeed, collaborative care programmes with a front-line lay health worker could be extended from CMD to other chronic diseases. We also need investments in research, notably in enhancing the acceptability and feasibility of lay counsellor-delivered psychosocial treatments, cost-effective methods for disseminating training for delivery of psychosocial interventions, and evaluating the scaling up of the integration of CMD care into routine health care.

References

1 **Bromet E, Andrade LH, Hwang I, Sampson NA, Alonso J, de Girolamo G, et al.** (2011) Cross-national epidemiology of DSM-IV major depressive episode. BMC Med, **9**:90.

2 **Lopez AD, Mathers CD, Ezzati M, Jamison DT, Murray CJL (eds)** (2006) Global burden of disease and risk factors. Washington, DC: World Bank.

3 **Mathers CD, Loncar D** (2006) Projections of global mortality and burden of disease from 2002 to 2030. PLoS Med, **3**(11):e442.

4 **Lund C, Breen A, Flisher AJ, Kakuma R, Corrigall J, Joska JA, et al.** (2010) Poverty and common mental disorders in low and middle income countries: a systematic review. Soc Sci Med, **71**(3):517–28.

5 Moussavi S, Chatterji S, Verdes E, Tandon A, Patel V, Ustun B (2007) Depression, chronic diseases, and decrements in health: results from the World Health Surveys. Lancet, 370(9590):851–8.

6 Prince M, Patel V, Saxena S, Maj M, Maselko J, Phillips MR, et al. (2007) No health without mental health. Lancet, 370(9590):859–77.

7 Hemingway H, Marmot M (1999) Evidence based cardiology: psychosocial factors in the aetiology and prognosis of coronary heart disease. Systematic review of prospective cohort studies. BMJ, 318(7196):1460–7.

8 Kuper H, Marmot M, Hemingway H (2002) Systematic review of prospective cohort studies of psychosocial factors in the etiology and prognosis of coronary heart disease. Semin Vasc Med, 2(3):267–314.

9 Anderson RJ, Freedland KE, Clouse RE, Lustman PJ (2001) The prevalence of comorbid depression in adults with diabetes: a meta-analysis. Diabetes Care, 24(6):1069–78.

10 Patel V, Kirkwood BR, Pednekar S, Pereira B, Barros P, Fernandes J, et al. (2006) Gender disadvantage and reproductive health risk factors for common mental disorders in women: a community survey in India. Arch Gen Psychiatry, 63(4):404–13.

11 Surkan PJ, Kennedy CE, Hurley KM, Black MM (2011) Maternal depression and early childhood growth in developing countries: systematic review and meta-analysis. Bull World Health Organ, 89(8):608–15.

12 Chung EK, McCollum KF, Elo IT, Lee HJ, Culhane JF (2004) Maternal depressive symptoms and infant health practices among low-income women. Pediatrics, 113(6):e523–9.

13 Galler JR, Harrison RH, Biggs MA, Ramsey F, Forde V (1999) Maternal moods predict breastfeeding in Barbados. J Dev Behav Pediatr, 20(2):80–7.

14 Patel V, Flisher AJ, Hetrick S, McGorry P (2007) Mental health of young people: a global public-health challenge. Lancet, 369(9569):1302–13.

15 Cavanagh JT, Carson AJ, Sharpe M, Lawrie SM (2003) Psychological autopsy studies of suicide: a systematic review. Psychol Med, 33(3):395–405.

16 Dua T, Barbui C, Clark N, Fleischmann A, Poznyak V, van Ommeren M, et al. (2011) Evidence-based guidelines for mental, neurological, and substance use disorders in low- and middle-income countries: summary of WHO recommendations. PLoS Med, 8(11):e1001122.

17 Wang PS, Aguilar-Gaxiola S, Alonso J, Angermeyer MC, Borges G, Bromet EJ, et al. (2007) Use of mental health services for anxiety, mood, and substance disorders in 17 countries in the WHO world mental health surveys. Lancet, 370(9590):841–50.

18 Abas M, Baingana F, Broadhead J, Iacoponi E, Vanderpyl J (2003) Common mental disorders and primary health care: current practice in low-income countries. Harv Rev Psychiatry, 11(3):166–73.

19 Cohen A. (2001) The effectiveness of mental health services in primary care: the view from the developing world. Geneva: WHO.

20 Patel V, Andrade C (2003) Pharmacological treatment of severe psychiatric disorders in the developing world: lessons from India. CNS Drugs, 17(15):1071–80.

21 World Health Organization (2008) The global burden of disease: 2004 update. Geneva: WHO.

22 Bolton P, Bass J, Neugebauer R, Verdeli H, Clougherty KF, Wickramaratne P, et al. (2003) Group interpersonal psychotherapy for depression in rural Uganda: a randomized controlled trial. JAMA, 289(23):3117–24.

23 Araya R, Rojas G, Fritsch R, Gaete J, Rojas M, Simon G, et al. (2003) Treating depression in primary care in low-income women in Santiago, Chile: a randomised controlled trial. Lancet, **361**(9362):995–1000.

24 Rahman A, Malik A, Sikander S, Roberts C, Creed F (2008) Cognitive behaviour therapy-based intervention by community health workers for mothers with depression and their infants in rural Pakistan: a cluster-randomised controlled trial. Lancet, **372**(9642):902–9.

25 Rojas G, Fritsch R, Solis J, Jadresic E, Castillo C, González M, et al. (2007) Treatment of postnatal depression in low-income mothers in primary-care clinics in Santiago, Chile: a randomised controlled trial. Lancet, **370**:1629–37.

26 Patel V, Weiss HA, Chowdhary N, Naik S, Pednekar S, Chatterjee S, et al. (2011) Lay health worker led intervention for depressive and anxiety disorders in India: impact on clinical and disability outcomes over 12 months. Br J Psychiatry, **199**(6):459–66.

27 Patel V, Chowdhary N, Rahman A, Verdeli H (2011) Improving access to psychological treatments: lessons from developing countries. Behav Res Ther, **49**(9):523–8.

28 Patel V, Chisholm D, Rabe-Hesketh S, Dias-Saxena F, Andrew G, Mann A (2003) Efficacy and cost-effectiveness of drug and psychological treatments for common mental disorders in general health care in Goa, India: a randomised, controlled trial. Lancet, **361**(9351):33–9.

29 Patel V, Araya R, Chowdhary N, King M, Kirkwood B, Nayak S, et al. (2008) Detecting common mental disorders in primary care in India: a comparison of five screening questionnaires. Psychol Med, **38**(2):221–8.

30 Lewis G, Pelosi AJ, Araya R, Dunn G (1992) Measuring psychiatric disorder in the community: a standardized assessment for use by lay interviewers. Psychol Med, **22**(2):465–86.

31 Ali BS, Rahbar MH, Naeem S, Gul A, Mubeen S, Iqbal A (2003) The effectiveness of counseling on anxiety and depression by minimally trained counselors: a randomized controlled trial. Am J Psychother, **57**(3):324–36.

32 Lara MA, Navarro C, Navarrete L, Mondragón L, Rubí NA (2003) Seguimento a dos anos de una intervencion psicoeducativa para mujeres con sintomas de depresion, en servicios de salud para poblacion abierta. Salud Mental, **57**:26–36.

33 Verdeli H, Clougherty K, Bolton P, Speelman L, Lincoln N, Bass J, et al. (2003) Adapting group interpersonal psychotherapy for a developing country: experience in rural Uganda. World Psychiatry, **2**(2):114–20.

34 Bower P, Gilbody S, Richards D, Fletcher J, Sutton A (2006) Collaborative care for depression in primary care. Making sense of a complex intervention: systematic review and meta-regression. Br J Psychiatry, **189**:484–93.

35 Chatterjee S, Chowdhary N, Pednekar S, Cohen A, Andrew G, Andrew G, et al. (2008) Integrating evidence-based treatments for common mental disorders in routine primary care: feasibility and acceptability of the MANAS intervention in Goa, India. World Psychiatry, **7**(1):39–46.

36 Patel V, Araya R, de Lima M, Ludermir A, Todd C (1999) Women, poverty and common mental disorders in four restructuring societies. Soc Sci Med, **49**(11):1461–71.

37 Patel V, Pereira J, Coutinho L, Fernandes R, Fernandes J, Mann A (1998) Poverty, psychological disorder and disability in primary care attenders in Goa, India. Br J Psychiatry, **172**:533–6.

38 Gerrity MS, Cole SA, Dietrich AJ, Barrett JE (1999) Improving the recognition and management of depression: is there a role for physician education? J Fam Pract, **48**(12):949–57.

39 Thompson C, Kinmonth AL, Stevens L, Peveler RC, Stevens A, Ostler KJ, et al. (2000) Effects of a clinical-practice guideline and practice-based education on detection and outcome

of depression in primary care: Hampshire Depression Project randomised controlled trial. Lancet, **355**(9199):185–91.

40 **World Health Organization** (2001) World Health Organization Disability Assessment Schedule II (WHODAS II). Geneva: WHO.

41 **Chisholm D, Sekar K, Kumar KK, Saeed K, James S, Mubbashar M, et al.** (2000) Integration of mental health care into primary care. Demonstration cost-outcome study in India and Pakistan. Br J Psychiatry, **176**:581–8.

42 **Shinde S, Andrew G, Bangash O, Cohen A, Kirkwood B, Patel V** (2013) The impact of a lay counselor led collaborative care intervention for common mental disorders in public and private primary care: a qualitative evaluation nested in the MANAS trial in Goa, India. Soc Sci Med, **88**:48–55.

43 **Pereira B, Andrew G, Pednekar S, Kirkwood BR, Patel V** (2011) The integration of the treatment for common mental disorders in primary care: experiences of health care providers in the MANAS trial in Goa, India. Int J Ment Health Syst, **5**(1):26.

Chapter 11

Trials of interventions for people with alcohol use disorders

María Elena Medina-Mora, Sairat Noknoy, Cheryl Cherpitel, Tania Real, Román Pérez Velasco, Rodrigo Marín Navarrete, Nancy Amador, and Viviana E. Horigian

This chapter was supported by a grant from the US Department of State (S-INLEC11GR020/S-INLEC11GR015) awarded to the Ramón de la Fuente National Institute of Psychiatry, Mexico, and to the Miller School of Medicine, Department of Public Health Sciences, University of Miami, US, and by a grant from the US National Institute on Alcohol Abuse and Alcoholism (RO1 AA013750) awarded to the Alcohol Research Group, Emeryville, California, US.

The opinions, findings, and conclusions stated herein are those of the authors and do not necessarily reflect those of the US Department of State.

Introduction

Alcohol use disorders AUD are a major contributor to the global burden of disease (GBD). According to the most recent publication of estimates, alcohol dependence was responsible for 1,111,000 deaths (0.21% of the total), an increase of 48.9% since 1990, and ranked 55th out of 106 causes of death (1). Overall, alcohol dependence accounted for 0.7% of the GBD due to premature mortality and disability (2), while alcohol use was the leading risk factor for deaths and DALYs in eastern Europe, most of Latin America, and southern sub-Saharan Africa in 2010 (3). Harmful use is also a significant problem in LAMIC (4) and a major cause of health inequalities, with poor populations and LIC having a higher burden of disease per unit of alcohol consumption than rich populations and HIC (5). The treatment gap for AUD is considerable; it has been estimated that up to 78% of those with AUD do not receive evidence-based treatments, with an expected wider gap in developing countries due to the unavailability of services (6), indicating the need to develop and evaluate efficient and culturally appropriate intervention models.

AUD are classified differently by the two most widely used classification systems, namely the ICD-10 (WHO) (7, 8) and DSM-V (American Psychiatric Association (APA)) (9). In the ICD-10, AUD are categorized into harmful use of alcohol and alcohol dependence (7). *Alcohol dependence* is diagnosed by a cluster of behavioural, cognitive, and physiological phenomena, which develop after repeated substance use and typically include 'a strong desire to drink, difficulties in controlling alcohol use, persisting in its use despite harmful consequences, a higher priority given to alcohol use than to other activities and obligations, increased tolerance, and sometimes physical withdrawal'. *Harmful use* is defined as 'a pattern of alcohol use that causes damage to health, which may be physical or mental, such as episodes of depressive disorder secondary to heavy alcohol consumption'. The WHO has conceptualized a third category of *hazardous use* defined as 'a pattern of substance use that increases the risk of harmful consequences for the user', which may include 'physical, mental health and social consequences of public health significance despite the absence of any current disorder in the individual user'. This term, which is useful for prevention purposes, is not included in the ICD-10 diagnostic classification (10).

DSM-V collapsed the two DSM-IV categories of substance abuse and substance dependence into a single continuum, defining it as 'substance use disorders' on a scale from mild to moderate to severe; the severity of the diagnosis depends on how many of the six criteria apply. Symptoms for dependence are similar to those included in ICD-10, but the criteria used to define *abuse* ('role impairment, hazardous use, legal and social problems') differ from those required by the ICD definition of *harmful use*, where actual damage must have been caused to the user's physical or mental health (8).

AUD is a priority condition identified by the WHO in the mhGAP (11) (see Table 11.1) as one of the disorders requiring urgent attention, for which three processes have been identified:

♦ *screening and brief interventions by trained primary health care professionals* aimed at those with a moderate risk to health and other problems derived from their drinking pattern, according to the screening. In this intervention, patients receive feedback on the results of the screening test using a simple structure of motivational interview (MI) with a duration of 5–15 minutes;

♦ *early identification and treatment of AUD in primary health care* aimed at those persons who have a high risk of dependence. Brief interventions can be used as a first step, but other interventions (i.e. behaviour/cognitive treatment) are also required;

♦ *referral and supervisory support by specialists* when the person has established alcohol dependence and adequate interventions are not available in the primary care (12, 13).

Table 11.1 WHO mhGAP (11)

Condition	Evidence-based interventions	Examples of interventions to be included in the package
Disorders due to alcohol use	Pharmacological and psychosocial interventions	♦ Early identification and provision of prevention and treatment ♦ Interventions for drug use disorders by trained primary health care professionals ♦ Referral and supervisory support by specialists

Brief intervention has been identified as one of the 11 'best practices' for reducing harmful alcohol use, based on effectiveness, scope of impact, quality of evidence, and cross-cultural testing (14). The rationale for brief intervention in primary care settings is compelling and studies have generally found brief intervention to be effective in reducing drinking and alcohol-related problems. Primary care and other such settings (e.g. emergency departments (EDs)) offer a window of opportunity for conducting brief interventions, especially if the reason for the visit to the clinic is in some way related to the patient's drinking (15, 16).

This chapter aims to analyse opportunities and barriers to conducting trials for interventions for AUD in clinical settings in the context of LAMIC. An overview of the literature on studies on the treatment of AUD in low-resource contexts is presented, followed by a case study of a trial conducted in Thailand that evaluated the effectiveness of MET for hazardous drinkers in rural primary care unit (PCU) settings (17) and which highlights the logistics and methodological considerations in undertaking such a study.

Intervention studies for AUD in low-resource contexts

Interventions for individuals with AUD can be divided into two groups: population-based (i.e. reduction of availability through taxation, control of marketing, and drink-driving countermeasures) and individual-based, which include brief intervention (14), with the evidence showing that early detection and intervention in primary care is feasible and effective in reducing harm related to alcohol misuse (16).

According to Babor and colleagues (14), population-based interventions are usually evaluated by survey research, analysis of archival and official statistics, time series analyses, qualitative research, and quasi experimental natural experiments. The latter involve before and after measurement of communities or jurisdictions exposed to the intervention compared with similar communities or jurisdictions where the intervention has not been implemented. Natural experiments take advantage of the implementation of a new policy to test the effects, and therefore lack the random assignment of communities to the interventions being tested. RCTs, considered a gold standard for evaluating the effect of health interventions, based on their persuasive evidence and superiority compared to other methods, are rarely used to test population-based interventions, although some attempts to randomize communities have been undertaken, showing the possible applicability of this methodology (14).

Individual-based interventions are more suitable for RCTs. However, their implementation poses significant challenges. First, methodologically, they need to meet required standards to be considered robust (Consolidated Standards of Reporting Trials (CONSORT) guidelines) (18). Second, in order to provide evidence that could be applicable in community settings, they must be implemented in the real world with a population that resembles treatment-seeking patients. Third, it is critical that, when using interventions developed in other contexts, these are adapted to the local culture. One approach for cultural adaptations of brief intervention in clinical settings that also included a capacity-building component has been the use of peer health promotion advocates (19). This strategy was implemented in an RCT of brief motivational intervention in an ED on the US–Mexican border among young Mexican-origin adults aged 18–30 years who screened positive for at-risk or dependent drinking (20). In this intervention, health promotion advocates, called '*promotores*' by the Mexican-origin population, were bilingual individuals (English/Spanish) from the community, previously employed in other health promotion activities, and hired and trained to deliver brief motivational intervention. Due to their established rapport in the community, *promotores* were viewed as culturally appropriate, low-cost, intervention models that not only successfully delivered the intervention, but also promoted the sustainability of the intervention in ED following the study.

Ultimately, translation of the results of trials into adoption, implementation, and sustainability in practice remains a challenge in all areas of medicine (21, 22), and particularly so in the field of substance abuse. Several literature reviews have pointed to two core challenges to achieving an impact on the population through evidence-based practices (23–26). The first core challenge is to build infrastructure and the capacity for broad translation of evidence-based interventions into community practices. It is therefore essential to develop infrastructure that is more capable of adoption, implementation, and sustainability of evidence-based practices. Also central to this requisite is the need for a dissemination and training platform that would facilitate adoption. The second core challenge is the development of conceptual frameworks that could prioritize research questions and are more suited to the real world and more likely to translate into sustainability of interventions. Additional barriers include the limited funding available for supporting such practice services and less regulated alcohol policies that result in a weaker population base impact.

The evidence from trials for AUD in LAMIC was recently reviewed by Patel and colleagues (27) who identified 11,501 trials worldwide assessing interventions for the treatment or prevention of mental disorders; only 0.9% were conducted in LIC and 12.3% in MIC, with over half published after the 2001 World Health Report on Mental Health (28). Only 11 trials (0.7%) dealing with alcohol dependence or harmful alcohol use were identified. The authors of this chapter updated this paper through a search of the literature including Cochrane, DARE (Database of Abstracts of Reviews of Effectiveness), PubMed, Scielo, the Association of Prevention Research, EBSCO Host (CINAHL, Health Business, MedicLatina, Medline, and News), Addiction Journal, Scholar Google, and WHO reports published between 2002 and 2013. The review by Patel and the one conducted by the authors of this chapter are described in Table 11.2 (17, 29–38) identified 11 RCTs meeting the CONSORT guidelines (18), and results support the usefulness of brief interventions in a variety of settings. However, definitions of brief interventions vary greatly, from simple suggestions for reducing drinking to a series of interventions provided within a treatment programme (11).

In general, the key elements of brief motivational intervention, as proposed by Miller and Sanchez, are summarized in the FRAMES acronym: Feedback, Responsibility, Advice, Menu of strategies, Empathy, and Self-efficacy (39). These six components remain consistent regardless of the number of sessions and length of interventions (40), and cumulative evidence has shown that the intervention has a clinically significant effect on drinking behaviour and related problems (41–44). The case study we describe next (17) is used to enrich and expand the discussion on the methodological challenges of

Table 11.2 RCTs for AUD in low-resource contexts

Country	Setting	Study design	Human resource used	Target sample	Type of intervention	Comparison group	Outcomes selected	Main findings
Kenya, 2011 (29)	HIV outpatient clinic	RCT, 30- and 90-day follow-up	Treatment was delivered by two counsellors with no prior CBT experience, one with a high-school diploma and no counselling experience and one with a 2-year post-high-school counselling diploma and minimal counselling experience. Supervision was conducted via telephone during the latter stages of trial. Data and Safety Monitoring Board with representatives from affiliated universities	75 HIV-infected patients who reported hazardous or binge drinking	CBT (six culturally adapted sessions)	Routine medical care provided in clinic	Percentage of drinking days and mean drinks per drinking days	Effect sizes of change in alcohol use since baseline between the two conditions at 30-day follow-up were large. Reported alcohol abstinence at 90-day follow-up was 69% (CBT) and 38% (usual care)
South Africa, 2012 (30)	Six primary care clinics and farms from a rural area	RCT, 3- and 12-month follow-up	Sessions were conducted by locally recruited and trained lay counsellors. MI trainer ensured quality control (regular meetings with lay interviewers). Fieldworkers were different from the counsellors and trained specifically to administer the questionnaire	165 women at risk for AEP (alcohol exposed pregnancy)	MI (five sessions)	No intervention (control group)	AEP at 2 and 12 months. Risky drinking and ineffective contraception use in non-pregnant women at 3 and 12 months	A difference in the decline of alcohol use in women in the MI group at 3 months (50% vs 24.59%; $p = 0.004$), maintained at 12 months (50.82% vs 28.12%; $p = 0.009$). Declines in both groups in risky drinking

Table 11.2 (continued) RCTs for AUD in low-resource contexts

Country	Setting	Study design	Human resource used	Target sample	Type of intervention	Comparison group	Outcomes selected	Main findings
Brazil, 2009 (31)	Unit of research on alcohol and drugs	RCT, double-blind	NA	71 alcohol dependent patients	Naltrexone with brief intervention	Placebo	Relapse rate and change in drinking behaviours	Naltrexone with brief intervention was not effective in decreasing drinking days, moderate drinking days, or heavy drinking days
México, 2010 (32)	Urban and rural zones	RCT, 3- and 6-month follow-up	Trained psychologists provided treatment	58 teenagers students screened for alcohol problems those who screened positive were	Evaluate effect of brief intervention programme for adolescents (PIBA, its acronym in Spanish) and brief advice (CB, its acronym in Spanish)	Control group. No treatment (waiting list)	Drinking pattern (quantity/frequency) and related problems. Risky drinking	PIBA and brief counselling significantly reduced consumption patterns in teenagers in follow-up at 3 and 6 months after completing treatment. Only PIBA reduced problems. 90% of those that received PIBA and 65% of those treated with CB at 6 months in follow-up were classified as at low risk

Table 11.2 (continued) RCTs for AUD in low-resource contexts

Country	Setting	Study design	Human resource used	Target sample	Type of intervention	Comparison group	Outcomes selected	Main findings
Brazil, 2010 (33)	Emergency rooms	RCT, 3-month follow-up	Three trained psychologist junior researchers (post-graduate or Master's students) and one senior psychologist. Junior researchers were responsible for screening and evidence-based intervention. Senior psychologist was previously trained according to MI principles. Junior researchers were responsible for selecting cases	175 patients treated for alcohol-related events	Brief MI	Educational brochure	Alcohol use days. Consequences	No significant difference between groups was observed. Significant reductions (p< 0.01) in related problems and alcohol abuse were found in both groups. However, a decrease in consumption was found at the 3-month follow-up
Thailand, 2010 (17)	PCUs	RCT, 6-week, 3-month, and 6-month follow-up (blood tests)	Trained nurses provided treatment	59 subjects identified using Alcohol Use Disorders Identification Test	MET delivered by nurses	Control group. No treatment	Drinks per drinking day, and frequency of daily and weekly hazardous drinking and of binge drinking sessions. Blood tests of GGT	Self-reported drinks per drinking day and frequency of hazardous drinking and of binge drinking sessions were reduced more in the intervention group than in the control group after both 3 and 6 months

Table 11.2 (continued) RCTs for AUD in low-resource contexts

Country	Setting	Study design	Human resource used	Target sample	Type of intervention	Comparison group	Outcomes selected	Main findings
México, 2011 (34)	Mental health and counselling centre	Efficacy of therapeutic interventions	Medical clinic within the university campus. Treatment was provided by trained professionals. Researchers	158 undergraduate students who received a diagnosis of alcohol disorders (ICD-10)	Individual or group MET	Individual or group CBT	Monthly frequency/ quantity of alcohol use. Number of drinks per drinking occasion	In the four interventions there was a reduction in the amount and in frequency and in number of drinks. There were no main effects of treatment (range of p 0.07–0.56). During the follow-up period, there was a reduction in the amount and frequency. During the following 6 months, there was a gradual increase
Iran, 2002 (33)	Urban outpatient clinic	RCT, double-blind, placebo-controlled, 12-week treatment period	Staff who conducted physical and psychiatric examinations, urinalysis, and urine toxicology screens	116 alcohol-dependent males	50 mg of naltrexone per day, including a weekly 30-minute individual counselling session	Placebo	Maintenance of abstinence and relapse to drinking	Completion rates for naltrexone-treated patients (79.3%) were significantly higher than the placebo group (43.1%). Fewer naltrexone-treated patients relapsed than placebo-treated patients

Table 11.2 (continued) RCTs for AUD in low-resource contexts

Country	Setting	Study design	Human resource used	Target sample	Type of intervention	Comparison group	Outcomes selected	Main findings
Brazil, 2003 (36)	Clinical hospital of the Medical School of the University of São Paulo	RCT, double-blind, placebo, 12-week period	Researchers and staff from the clinic	75 men, with a diagnosis of alcohol dependence according to the ICD-10	Efficacy and security of acamprosate	Placebo	Continued abstinence	39% of patients from the acamprosate group and 17% from the placebo group were abstinent ($p = 0.003$)
Korea, 2003 (37)	Outpatient clinics of university general hospitals and psychiatric hospitals	Multicentre RCT, double-blind, placebo-controlled trial	Researchers and staff from the clinic	142 alcohol-dependent patients in 12 centres	Efficacy and safety of acamprosate over 8 weeks	Placebo	Length of time to first drink and to first relapse. Percentage of days abstinent, without heavy drinking, and mean consumption per drinking occasion	Days abstinent (81.2% acamprosate treated vs 78.5% placebo) and mean amount drunk per drinking occasion (7.2 vs 8.6 standard drinks) differed, but no differences were found in serum GGT level or craving scores. Acamprosate was ineffective in reducing drinking in this Korean sample
Brazil, 2008 (38)	University of São Paulo	RCT, double-blind, placebo-controlled study	Researchers and staff from the clinic	155 patients, 18–60 years of age, alcohol dependent	Efficacy of topiramate with naltrexone	Placebo	Time to first relapse (consumption of > 60 g ethyl alcohol), cumulative abstinence duration, and weeks of heavy drinking	Results of this study support the efficacy of topiramate in relapse prevention of alcoholism

conducting clinical trials of brief interventions for AUD in LAMIC. In addition, several ongoing projects meeting the CONSORT criteria were identified (20, 45, 46). From these projects we can learn ways to address significant challenges such as the cultural adaptation of interventions, develop infrastructure to meet the complex requirements of RCTs in underresourced settings, and the need to develop strategies to make the tested interventions sustainable after the research project ends. These findings are described in more detail in the final section of the chapter.

Case study: brief interventions for harmful drinking in primary care in Thailand

Thailand has seen a rapid increase in alcohol consumption since the approval of the national policy on liberalizing the production and distribution of alcohol in 1998, which resulted in a growing number of alcohol-producing establishments, particularly in the north and north-east regions where agricultural products for alcohol production are largely grown (47). In addition, availability of informally produced rice-derived alcohol has increased (48). Drinking in the north-east region or *Isaan* is embedded in everyday life and explicitly accepted with positive attitudes, and drinking is not usually linked with alcohol-related social problems (49). Morbidity and mortality from alcohol-related problems in Thailand are high and increasing over time (50–52), indicating the need for early detection and intervention with problem drinkers. As brief interventions in primary care were a policy option, a study was designed to test their effectiveness among people with an early-stage AUD.

Design

A single blind RCT with two arms (experimental and control groups) was conducted between July 2003 and April 2004. The study sought to randomize 128 participants with harmful and hazardous drinking within seven rural PCUs to a brief intervention of adapted MET over a 6-week period (experimental arm) or health information only (control arm). Participants were assessed for their amount of alcohol use at baseline, at 3 months and 6 months post randomization by self-report, and by serum levels of GGT (a biomarker for AUD) at baseline and 6 months post randomization.

Setting

PCUs in resource-poor settings with three to four staff members each were targeted. At the district level, the health system in Thailand consists of a community hospital and a network of PCUs. Seven rural PCUs from four districts known to the principal investigator (PI) were selected according to the availability of nurses and the staff's previous performance. Site feasibility assessment was facilitated by approaching the directors of five community hospitals who coordinate PCUs within each district. Site feasibility assessment included site demographics, the availability and competence of study coordinators and nurses, infrastructure required for blood sample collection such as refrigerators, and access to transportation. Readiness and acceptance of the project as well as recruitment potential and the possibility of ensuring high retention were assessed.

Sample description

The sample size calculation was based on a previous study in Thailand (53), which examined the effect of a brief intervention on hazardous and harmful drinking patients admitted to a provincial hospital, finding that 66.3% of the treatment group changed their drinking behaviour in comparison to 32% in the control group, thus providing a base for the estimation of the sample size required to detect the effect of the intervention. To provide power of 80% at a 5% level of significance, it was estimated that at least 76 patients were required to be recruited and retained at 6-month follow-up (98 patients for a 90% power). Based on evidence (53, 54) and anticipating an attrition rate of between 10 and 35%, a target of 128 subjects was selected.

The study sought to enrol patients with AUD at the hazardous/harmful level, excluding alcohol dependence, since brief intervention have been found to be effective for the former group of drinkers. All patients coming to PCUs during the recruitment period were screened using the self-completed AUDIT questionnaire (Thai version) (50), and those with a score of ≥ 8 were invited to participate in a study designed to examine lifestyle change over a 6-month period. Exclusion criteria applied after this initial selection included:

+ alcohol-dependent persons (DSM-IV criteria, as applied by a physician);
+ persons with a history of regular alcohol drinking starting early in the morning;
+ recent consumption of extremely high amounts per day (> 120 g for men or > 80 g for women);
+ persons with neurological disease and psychiatric disorders;
+ pregnant women;
+ age < 18 years or > 65 years.

Persons suspected of being alcohol dependent were referred to community hospitals for appropriate diagnosis and treatment. Persons screening positive on the AUDIT were interviewed by a trained health care worker who helped the person complete a health survey questionnaire, including baseline questions related to smoking, exercise, eating behaviour, weight control, and alcohol use, and then scheduled an appointment for the patient to see a nurse the following day. The health survey questionnaire was transferred to nurses at the PCU, who re-evaluated patients for eligibility for the study during the scheduled appointment.

Randomization

Randomization of subjects was carried out at the coordinating centre in Pragmongkutklao Hospital. Each PCU was instructed to randomize persons to either the intervention or control arms. A standard randomization table was used, and in order to keep both groups a similar size, random allocation was carried out in blocks. Randomization codes were distributed to each PCU in opaque, sealed envelopes. The process was monitored by requesting sites to submit a form to the coordinating centre, including details on screening, participants randomized to each arm, recruitment dates, appointment dates for follow-up, and baseline assessment. Participants were blinded to condition assignment by informing them that the trial focus was on health behaviours, including questions on smoking, exercise, eating behaviour, weight control, and alcohol use. Assessors for the primary and secondary outcomes were also blind to condition.

Study preparation and training

A survey on alcohol consumption in the selected communities was conducted as a basis for the development of an instrument to measure drinking levels, and included patterns of drinking, the size of the container used to drink alcohol, and alcohol concentrations from locally produced alcohol. This information was subsequently used for the development of the case report form and educational materials that provided knowledge on standard drinks, low-risk, and hazardous and harmful drinking patterns, as adapted to the local context. Alcohol beverages were divided into beer, wine, marketed spirit, and informally made local beverages, with one drink defined as containing 10 g of alcohol, equivalent to an Australian standard drink, as adopted by many countries including Thailand (52).

A 1-day meeting with hospital directors, nurses, and health care workers was held to present the protocol to PCU staff agreeing to collaborate in the trial. Randomization and blinding procedures were emphasized, together with instructions on how these procedures would be applied. During this meeting, the research team also introduced the study background, the instruments, and the process for obtaining informed consent. Training in the use of the health survey questionnaire was provided through a half-day training course.

The research team travelled to each of the participating PCUs to gain further trial ownership from PCU heads and local staff, as well as to ensure study feasibility by rehearsing pre-trial procedures. The responsibilities of the staff and nurses involved were reviewed and trial materials distributed, with instructions for use given directly to the staff involved. The research team evaluated the level of understanding of data collection procedures, including the collection of blood samples for serum GGT (i.e. the serum needed to be separated after the blood sample was collected and subsequently frozen and transferred to a container that would keep the sample frozen). The research team developed an understanding of the practical issues involved in trial procedures and identified potential obstacles (related to recruitment, participant appointments, integration in routine practice) in successfully conducting the trial. These visits also enhanced communication between the research team and local staff, facilitating problem-solving during the trial.

The intervention arm

The intervention comprised a brief motivational intervention comprising four steps: Ask, Assess, Advise, and Monitor a person's progress (55). The Ask and Assess phases were conducted using the validated AUDIT screening test (50) and the health survey questionnaire, after which those identified as problem drinkers received advice and assistance on behavioural change, based on the six critical elements summarized in the FRAMES acronym, as discussed in the section 'Intervention studies for AUD in low-resource contexts' (34). The intervention was adapted and integrated with MET, originally developed from the project MATCH (56). In particular, the assessment, advice, feedback, and materials to provide information on alcohol use were tailored to the local context, by using appropriate language expressions and bringing them into line with common practices. MET is an adaptation of MI (57), grounded in Prochaska and Diclemente's transtheoretical model which uses patient-centred interviewing techniques to enhance people's motivation to change their behaviour (58, 59). The manual from MATCH (57) was translated into Thai by two trial investigators. MET, originally consisting of four brief sessions, was adapted into three 15-minute counselling sessions, which was considered more practical for maintaining intervention fidelity in the low-resource primary care setting in Thailand. The follow-through session at 12 weeks was not included in this trial due to the length of time between the initial and the fourth sessions, making it harder to keep the quality of the intervention at the same level. The first counselling session was scheduled for the day following screening, while the second and third sessions were scheduled for 1 week and 6 weeks later.

The intervention was delivered by nurses at PCUs. Nurses attended a 1-day training course, including a lecture, practical exercises, and role-play session on how to perform the intervention. The outcome of training was evaluated using pre-test and post-test questionnaires. A set of materials was developed to facilitate the intervention, including the translated version of the MET manual, a booklet for participants, coloured flip charts, and record forms. A record form for nurses was also developed to assist in counselling, including the stage of change of the participant, and to enable nurses to provide interventions in the follow-up sessions.

The control arm

At the initial appointment with nurses, participants received a booklet with feedback on findings from the health survey questionnaire and general information on health care, before being scheduled for subsequent visits at which drinking patterns were monitored.

Outcomes

The primary outcome measure was the amount of alcohol consumption during the previous week. Secondary outcomes included serum GGT, alcohol consumption during the previous month, number of episodes of binge drinking in the past 7 days, number of episodes of drunkenness in the previous month, and frequency of traffic accidents and traffic accidents due to drinking during the previous 6 months. A history of drinking was systematically obtained, using different but related questions to examine the coherence of responses. Outcomes were measured through a health survey questionnaire at baseline evaluation, and then at 6-week, 3-month, and 6-month follow-up. If participants failed to keep a follow-up appointment, they were followed up by telephone and home visits when needed.

To minimize bias related to self-report data, with the participants' consent, parallel interviews with collateral informants (e.g. spouses and other family members) were used to check for the validity and accuracy of the information. In addition, blood samples were collected for estimation of serum GGT as an objective measure of change in drinking between baseline and 6-month follow-up. Materials for blood sample collection were distributed to all PCUs. Nurses were instructed on how to collect and transfer samples. Blood samples were collected in special tubes provided by the research team, then frozen and transferred in a container with cold packs to remain frozen, before being sent to Phragmongkutklao Hospital's central laboratory.

Ethical issues

Ethical approval was granted by Royal Thai Army Medical Department Ethics Review Committee Phragmongkutklao Hospital and the College of Medicine, Bangkok, one of the eight Ethical Committees (Ecs) that is accredited by the Ministry of Public Health. Formal permission was also sought from the respective chief provincial officers. The written consent form contained detailed information including the trial processes and assurance of anonymity, as well as the name and telephone of the PI for contact in the event that further information was required. Each subject was informed by a PCU staff regarding eligibility for the study and, after agreeing to participate, was asked to sign two copies of the consent form, one for the central research team and another for the participant. There was no significant ethical challenge, though as will be described in the Conclusion, answers to questions on alcohol intake might have been derived from social desirability or the person's wiliness to please, more than reflecting actual behaviour.

Although there are limited adverse events in behavioural intervention, the issue of the possibility of anxiety was raised. Therefore reasons for dropping out of the trial, due to anxiety or other motives linked to the intervention, were asked to be immediately reported to the research coordinating centre. The procedure indicated that persons with this condition should be referred to evaluation and, if required, treatment.

Key findings

Of the 126 persons enrolled, nine were excluded due to lack of data or failure to meet the exclusion criteria. The intervention group included 59 persons: 50 were reinterviewed 6 weeks after and 55 at the 3-month follow-up interview; comparable data for the control group were 58, 48, and 53. Overall, there was an attrition rate of 7% in the experimental group and 9% in the control group; the overall follow-up rate was 92% (108 persons). There was no significant difference between the intervention and the control groups in age, sex, or marital status; 107 (91%) participants were male. The mean age was 37 ± 10 years old. The amount of drinking during the previous month was 6.39 ± 3.97 drinks/drinking day or 15.15 ± 17.74 drinks/week. The amount of drinking in the previous week was 4.75 ± 4.27 drinks per drinking day or 11.92 ± 16.17 drinks per week, and the AUDIT score was 17.4 ± 6.5. Generally, 59% of participants had hazardous drinking behaviour (men > 4 drinks/day, women > 3 drinks/day) during the previous month, while 43% of the participants had hazardous drinking behaviour above this threshold during the previous week.

There was a significant reduction in the frequency of daily and weekly hazardous drinking and of binge drinking sessions, from self-reported drinks per drinking day in the intervention group as compared to the control group ($p < 0.05$ in 9/10 outcomes assessed) at both 3 and 6 months. There was no difference in the self-reported frequency of being drunk at either of the follow-up periods. The incidence of alcohol-related consequences in the 6-month period was low in both groups, and the difference was not statistically significant. There was one accident in the intervention group compared to four in the control group; three traffic accidents in the intervention group compared to five in the control group. There were no visits to PCUs due to alcohol consumption in the intervention group compared to three in the control group. At 6-month follow-up, blood samples were obtained from 96 participants (51 in the intervention group and 45 in the control group) who provided GGT data at both study entry and follow-up. GGT levels were higher in both the intervention and control groups at 6-month follow-up than those observed at baseline and there was no difference between the two groups.

These results suggest that brief interventions based on MET decreased self-reported drinking levels in persons seeking primary care in Thailand. In contrast with self-reported alcohol consumption, however, an increase was found in mean GGT levels at follow-up in both study groups, suggesting an increase in alcohol consumption during this period. While improvement in drinking found from the self-reports may be the result of a social desirability bias (i.e. the participant's desire to please), which is especially relevant in a patient–provider relationship, another key factor of this study was that baseline data collection occurred just after *Kao Pansaa*, the 3-month Buddhist Lent, during which people avoid unhealthy behaviours, including alcohol consumption. Normal drinking patterns are usually resumed following this and are likely reflected in the overall GGT increase found in this study. Data from this study support further investigation of the measurement of alcohol consumption with biological measures in heavy drinking populations to determine the validity of self-reported outcomes.

Strengths and limitations

This study is one of the very few RCTs of brief interventions for AUD in primary care in LAMIC. The sites were known to the PI, enhancing the cooperation of staff, which helped ensure the success of implementing a complex intervention. There were clear participant recruitment criteria designed to include persons at the early stages of AUD and exclude those with alcohol dependence. The educational materials and knowledge on drinking obtained from local surveys were adapted to the local context, enhancing the appropriateness of the intervention (60–65). However, the high mean AUDIT scores suggested that exclusion might not have been fully achieved.

The investigators developed a protocol with clearly defined primary and secondary outcomes, the research process was described, sites were selected according to research requirements, and training in both the research methodology and the interventions was provided and its success evaluated through pre- and post-training questionnaires. Thus, the interventionists were certified as demonstrating competence in delivering the intervention. This is one of the steps to ensure that the intervention is delivered adequately in the trial. Although the intervention sessions were not recorded and a clinical research associate to perform source data verification was not included, quality assurance was monitored using a record form for nurses to monitor how the intervention was provided. Efforts to ensure retention of persons included the selection of sites with enthusiastic staff members and providing training and supervision for the staff members involved. Flexibility in the appointment schedules was allowed in order to increase the follow-up rate. Frequent contact and monitoring were also included to increase retention. Local staff contacted participants by telephone to ensure the follow-up visits.

The study strictly applied standard randomization procedures and allocation concealment as well as blinding participants and outcome assessors to minimize bias. The subjects randomized into the control condition were told that the trial would focus on health behaviours, which included questions on smoking, exercise, eating behaviour, weight, and alcohol use. In the consent form, they were told that there would be two different forms of the intervention but were not specifically informed whether they would receive MET or the booklet (17). Findings on drinking were fairly robust across various sensitivity analyses for the primary outcome measure and, coupled with the low attrition rate at 6 months, provide confidence in the internal validity of the study.

There are, however, certain limitations to the study. Fidelity was not fully assessed. Fidelity, along with the demonstration of competence in delivering the intervention, is a key aspect ensuring that the intervention is adequately delivered. However, nurses were requested to complete a form for each intervention session delivered, and the research team visited each site two or three times throughout the entire trial to monitor progress and intervention fidelity. The number of persons screened, those screening positive, and those refusing to participate in the study was not recorded, leading to uncertainty about the generalizability of study findings.

It proved impossible to measure a gender effect on outcomes, given the small number of women recruited, reflecting the low prevalence of drinking among women in the country. The challenges in conducting this study include the distance between the eight PCUs, making coordination more difficult. Furthermore, the logistics of sending blood samples for analysis was complicated by the distance between certain PCUs and the laboratory. However, these problems were overcome through the contact the PI had already established with the community hospital directors who were instrumental in the project logistics. Another challenge was related to the actual implementation of the trial procedures, including making the staff understand the importance of randomization to minimize bias, as health care workers and nurses in primary care were unfamiliar with the concept.

Conclusion

Several lessons can be drawn from the literature review and the case study included in the chapter. Like other studies conducted in LAMIC contexts (Table 11.2), this RCT conducted in Thailand demonstrated the effectiveness of a brief intervention and its impact on alcohol use in a primary care setting. The study was undertaken in rural, low-resourced primary care centres and the intervention delivered by nurses. The findings support the WHO recommendations of introducing psychosocial interventions for AUD into primary care settings. The increase in GGT levels at follow-up, in both the experimental and control groups, however, highlights the need to time AUD trials so that findings are not affected by contextual factors that may affect alcohol consumption and to use objective indicators of alcohol use where possible. The trial also follows the Institute of Medicine (IOM)'s recommendations (66) regarding the need to narrow the communication gap between the research community and community-based treatment programmes by maintaining two-way communication between public policy requirements and community care needs. In this relationship, clinical research plays a dual role, first as a vehicle for improving clinical practice and second as an instrument for the implementation of public policies on treatment based on community needs. Due to the fact that the intervention was tested directly in the community centres targeted by the public policy designed to develop interventions for primary care environments, it also overcomes the difficulties inherent in efficacy or explanatory trials conducted in specialized research settings regarding issues such as: lack of fit between the characteristics of subjects included in the trial and those in the community where the tested intervention is to be implemented (67, 68); the divergence between the felt needs of the community and the intervention implemented; and the considerable lag between the time when evidence is obtained from the study and when it is applied in the community.

This trial included an adaptation and previous testing of the instruments to the local setting, but the intervention was not piloted in these communities prior to the implementation of the trial. Other studies have shown how to adapt interventions tested in developed countries to LAMIC contexts (Table 11.2). One challenge addressed in this project is the sustainability of a brief intervention in a clinical setting and the fact that the intervention and related factors, including the personnel delivering the intervention, must be appropriate to the specific cultural milieu of the setting. The trial conducted in Thailand took care to involve the persons in charge of the jurisdiction where the study was implemented and to train routine staff to implement the intervention. Another example of a trial that sought to develop a brief intervention which can be scaled up is a study from Poland which used focus groups with those screening eligible for the intervention, prior to the initiation of the RCT (19).

The focus group participants (persons seen in emergency rooms and staff) concluded that nurses were the most suitable candidates for providing the brief intervention, rather than physicians, as this was more likely to be seen by patients as normal and acceptable in this setting and also because nurses normally devote more time to patients than physicians. A second focus group explored the specific context of Polish drinking and informed the actual content of the brief intervention, including barriers to changing drinking behaviour and/or obtaining alcohol treatment, identifying opportunities for excess drinking as a major reason for drinking and a barrier to changing drinking patterns. Reasons given for failing to seek treatment included lack of familiarity with treatment resources and stigma. The group recommended moderation rather than abstinence as a negotiation goal, with a separate (higher) norm for special celebrations lasting over 6 hours. This example highlights the usefulness of involving prospective recipients of a brief intervention in assuring that the intervention and its implementation are contextually appropriate and will be well received, thereby increasing the likelihood of its effectiveness and the potential sustainability of the ongoing implementation of the brief intervention in a particular setting.

The increasing involvement of women in alcohol intake requires ensuring their participation in clinical trials. Significant challenges are posed by their lower prevalence of problem drinking, along with cultural factors that increase the likelihood of failing to report their problems with alcohol (69) when they attend clinical centres. In our case study, an a priori stratification of arms by gender would have provided enough women to adequately test the intervention. The important role of alcohol in local cultures in LAMIC (70), with periods of abstinence or excessive intake at local festivities, makes the case for planning trials at a time when such events do not alter the results of the trials.

The need for an informed consent, a challenge for clinical studies in many cultures, is another lesson learned. There is a need for better ways to ensure that those persons involved in the studies and less familiar with this procedure understand the implications and ethics of human subjects research (71). The social desirability bias found in this study provides an opportunity to understand the need for explaining the importance of equipoise to prospective participants during the consent process.

Sustainability of brief interventions in clinical practice is a long-term challenge in most countries, requiring strong local support. While capacity building with routine implementation of brief intervention in these settings is recommended, time constraints and staffing resources are common barriers to this form of implementation, as are clinic staff attitudes regarding their ability to conduct a brief intervention and their beliefs regarding the efficacy of such an intervention for problem drinking (14).

Sustainability requires an effective administrative and scientific structure. In Mexico, interventions tested through efficacy clinical trials as part of a university programme (72, 73) were subsequently replicated in 320 community centres in order to identify and intervene with hazardous and harmful substance users. The National Autonomous University of Mexico (UNAM) was also involved in training the professionals who delivered the services and testing their intervention abilities by monitoring their daily work along with the fidelity of treatment. Also in Mexico, the Ramón de la Fuente National Institute of Psychiatry, in collaboration with the University of Miami and the Clinical Trials Network of the National Institute of Drug Abuse (NIDA CTN), successfully established a clinical trial network as an adaptation of the CTN programme established in the US, through a technology transfer grant.

This collaborative project followed the IOM 1998 recommendations regarding the need to develop strategies and infrastructure to link research and practice. The first randomized clinical trial (45, 46, 74, 75) supported by the newly created Mexican CTN was conducted in the treatment sites that form part of the main treatment institutions in the country, with a mandate and an active role in informing policy makers. The formation of the Mexican network also followed recommendations regarding consumer participation and community-based centres and envisioned the creation of an infrastructure for dissemination and technology transfer. The network was designed to include new projects as a means of sustaining the programme and sought to overcome the lack of a trial oversight committee to guarantee quality control. This type of organization may be required to provide accreditation of sites and personnel, report on adverse events, and guarantee the protection of the human rights of persons in treatment. The network can also implement the IOM (66) recommendation of integrating community treatment agencies for the development of concepts and research protocols with the objective of responding to the requirements of real-world practice. This network could also meet the state's need to implement public polices and narrow the research and practice gap by considering the principles of cost-effectiveness and the cost-benefit of such an action. The creation of this infrastructure makes it possible to address barriers to sustainability through the implementation of clinical trials in real-world settings, with the involvement of practitioners in the development and implementation of these trials.

Success in the implementation of RCTs is based on: (1) establishing clear goals and planning accordingly; (2) the development of a plan to attain goals that take into account process mapping and manualization; and (3) the consolidation of a structure/ organization, including the procurement of resources, and the formation of a team with clear roles and responsibilities with a clear distribution of activities. This can only happen with clear leadership and direction, effective communication with teams that are motivated and open to learning and changing with proper conflict resolution, and adequate monitoring of the goals established that would permit corrective action when deviations occur. Since RCTs show the effectiveness of an intervention, a platform is needed for training and the dissemination of these practices. Adoption of evidence-based practices by newly trained organizations incorporates adequate attention to the process of change. A pilot implementation phase could shed light on the potential barriers that must be addressed for successful scale-up. Once this infrastructure is in place, studies could be undertaken to assess and control for community readiness to change and test the cultural appropriateness of the intervention before the clinical trial is implemented.

Looking ahead, intervention research to generate policy-relevant evidence for AUD in LAMIC should seek to evaluate pharmacological and non-pharmacological treatments for alcohol dependence; provide alternative interventions better suited to women, youths, the elderly, or indigenous communities to enhance the effectiveness of available interventions; estimate the cost-effectiveness of interventions; adapt interventions to a rapidly changing environment and expectations in relation to alcohol consumption; and use appropriate designs for evaluating population-based interventions.

References

1 Lozano R, Naghavi M, Foreman K, Lim S, Shibuya K, Aboyans V, et al. (2013) Global and regional mortality from 235 causes of death for 20 age groups in 1990 and 2010: a systematic analysis for the Global Burden of Disease Study 2010. Lancet, **380**(9859):2095–128.

2 Murray C, Vos T, Lozano R, et al. (2012) Disability-adjusted life years (DALYs) for 291 diseases and injuries in 21 regions, 1990–2010: a systematic analysis for the Global Burden of Disease Study 2010. Lancet, **380**(9859):2197–223.

3 Lim SS, Vos T, Flaxman AD, Danaei G, Shibuya K, Adair-Rohani H, et al. (2012) A comparative risk assessment of burden of disease and injury attributable to 67 risk factors and risk factor clusters in 21 regions, 1990–2010: a systematic analysis for the Global Burden of Disease Study 2010. Lancet, **380**(9859):2224–60.

4 Rehm J, Rehnd N, Room R, Monteiro M, Gmel G, Jernigan D, et al. (2003) The global distribution of average volume of alcohol consumption and patterns of drinking. Eur Addict Res, **9**:147–56.

5 **Beaglehole R, Bonita R** (2009) Alcohol: a global health priority. Lancet, **373**(9682): 2173–4.

6 **Kohn R, Saxena S, Levav I, Saraceno B** (2004) The treatment gap in mental health care. Bull World Health Organ, **82**(11):858–66.

7 **WHO** (2013) ICD-10 Diagnostic criteria for research. <http://www.who.int/substance_ abuse/terminology/icd_10/en/index.html last open 16062013>.

8 **WHO** (1992) The ICD-10: classification of mental and behavioural disorders, clinical description and diagnostic guidelines. Geneva: WHO.

9 **American Psychiatric Association** (2013) DSM V. Substance-related and addictive disorders. <http://www.dsm5.org/Documents/Substance%20Use%20Disorder%20Fact%20Sheet.pdf>.

10 **WHO** (1960) Lexicon of alcohol and drug terms published by the World Health Organization. <http://www.who.int/substance_abuse/terminology/who_lexicon/en/>.

11 **WHO** (2008) mhGAP Mental Health Gap Action Programme. Scaling up care for mental, neurological and substance use disorders. Geneva: WHO.

12 **Humeniuk RE, Henry-Edwards S, Ali RL, Poznyak V, Monteiro M** (2011a) Intervención breve vinculada a ASSIST para el consumo riesgoso y nocivo de sustancias: manual para uso en la atención primaria. Ginebra: Organización Mundial de la Salud.

13 **Humeniuk RE, Henry-Edwards S, Ali RL, Poznyak V, Monteiro M** (2011b) La prueba de detección de consumo de alcohol, tabaco y sustancias (ASSIST): manual para uso en la atención primaria. Ginebra: Organización Mundial de la Salud.

14 **Babor T, Caetano R, Caswell S, Edwars G, Giesbrecht N, Graham J, et al.** (2010) Alcohol. No ordinary commodity. Research and public policy. Oxford: Oxford University Press.

15 **Bernstein E, Bernstein J** (2008) Effectiveness of alcohol screening and brief motivational intervention in the emergency department setting. Ann Emerg Med, **51**(6):751–4.

16 **Kaner EF, Dickinson HO, Beyer F, Pienaar E, Schlesinger C, Campbell F, et al.** (2009) The effectiveness of brief alcohol interventions in primary care settings: a systematic review. Drug Alcohol Rev, **28**(3):301–23.

17 **Noknoy S, Rangsin R, Saengcharnchai P, Tantibhaedhyangkul U, McCambridge J** (2010) RCT of effectiveness of motivational enhancement therapy delivered by nurses for hazardous drinkers in primary care units in Thailand. Alcohol Alcohol, **45**(3):263–70.

18 **Mohr D, Hopewell S, Kenneth F, Schulz F, Montori V, Gotzsche P, et al.** (2010) CONSORT 2010 explanation and elaboration: updated guidelines for reporting parallel group randomized trials. J Clin Epidemiol, **63**(2010):e1–37.

19 **Cherpitel CJ, Bernstein E, Bernstein J, Moskalewicz J, Swiatkiewicz G** (2009) Screening, brief intervention and referral to treatment (SBIRT) in a Polish emergency room: challenges in cultural translation of SBIRT. J Addiction Nurs, **20**:127–31.

20 **Cherpitel CJ, Woolard R, Ye Y, Bond J, Bernstein E, Bernstein J, et al.** (2013) Screening, brief intervention and referral to treatment (SBIRT) in an emergency department: three-month outcomes of a randomized controlled clinical trial among Mexican-origin young adults. Proc Meeting International Network on Brief Interventions for Alcohol and Drugs, Rome, 19–20 September.

21 **Balas EA, Boren SA** (2000) Managing clinical knowledge for health care improvement. In: Bemmel J, McCray AT (eds) Yearbook of medical informatics 2000: patient-centered systems, pp. 65–70. Stuttgart: Schattauer.

22 **Green LW, Ottoson JM, Garcia C, Hiatt RA** (2009) Diffusion theory and knowledge dissemination, utilization, and integration in public health. Ann Rev Public Health, **30**:151–74.

23 **Backer T, Guerra N** (2011) Mobilizing communities to implement evidence-based practices in youth violence prevention: the state of the art. Am J Commun Psychol, **48**:31–42.

24 Fixsen D L, Naoom SF, Blase KA, Friedman RM, Wallace F (2005) Implementation research: a synthesis of the literature (FMHI Pub. No. 231). Tampa: National Implementation Research Network, University of South Florida.

25 Glasgow RE, Green LW, Klesges LM, Abrams DB, Fisher EB, Goldstein M, et al. (2006) External validity: we need to do more. Annal Behav Med, **31**:105–8.

26 Spoth R, Rohrbach LA, Greenberg M, Leaf P, Brown CH, Fagan A, et al. (2013) Addressing core challenges for the next generation of type 2 translation research and systems: the translation science to population impact (TSci Impact) framework. Prev Sci, **14**(4):319–51.

27 Patel V, Araya R, Chatterjee S, Chisholm D, Cohen A, De Silva M, et al. (2007) Treatment and prevention of mental disorders in low-income and middle-income countries. Lancet, **370**:991–1005.

28 WHO (2001) The World Health report 2001: mental health: new understanding, new hope. Geneva: WHO.

29 Papas R, Sidle J, Gakinya B, Baliddawa J, Martino S (2011) Treatment outcomes of a stage 1 cognitive-behavioral trial to reduce alcohol use among human immunodeficiency virus-infected out-patients in western Kenya . Addiction, **106**:2156–66.

30 Rendall-Mkosi K, Morojele N, London L, Moodley S, Singh C (2012) A randomized controlled trial of motivational interviewing to prevent risk for an alcohol-exposed pregnancy in the western Cape. S Afr. Addiction, **108**:725–32.

31 Castro LA, Laranjeira R (2009) Ensaio Clínico dupli-cego randomizado e placebo-controlado com Naltrexona e intervencao breve no tratamento ambulatorial da dependencia de alcool. J Bras Psiq, **58**(2):79–85.

32 Martínez K, Pedroza FJ, Salazar ML, Vacío MA (2010) Evaluación experimental de dos intervenciones breves para la reducción del consumo de alcohol en adolescentes. Rev Mex Anál Conducta, **36**(3):35–53.

33 Segatto ML, Andreoni S, De Souza R, Diehl I, Pinsky I (2011) Brief motivational interview and educational brochure in emergency room settings for adolescents and young adults with alcohol-related problems: a randomized single-blind clinical trial. Rev Brasil Psiq, **33**(3):225–33.

34 Díaz A, Díaz LR, Rodríguez AC, Díaz A, Fernández H, Hernández C (2011) Eficacia de un programa de intervenciones terapéuticas en estudiantes universitarios diagnosticados con dependencia al alcohol. Salud Mental, **11**(34):185–94.

35 Ahmadi J, Ahmadi N (2002) A double-blind controlled study of naltrexone in the treatment of alcohol dependence. German J Psychiatry, **5**:85–9.

36 Baltieri DA, de Andrade AG (2003) Efficacy of acamprosate in the treatment of alcohol-dependent outpatients. Rev Bras Psiq, **25**:156–9.

37 Namkoong K, Lee B-O, Lee Ch, Korean Acamprosate Clinical Trial Investigators (2003) Acamprosate in Korean alcohol dependent patients: a multi-centre randomized, double bind, placebo-controlled study. Alcohol Alcohol, **38**(2):135–41.

38 Baltieri DA, Daro FR, Ribeiro PL, de Andrade AG (2008) Comparing topiramate with naltrexone in the treatment of alcohol dependence. Addiction, **103**(12):2035–44.

39 Miller WR, Sanchez VC (1994) Motivating young adults for treatment and lifestyle change. In: Howard GS, Nathan PE (eds) Alcohol use and misuse by young adults. Notre Dame: University of Notre Dame Press.

40 NIAAA (1999) No. 43. Brief intervention for alcohol problems. Alcohol alert (serial on the Internet). <http://pubs.niaaa.nih.gov/publications/aa43.htm>.

41 Bien TH, Miller WR, Tonigan JS (1993) Brief interventions for alcohol problems: a review. Addiction, **88**(3):315–35.

42 Poikolainen K (1999) Effectiveness of brief interventions to reduce alcohol intake in primary health care populations: a meta-analysis. Prev Med, **28**(5):503–9.

43 Kahan M, Wilson L, Becker L (1995) Effectiveness of physician-based interventions with problem drinkers: a review. CMAJ, **152**(6):851–9.

44 Wilk AI, Jensen NM, Havighurst TC (1997) Meta-analysis of randomized control trials addressing brief interventions in heavy alcohol drinkers. J Gen Intern Med, **12**(5):274–83.

45 Marín-Navarrete R, Horigian VE, Verdeja RE, Alonso E, Perez M, Berlanga-Cisneros C, et al. (2013) Development of a clinical trial network to test and disseminate evidence-based practices to treat addictions and mental disorders in Mexico (poster). Abstracts of the NIDA International Forum, San Diego, CA.

46 Horigian VE, Marín-Navarrete RA, Verdeja RE, Alonso E, Perez M, Berlanga C, Medina-Mora ME, et al. (Unpublished results) Technology transfer for the implementation of a clinical trials network on drug abuse and mental health in Mexico.

47 Assanangkornchai S, Sam-Angsri N, Rerngpongpan S, Lertnakorn A (2010) Patterns of alcohol consumption in the Thai population: results of the National Household Survey of 2007. Alcohol Alcohol, **45**(3):278–85.

48 WHO (2004) Country profiles: Thailand global status report on alcohol 2004 (serial on the Internet). <http://www.google.co.th/url?sa=t&rct=j&q=&esrc=s&source=web&cd=1&ved=0CDEQFjAA&url=http%3A%2F%2Fwww.who.int%2Fsubstance_abuse%2Fpublications%2Fen%2Fthailand.pdf&ei=l2VwUcKRFsavkgWi6IGwDQ&usg=AFQjCNHC7P2hLpfRlStkFXua-XwdjarxEA&sig2=YwVs3dcW9w4rL8vMQTx-aQ&bvm=bv.45373924,d.dGI>.

49 Moolasart J, Chirawatkul S (2012) Drinking culture in the Thai-Isaan context of northeast Thailand. Southeast Asian J Trop Med Public Health, **43**(3):795–807.

50 Assanangkornchai S, Pinkaew P, Apakupakul N (2003) Prevalence of hazardous-harmful drinking in a southern Thai community. Drug Alcohol Rev, **22**(3):287–93.

51 Siviroj P, Peltzer K, Pengpid S, Morarit S (2012) Non-seatbelt use and associated factors among Thai drivers during Songkran festival. BMC Public Health, **12**:608.

52 Thai Foundation for Responsible Drinking (2011) Know your limit. <http://www.thinkb4drink-tfrd.com/en/campaigns_know_your.php>.

53 Chavengchaiyong W, Foncom A, Chockeard N (2000) The effect of brief intervention to changing behaviour of alcohol disorder patients at Lamphun Hospital. Bull Dept Med Serv, **25**:87–95.

54 Hallgren KA, Witkiewitz K (2013) Missing data in alcohol clinical trials: a comparison of methods. Alcohol Clin Exp Res, **37**(12):2152–60.

55 Graham AW, Fleming MS (1998) Brief Intervention. In: Graham AW, Schultz TK (eds) (2009) Principles of addiction medicine, 2nd edn, pp. 615–30. Chevy Chase: American Society of Addition Medicine.

56 Miller WR, Zweben A, Diclemente CC, Rychtarik RG (eds) (1992) Project MATCH: motivational enhancement therapy manual. Bethesda: NIAAA.

57 Miller WR (ed.) (1991) Motivational interviewing: preparing people to change addictive behavior. New York: Guildford Press.

58 DiClemente CC, Prochaska JO (1982) Self-change and therapy change of smoking behavior: a comparison of processes of change in cessation and maintenance. Addict Behav, **7**(2):133–42.

59 Prochaska JO, DiClemente CC (1982) Transtheoretical therapy toward a more integrative model of change. Psychother Theory Res Practice, **19**:276–88.

60 Ball SA, Martino S, Nich C, Frankforter TL, Van Horn D, Crits-Christoph P, et al. (2007) Site matters: multisite randomized trial of motivational enhancement therapy in community drug abuse clinics. J Consult Clin Psychol, **75**:556–67.

61 Carroll K, Ball S, Nich C, Martino S, Frankforter T, Farentinos C, et al. (2006) Motivational interviewing to improve treatment engagement and outcome in individuals seeking treatment for substance abuse: a multisite effectiveness study. Drug Alcohol Depend, **81**(3):301–12.

62 Carroll KM, Farentinos C, Ball S, Crits-Christoph P, Libby B, Morgenstern J, et al. (2002) MET meets the real world: design issues and clinical strategies in the clinical trials network. J Subst Abuse Treat, **23**:73–80.

63 Carroll KM, Martino S, Ball SA, Nich C, Frankforter T, Anez LM, et al. (2009) A multisite randomized effectiveness trial of motivational enhancement therapy for Spanish-speaking substance users. J Consult Clin Psychol, **77**(5):993–9.

64 Carroll K, Martino S, Rounsaville B (2010) No train, no gain? Clin Psychol Sci Pract, **17**:36–40.

65 Martino S, Ball S, Tami C, Frankforter T, Carroll K (2009) Correspondence of motivational enhancement treatment integrity ratings among therapists, supervisors. HYPERLINK "http://www.ncbi.nlm.nih.gov/pubmed/?term=Correspondence+of+motivational +enhancement+treatment+integrity+ratings+among+therapists%2C+supervisors" \o "Psychotherapy research : journal of the Society for Psychotherapy Research." Psychother Res, **19**(2):181–93.

66 Lamb S, Greenlick M, McCarty D, Institute of Medicine (1998) Bridging the gap between practice and research: forging partnerships with community-based drug and alcohol treatment. Washington, DC: Committee on Community-Based Drug Treatment, Institute of Medicine, National Academy Press.

67 Humphreys K, Horst D, Joshi AA, Finney JW (2005) Prevalence and predictors of research participant eligibility criteria in alcohol treatment outcome studies, 1970–98. Addiction, **100**(9):1249–57.

68 Humphreys K, Weingardt K, Harris AH (2007) Influence of subject eligibility criteria on compliance with National Institutes of Health guidelines for inclusion of women, minorities, and children in treatment research. Alcohol Clin Exp Res, **31**(6):988–95.

69 Berenzon S, Robles R, Reed GM, Medina-Mora ME (2011) Gender-related issues in the diagnosis and classification of alcohol use disorders among Mexican patients seeking specialized services. Rev Bras Psiq, **33**(1):S109–24.

70 Room R, Jerningan D, Carlini B, Gureje O, Mäkelä K, Marshal M, et al. (2002) Alcohol in developing societies: a public health approach. Finnish Foundation for Alcohol Studies. Geneva: WHO.

71 Aguilera RM, Mondragón L, Medina-Mora ME (2008) Consideraciones éticas en intervenciones comunitarias: la pertinencia del consentimiento informado. Salud Mental, **31**(2):129–38.

72 Rojas E, Real T, García-Silberman y Medina-Mora ME (2011) Revisión sistemática sobre tratamiento de adicciones en México. Salud Mental, **32**:351–65.

73 Echeverría SL, Carrascoza VC, Reidl ML (2007) Prevención y Tratamiento de Conductas Adictivas. Mexico City: UNAM, Facultad de Psicología.

74 **Marin-Navarrete R** (2012) Developing collaborative networks across international borders: the CTN Florida node alliance collaboration with the National Institute of Psychiatry in Mexico (oral presentation). Abstracts from the ICBM 2012 Meeting. Int J Behav Med, **19**:S1–24.

75 **Marín-Navarrete R, Horigian VE** (2013) Development of a clinical trial network in Mexico to test and disseminate evidence based practices for addiction and mental disorders: a binational collaboration for transfer of technology (oral presentation). Breakout: using the CTN model to improve treatment in the NIDA International Forum 2013, San Diego, CA.

Chapter 12

Trials of interventions for people with dementia

Amit Dias, Dilip Motghare, Daisy Acosta, Jacob Roy, A.T. Jotheeswaran, and Ralph N. Martins

Introduction

Ever since Alois Alzheimer first described Alzheimer's disease in 1906, a condition that was later named after him, there has been a growing body of research to understand its causes and treatment. However, we are still in the process of understanding dementia and developing strategies to combat this condition. Dementia is a syndrome due to a progressive brain condition leading to the disturbance of multiple higher cortical functions such as memory, orientation, thinking, comprehension, calculation, capacity for learning, judgement, and language. Dementia is referred to as a major neurocognitive disorder (NCD) in the DSM-V (1, 2). They even recognize the milder form of cognitive impairment as mild NCD, which has been the subject of research in recent times. The DSM-V specifies the criteria to differentiate between the several aetiological subtypes of dementia. Dementia is not a single entity and refers to conditions such as Alzheimer's disease, which is the most common form, contributing to almost 60% of all the cases, as well as vascular dementia, dementia with Lewy bodies, frontotemporal dementia, dementias due to vitamin deficiencies, hypothyroidism, and a host of other conditions which come under this umbrella. People often have a mixed pathology, such as a combination of Alzheimer's disease and vascular dementia. In most cases, the disease is irreversible and there is no known cure as of now. However, symptomatic treatment and support is helpful (3).

The WHO has recently declared dementia as a public health priority (4). It is estimated that there are around 35.6 million people with this condition around the world. Studies indicate that the numbers are expected to double every 20 years, reaching 65.7 million in 2030 and 115.4 million in 2050 when the global population over the age of 60 years is expected to reach 2 billion (5). What is of greater concern is that given the rapid demographic transition in the LAMIC, the majority of people with dementia will be living in these regions. In 2010 it was estimated that 57.7% of all people with dementia lived in LAMIC, which is expected to rise to 63.4% in 2030 and 70.5% in 2050, and this clearly highlights the need for more research and services for people with dementia in these regions (4, 6). Dementia accounts for 11.9% of years lived with disability due to a non-communicable disease (7). This is a higher proportion than that for stroke (9.5%), musculoskeletal disorders (8.9%), cardiovascular disease (5.0%), and cancer (2.4%), making it a leading cause of disability and dependency in later life. In 2010, the

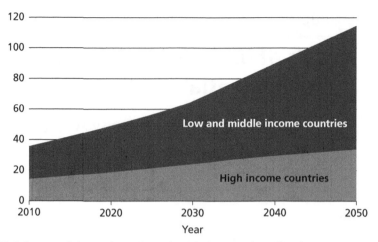

Fig. 12.1 The growth in numbers of people with dementia (in millions) in LAMIC as compared with HIC.

worldwide cost of dementia was estimated to be US $604 billion (8). Dementia has an enormous impact on the person with this condition as well as their caregiver (9, 10). The major cost in the HIC is due to formal care costs and institutionalization, which accounts for almost 77% of the costs (11). In contrast, family care is more important in resource-poor settings, accounting for 56% in LIC and 42% in MIC (12). In the area of mental health research, there is an increasing interest in recognizing the public health challenges posed by dementia in LAMIC (12). At the same time, there is a need to understand the several challenges that one would face while conducting research, especially RCTs in these regions (13, 14) (see Fig. 12.1).

The treatment gap for dementia research and care in LAMIC

The treatment gap for dementia, which refers to the gap between those who need and get evidence-based care for the condition, varies from around 90% in India (15) to 70% in China (16). This again highlights the need to evolve and evaluate innovative strategies to overcome the barriers and provide evidence-based, cost-effective quality care to all people with dementia and their families. In this chapter we highlight the tremendous scope for well-designed RCTs to test innovative interventions that would be affordable and effective for the people in low-resource settings.

There has been considerable interest in trying to understand the treatment gap for dementia in LAMIC in the past decade (17). Two major initiatives undertaken by Alzheimer's Disease International and the WHO have changed the way we look at dementia in LAMIC. The first is the 10/66 Dementia Research Group, which was established in India in 1998 with the objective of encouraging research in LAMIC. Much of the research on dementia conducted till recently has been in the HIC (3, 18). Less than 10% of funds for research were diverted to LAMIC where nearly two-thirds of the people

Table 12.1 Recommended interventions for people with dementia in LAMIC (adapted from the mhGAP initiative and the packages of care for dementia in LAMIC) (3, 19)

	Recommended interventions	Caution in LAMIC	Supporting evidence from LAMIC
Pharmacological interventions	Dementia-specific medication such as anticholine-esterase inhibitors (donepezil, rivastigmine, galantamine) and N-methyl-D-aspartate (NMDA) inhibitor (memantine) (21)	Should only be considered if there is adequate supervision by specialists. Should be avoided in a non-specialist setting in LAMIC	Several industry-sponsored trials have been conducted in LAMIC on dementia-specific medication (13). All the approved drugs are available in several LAMIC. However, lack of specialists is a major barrier to providing medical management (22)
	Antidepressants	Moderate to severe depression could be treated with SSRIs. Patients have to be referred to a specialist if no improvement is noticed in 3 weeks	
	Antipsychotics	Antipsychotics are not routinely recommended for the management of behavioural and psychological symptoms of dementia (BPSD). They may be considered in special situations under strict specialist monitoring. Care should be taken to limit the duration of such treatment. Meta-analysis has shown that antipsychotics are associated with an increased risk of death and cerebrovascular adverse events (23). Non-pharmacological interventions are recommended for BPSD and should be the first choice	
Non-pharmacological interventions	Cognitive and psychological interventions	Various therapies such as reality orientation and reminiscence therapy may be considered. Therapy needs to be adapted to LAMIC, and adequate training of personnel is necessary	There is work on psychosocial interventions for people with dementia and their caregivers; however, there is a need to gather robust evidence on cognitive stimulation interventions. A small trial on cognitive stimulation was reported from Brazil (24)
	Diagnosis of dementia	Non-specialist health care providers should seek to identify possible cases of dementia in the primary health care setting. Brief informant assessment and cognitive tests should be used to assist in confirming these cases	Community health workers, after a few hours of training, could detect dementia with a positive predictive value of 66% (25, 26)
	Medical review and follow-up	People with dementia should receive an initial and a regular medical review (at least every 6 months) and appropriate care. Caregivers should also receive attention as they often tend to have poor mental health	Some trials show evidence of benefit on caregiver outcomes (27–29)
	Psychoeducation	Should be offered to the family and caregivers of people with dementia. Home-based care should be encouraged	

with dementia live. This prompted the formation of the 10/66 Dementia Research Group aimed at bridging the research gap and developing evidence-based strategies in LAMIC. The 10/66 Dementia Research Group findings have helped in closing much of the gaps in our understanding of the burden of dementia and its impact in LAMIC, thus laying the foundation for developing needs-based interventions to improve the quality of care for people with dementia in these regions.

The second major step in this regard has been the mhGAP, which is an initiative of the WHO with the objective of scaling up care for mental, neurological, and substance use disorders in LAMIC (19, 20). Dementia is one of the priority conditions under this programme. Through this initiative the WHO has provided evidence-based recommendations and prepared a model intervention guide for the management of dementia. Table 12.1 provides a summary of the recommendations for LAMIC and the evidence to support the same. The recommendations echo the suggested 'packages of care' for dementia in LAMIC published in *PLOS Medicine* (3). They highlight the need for a combination of treatments aimed at improving the recognition and management of the condition to achieve optimal outcomes.

Not every person with dementia will present in the same way. They could have a range of behavioural problems to a varying degree. An intervention, to be effective, would have to be designed to manage the whole complex spectrum of dementia care, ranging from the diagnosis, improving cognition, managing BPSD, support to caregivers, and improving physical health and quality of life. There have been several studies in this regard, but most of the evidence has been from the HIC.

Challenges to conducting trials involving people with dementia in LAMIC

The majority of people with dementia live in LAMIC and the numbers are expected to rise rapidly. It is necessary to encourage research in this region to gather the evidence of what works in this setting. A trial on dementia could be designed with several aims targeting both the caregiver as well as the person with dementia. Depending on the research question, one could choose several outcomes for the intervention, such as: increase the caregiver knowledge on dementia care, reduce caregiver burnout or stress, improve the functional ability of the person with dementia, improve cognition in the person with dementia, delay the progression of the disease, prevent a particular type of dementia, or even cure or prevent the condition. There are several advantages to conducting trials in LAMIC, such as low cost and faster recruitment of participants. A number of industry-driven drug trials have been started in LAMIC due to these advantages (13). Globalization of drug trials is a welcome step and increase the chances of bringing a new product to the market. However, on the flip side, there is a possibility of industries resorting to dubious unethical practices, taking advantage of the vulnerability of people living in this region where the participants are more likely to be illiterate and poor and in a scenario where institutions ensuring ethical procedures may not be well established (30–32). It also raises the ethical question around justice; how many drugs tested on people in LAMIC will be made available to them at a cost that they can afford? A number of new promising treatments have reached phase 3 trials (4, 33);

however, there are still no promising, cost-effective, pharmacological interventions for dementia, particularly for use in routine health care settings, and the focus of care, as of now, is on psychosocial interventions.

While designing a trial in this region, one has to carefully consider the culture and the ground reality in LAMIC. Several studies in the HIC, for example, have considered a delay in the admission into a long-term care facility as the primary outcome (34). However, this would be inappropriate in LAMIC as long-term care homes often ironically deny admission to people with dementia. According to the Dementia India report, there were only ten residential homes for people with dementia in India in 2010 (35). There are several other challenges to conducting trials in LAMIC. Dementia, as mentioned in the Introduction, is not a disease entity by itself; it is a syndrome consisting of multiple conditions— each of which is unique and has a unique pathology and risk factors. Trials designed to look into treatment should therefore be able to select the specific type of dementia for the study. The major hurdle in dementia research is that assessment of dementia and diagnosing the type is challenging, and more so in LAMIC where diagnostic facilities for neuroimaging and testing biomarkers are in their infancy, if at all available (36). The diagnostic methods also need to be standardized and require trained personnel. There is increasing evidence to support the need to stratify for the apolipoprotein E4 (ApoE4) genotype in the trials for Alzheimer's disease. There could be a differential response probably due to the fact that those with ApoE4 get the disease earlier and tend to develop more amyloid in the brain known to be responsible for the condition. Trials involving drugs such as docosahexaenoic acid (DHA), an omega 3 fatty acid, and bapineuzumab, an antiamyloid molecule, have shown better response in those who do not carry the ApoE4 gene (33). Some countries in LAMIC prohibit genotyping in trials and have strict regulations prohibiting the transfer of genetic material across borders. This makes it necessary to establish a fully equipped laboratory or diagnostic centre and have trained staff at the site itself.

The psychometric assessments for dementia could be very time-consuming and laborious. Conducting such assessments repeatedly could be a challenge. Moreover, dementia assessments often require the assessment or inputs from the caregiver as well, which adds to the complexity. To make matters worse, there are several languages spoken in the region and each language may have several dialects. Getting the instruments for assessment and diagnosis adequately translated and validated is a challenging exercise in itself. India, for example, has 447 currently spoken languages and many more dialects. The 10/66 Dementia Research Group has done considerable work in this area and has developed instruments for evaluation and assessment in the local language.

People with dementia do not visit a health facility. If at all they do, they usually present in an advanced stage with severe BPSD. Most of the trials need to recruit mild to moderate stages of the condition. Recruitment from a hospital setting may therefore not be representative of the people in the community and recruitment from the community may be a challenge as most of the people are not aware of the diagnosis.

In this chapter, we focus on the trials involving non-pharmacological interventions for families of people with dementia in LAMIC as they have a greater potential for scaling up in this region in the current scenario. Though we did not perform a systematic literature review, we contacted several researchers involved in dementia research in LAMIC for information regarding trials. The three well-conducted trials on

Table 12.2 RCTs involving psychosocial interventions for people with dementia in LAMIC

Country	Interventions	Provided by	Key findings
Moscow (29) $N = 60$	Caregiver education and training using modules	Newly qualified doctors, as it was not possible to recruit NSHWs	Improvements in caregiver perception of burden in 6 months. However, no effect on caregiver distress and patient and caregiver quality of life
Peru (28) $N = 47$	Caregiver education and training using modules	Junior psychologists and social workers, as it was not possible to recruit NSHWs	Caregivers reported a significant decrease in strain at the end of 6 months. However, there was no effect on psychological distress and quality of life of both caregivers and people with dementia
Goa (27) $N = 81$	Psychosocial education using ten simplified steps including one initial visit to a specialist	Specially recruited NSHWs under the supervision of a counsellor and psychiatrist	Significant reduction in caregiver stress and distress due to BPSD. No significant improvement in the functional ability of the person with dementia Demonstrated the feasibility of using NSHWs to provide support

N indicates the total number of participants randomized in each of the studies.

psychosocial interventions in LAMIC have been summarized in Table 12.2. We have considered the Dementia Home Care Project as the case study to illustrate the challenges in conducting such a trial in India.

Case study: the Dementia Home Care Project, Goa, India (27)

Background

Goa is a relatively small state on the west coast of India. The state has better health care facilities resulting in better health outcomes and a life expectancy that is a decade higher than the rest of the country. Awareness about dementia is poor and loss of memory in older people is often misconstrued to be part of normal ageing. The health services are ill-equipped to meet the needs of older people with such conditions (37). Care is typically facility based and often involves a long journey and waiting time, which discourages family members from taking a person with dementia to a clinic. Only people with severe BPSD would visit a clinic and their management is often focused on the acute condition (15). Most care of people with dementia in this region is informal with hardly any support from the health and social services (9). Our earlier research further showed that caring for people with dementia is associated with significantly worse mental health scores, higher perceived burden by caregivers, and greater out-of-pocket health care costs due to reliance on private GPs who make home visits (10). Given this background, we sought to develop a complex intervention using locally available resources and targeting the dyad of the person with dementia and the caregiver. The trial was conducted under the Dementia Society of Goa, an NGO working in the field of dementia, based in the state of Goa.

The steps laid down in the CONSORT guidelines were followed in designing the trial. The trial protocol was registered at <http://www.clinicaltrials.gov> (NCT 00479271). There were no protocol violations.

Sampling

The study was carried out in two large administrative blocks in the state with a population of 340,000. We preferred not to recruit cases who visit the clinics as they would more likely be severe cases or those with severe BPSD and would not be representative of people in the community. This would have had an impact on the external validity of the trial. However, finding cases in the community was a major challenge as most of them were never diagnosed. We used the snowballing technique to identify probable cases. This is a sampling technique where the family members of people identified with a person with dementia helped us identify other probable cases in the community. We also took the help of the local leaders, religious leaders, doctors, health workers, and anganwadi workers (local community workers for a nutrition initiative for women and children). A total of 146 people were identified as probable cases, of which 89 were diagnosed as having dementia, 83 met the inclusion criteria, two refused consent, while 81 were enrolled and were randomized.

Diagnosis

Diagnosis of dementia can be influenced by education and culture. Fortunately, the 10/66 Dementia Research Group had extensively looked at this aspect while attempting to develop an education and culture fair tool for assessment of dementia in LAMIC (38). Tests that depend on the ability to spell or write, as is most often the case, cannot be used with illiterate people and such items need appropriate modification. For example, one cannot ask the participants to spell the word 'WORLD' backwards as a measure to test the memory if they are illiterate or do not speak English. In this study, for example, 43% of the people with dementia had education below primary level and most of them were educated in Portuguese, as Goa was a Portuguese colony until 1961. All the probable cases, detected by snowballing in the community, were subject to a clinical evaluation by a trained primary care physician. Diagnosis was confirmed according to the DSM-IV criteria (39) and graded using the Clinical Dementia Rating (CDR) scale (40). Only those with mild to moderate dementia were included; those with severe dementia on the CDR and with a severe life-threatening co-morbid condition were excluded from the trial. The reason for excluding those with severe dementia or co-morbid condition was to allow us to follow them up over time. Severe co-morbid conditions could also confound the study. The principal caregiver as identified by the family was also included in the study.

Randomization

Randomization of the dyads comprising of the person with dementia and their principal caregiver was carried out by an independent person based on simple random number tables, either to the intervention or to a waiting list group, who received the intervention after 6 months.

Intervention

The intervention was developed from a systematic literature review and meetings with experts in the field of dementia in India and abroad. It was designed with the principle that it should utilize locally available health and human resources so that there was a good probability that it might be affordable for further scaling up. Moreover, since a majority of the population had difficulty in accessing the public health service, the intervention had to be delivered in the community at the homes of the people with dementia. The intervention was a stepped-care psychosocial model primarily aimed at improving the awareness and knowledge of family caregivers regarding dementia, and providing emotional support to the caregivers, maximizing their caregiving resources, and improving their caregiving skills. The intervention was delivered by a team consisting of a NSHW under the guidance of a psychiatrist attached to the local health services and a trained lay health counsellor. In this study the lay health counsellor was a person who was the primary caregiver for her mother who died after living with dementia for 8 years. The role of each of the team member is described in Table 12.3. The NSHW acted as a link worker between the family and the specialist. The minimum qualification required of the NSHW was knowledge of the local language; they should also have passed higher secondary examinations (10 years of schooling) and be motivated to be involved in community care. Figure 12.2 provides a schematic representation of the six steps followed by the dementia home care team and how they collaborated to provide the service.

Table 12.3 The role of dementia home care team members

Team member	Role
Primary care physician (one)	Diagnose and provide basic education to the family
Psychiatrist (one)	Meet the NSHWs every 2 weeks and supervise the medical needs of the person with dementia and the caregiver. Participants were encouraged to meet the psychiatrist once at the start of the trial
Counsellor (one)	Meet the NSHWs every 2 weeks and supervise the non-pharmacological components of the intervention
NSHWs (four)	NSHWs were trained in listening skills and counselling skills, bereavement counselling, stress management, health advice for common health problems, and specific components of the intervention involving understanding dementia, using a person-centred approach to identifying problem behaviours, and reaching a working solution with the help of the caregiver and in consultation with the specialists. They used the snowballing technique with the help of key informants in the community to identify the probable cases to be referred to the primary care physician for diagnosis. They delivered the flexible stepped-care intervention to the family at their residence under the supervision of the psychiatrist and counsellor

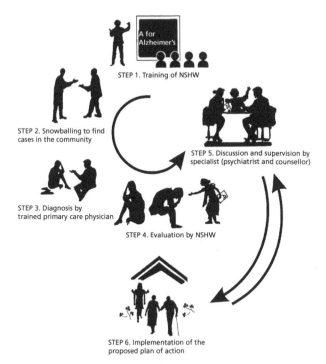

Fig. 12.2 The team approach to dementia in the community.

Specific components of the intervention involved the following:

- Identify caregiver burnout and help the caregiver deal with it.
- Balance family support, which involves trying to get other family members to help in the care, either directly or indirectly.
- Provide basic education of dementia.
- Provide education about common behavioural problems and how to prevent and manage them.
- Help caregivers assist the person with dementia with their activities of daily living.
- Advise referral when the problem behaviour needs medical attention.
- Network with other family members to form support groups.
- Provide advice regarding management of other associated health conditions.
- Provide advice on making the home environment safe for the person with dementia.
- Provide advice on existing government welfare schemes for support.

The minimum frequency of visits was at least once a fortnight for 6 months. The maximum was based on the need as assessed by the NSHW. The person with dementia was encouraged to visit the psychiatrist once in the beginning. Home visits were arranged only if this was not possible. The intervention was provided by the NSHW in the community under the supervision of the psychiatrist and counsellor.

The control arm

Participants in the control arm received enhanced usual care. The family was given education and information regarding dementia and were placed on a waiting list to receive the intervention in 6 months time. They were free to seek or continue any other treatment.

Outcomes

Our primary outcome was caregiver mental health as measured by the General Health Questionnaire (GHQ). Secondary outcomes were the perceived burden by the caregiver as measured on the Zarit Burden Scale (ZBS) (41), distress due to problem behaviours measured by the Neuropsychiatric Inventory (NPI-D) Questionnaire, severity of the behavioural problem as assessed by the caregiver (NPI-S) (42), and functional ability as assessed by the Everyday Ability Scale for Dementia in India (EASI) (43). Cause of death was recorded for those who died during the trial.

The challenge in mental health evaluation is that we do not have a biological marker and we need to rely on questionnaires to assess the health condition or outcome. These questionnaires have to be adapted and standardized for the region in which the data are collected. In this case, the 10/66 Dementia Research Group had translated, standardized, and used these instruments in this region prior to the study (44).

Blinding

Assessments were carried out at the baseline, followed by 3 and 6 months, by researchers who were masked to the allocation status of the participant. The outcome evaluation team (researchers) functioned independently of the intervention team. Families were instructed not to divulge information to the researchers. We did expect some amount of unmasking to occur, due to the nature of the intervention and given the fact that both the intervention and outcome evaluation were home based.

Ethical issues

The proposal was approved by the local ethics committee of the Dementia Society of Goa. Informed consent was taken from the primary caregiver and the head of the family. Assent was taken from the person with dementia as well, in the presence of the caregiver, and the same was recorded. Though the literacy rate in these regions as a whole is on the rise, there is still considerable illiteracy in the older adults, and consent was taken by reading out the information in front of a witness if this was the case. The majority of the families were getting the diagnosis for the first time and we were conscious of the possibility that breaking the news of a chronic progressive mental health problem could lead to emotional distress and social stigma for the family members. We were of the opinion that people with dementia and their families must be given the diagnosis, as this is in keeping with the ethical principles of beneficence, autonomy, and justice (45). Care was taken to ensure that the news was broken by a trained physician and the family was adequately counselled about it. No untoward incident was reported in this trial.

Medical professionals are generally given a lot of respect and people generally cooperate with them. There is a culture of trust especially in the rural areas of India. People will come forward to get treated and may not fully understand the concept of a research trial and the uncertainty that is associated with the new intervention. In fact, the process of getting a person to sign an informed consent form is sometimes viewed with suspicion. The families were enthusiastic and thankful for selecting them for the trial. This is evident from the fact that only two families refused consent. In both the cases, the caregivers and the person with dementia had agreed but a relative who does not live with them, but supports them financially, advised them against the consent and the families had to reluctantly refrain from giving consent.

Key findings

The evaluation was performed at the residence of the participant. There was no baseline difference in the sociodemographic profile, psychiatric co-morbidity, and socioeconomic status between the two arms. Outcome measures were similar at baseline except that the GHQ scores were higher in the intervention arm. This difference was adjusted for in the analysis. Each of the outcome measures (GHQ, ZBS, EASI, NPI-S, NPI-D) were analysed using a mixed effects model (46). The estimated coefficients were reported with their 95% confidence intervals. The effect of the treatment on mortality was analysed using logistic regression, with age and sex as the covariates. Eighty one families enrolled for the trial, 41 were randomly allocated to receive the intervention, 59 completed the trial, while 18 died during the period of the trial. There was no significant difference in the baseline characteristics of those who died and those who survived till the end of the trial period. The intervention led to a significant reduction in the GHQ (–1.12; 95% CI –2.07 to –0.17) and NPI-D scores (–1.96; 95% CI –3.51 to –0.41) and non-significant reductions in the ZBS, EASI, and NPI-S scores. We also observed a non-significant reduction in the total number of deaths in people with dementia in the intervention arm (OR 0.34; 95% CI 0.01–1.03).

Strengths and limitations

The trial was the first to describe the effectiveness of a community-based intervention for people with dementia and their caregivers in LAMIC. Until then such trials were only described in the HIC (18). Through this trial we were able to demonstrate that locally available resources could be utilized to decrease the burden and burnout associated with looking after a person with dementia. The instruments for assessment were translated and validated in the region in the previous 10/66 Dementia Research Group studies. The NSHWs were selected from the local community and were trained locally by experts in the region. The intervention was modelled on the evidence from the developed settings but was carefully adapted to address the local health needs, systems, and realities, and use local resources. It included mainly psychosocial interventions to address the health needs of the caregiver and the person with dementia in the comfort of their home environment.

The key limitations were, first, that it had a relatively small sample size and was probably not adequately powered to detect significant reductions in the behaviour problems and functional disabilities of the person with dementia. The sample was selected based on our estimate of how many individuals we would be able to enrol given the geographic area and the time and resources at our disposal. Second, we only followed up for 6 months, anticipating a high mortality. The short follow-up might have prevented us from demonstrating greater effects. Snowballing as a sampling technique might not have given the most representative sample in the region, but it was the most pragmatic and cost-effective technique in a low-resource setting (25).

Challenges in conducting the study

To begin with, nothing was known about the extent of dementia in the region and it was difficult to get financial support for dementia research as it was not considered a public health problem. We were fortunate that our engagement with the 10/66 Dementia Research Group helped us understand the burden of dementia in the region and the existing care arrangements and the needs for care. We were also fortunate to get funding from the WHO through the Ministry of Social Justice and Empowerment, Government of India, for conducting this trial. There were several challenges in planning and conducting the study. We had to begin with a clearly defined research question and knowledge of the ground realities of the condition in the area before conducting a trial. We also had to clearly define the population, intervention, controls, outcome, and time. The intervention was complex in nature and care had to be taken to define and also simplify it so that it could be implemented by non-specialists.

In the field, most medical doctors were ill-equipped in recognizing dementia and would hardly see people with dementia in their clinics. People with dementia and their family did not realize that the memory problems and confusion in their loved one was due to a disease. There was stigma associated with the condition and people would prefer not to speak about it to anyone—this is also the case with other conditions affecting mental health in LAMIC. The NSHWs had no health training and they needed to be systematically trained to provide the interventions. A week-long training was specially designed for them using role play and interactive lectures. Their training helped them understand dementia and the behavioural problems that accompany it. They were able to recognize and address caregiver burnout. It also helped them provide the necessary advice to the caregivers for managing BPSD and assisting in the activities of daily living. They were trained in skills such as listening and counselling. The catchment area for the study was very large, encompassing two large talukas (administrative blocks) in the State. Travelling to visit the person with dementia and their family in their homes accounted for a major part of the recurring costs. Moreover, since the study was spread over a large area and the interventions were based in the homes, we were concerned about the security of the home care advisors and we decided to send them in pairs. We had to do the same with the researchers to ensure security. There was only one untoward incident, where the person with dementia happened to be with her son who was in an inebriated state due to alcohol in the afternoon and the counsellors had to return without providing the intervention.

Conclusion

The results of the study showed that community-based interventions with locally available manpower and resources can make a difference to the families of people with dementia. The results of the community-based research in Goa began to create a lot of awareness in the region regarding dementia. The print media would report news on dementia, urging the local government to take action. People began to be aware that memory problems in late life could be signs of dementia and would come forward for examination as they realized that help was available. This intervention won the Alzheimer's Disease International and Fondation Médéric Alzheimer award for being the best evidence-based psychosocial intervention for people with dementia in 2010. This further raised awareness of the condition and the hopes in the people far and wide that help is available and that there is life after the diagnosis of dementia. The Rotary Club of Crosby, UK, came forward to support Sangath (an NGO based in Goa working towards bridging the gap in mental health services) to extend the services free of cost to the people in the entire State.

The Alzheimer's and Related Disorders Society of India (ARDSI), in the Dementia India Report presented to the Government of India, has acknowledged this model to be a possible solution to the problem of an estimated 3.7 million people with dementia in India (35). In LAMIC there is always a challenge of sustainability and this can happen if there is political will and commitment. Conditions such as dementia have long been neglected by the government, which has always felt the pressing need to combat issues such as malnutrition and infectious disease which continue to pose a significant burden of disease in LAMIC. This is compounded by the fact that due to the lack of local research, they are often not aware of the growing epidemic of dementia and do not know what steps to take to address this burden. The step taken by ARDSI in gathering the evidence on dementia and providing a roadmap for the government to act is a welcome one (35). Encouraging research and building capacity is one of the important policy prescriptions provided in the report.

The interventions in Peru (28) and Moscow (29) were based on the same principle as the one in Goa. They planned to use locally available resources and community health workers, but they were not able to recruit them and settled for junior doctors in Moscow and junior psychologists and social workers in Peru. It may not be a good idea to utilize the existing multipurpose health workers for providing dementia services at the primary health centre as they are already burdened with infectious disease and maternal and child health programmes. We propose that the dementia NSHW should be specially recruited and based at the primary health centre to provide services for people in the catchment area of the centre. A primary health centre in India caters for a population of 30,000 and would be within the reach of the NSHW and avoid the recurring travel costs. It may be worthwhile extending their services to all other frail adults, such as those with a chronic disability such as stroke or Parkinson's disease, as they too can benefit from the flexible stepped-care intervention provided by a locally trained counsellor under the supervision of a specialist.

Good quality research raises awareness and helps influence policy. This has been the motto of the 10/66 Dementia Research Group. There is a need to build research capacity, interest, and infrastructure for dementia research. Not all LAMIC are in the same stage of growth and not all regions in the particular country have the same capacity. The situation is rapidly changing; China, for example, has rapidly responded to the growing dementia epidemic and has set up several centres for neurological research and advanced positron emission tomography (PET) scans for evaluation (13). Conducting trials on Alzheimer's disease and dementia in LAMIC has a number of challenges, but at the same time they are necessary to bridge the gap in our knowledge and develop sustainable, locally relevant initiatives in the region. With rising awareness in this region there will be a greater demand for such research in the years to come. We need not only mental health workers but also mental health leaders who can face the challenges and put conditions such as dementia on the public health agenda where it rightfully belongs.

Acknowledgements

We are deeply indebted to Jean D'Souza who was the lay health counsellor on the project. She died in 2010 but continues to inspire our work. We thank Prof Martin Prince for his contribution to this chapter. We appreciate the contributions from Cleusa Ferri and Prathap Tharyan. We also thank the World Health Organization and the Ministry of Social Justice and Empowerment, Government of India, for financially supporting the trial.

References

1 **American Psychiatric Association** (2013) Diagnostic and statistical manual of mental disorders, fifth edition (DSM-5). Arlington: American Psychiatric Association.

2 **American Psychiatric Association** (2013) Highlights of changes from DSM-IV-TR to DSM-5. Arlington: American Psychiatric Association.

3 **Prince MJ, Acosta D, Castro-Costa E, Jackson J, Shaji KS** (2009) Packages of care for dementia in low- and middle-income countries. PLoS Med, **6**:e1000176.

4 **World Health Organization, Alzheimer's Disease International** (2012) Dementia: a public health priority. Geneva: WHO.

5 **Prince M, Jackson J** (2009) World Alzheimer report 2009. London: Alzheimer's Disease International.

6 **Prince M, Bryce R, Albanese E, Wimo A, Ribeiro W, Ferri CP** (2013) The global prevalence of dementia: a systematic review and metaanalysis. Alzheimers Dement, **9**(1):63–75.

7 **World Health Organization** (2010) The global burden of disease: 2004 update. Geneva: WHO.

8 **Alzheimer's Disease International** (2010) World Alzheimer report 2010. London: Alzheimer's Disease International.

9 **10/66 Dementia Research Group** (2004) Care arrangements for people with dementia in developing countries. Int J Geriatr Psychiatry, **19**:170–7.

10 **Dias A, Samuel R, Patel V, Prince M, Parmeshwaran R, Krishnamoorthy ES** (2004) The impact associated with caring for a person with dementia: a report from the 10/66 Dementia Research Group's Indian network. Int J Geriatr Psychiatry, **19**(2):182–4.

11 **Wimo A, Winbald B, Jonsson L** (2005) An estimate of the total worldwide societal costs of dementia in 2005. Alzheimers Dement, **3**(2):81–91.

12 **World Health Organization** (2006) Neurological disorders: public health challenges. Geneva: WHO.

13 **Doody RS, Cole PE, Miller DS, Siemers E, Black R, Feldman H, et al.** (2011) Global issues in drug development for Alzheimer's disease. Alzheimers Dement, **7**:197–207.

14 **Prince M** (2000) Methodological issues for population-based research into dementia in developing countries. A position paper from the 10/66 Dementia Research Group. Int J Geriatr Psychiatry, **15**:21–30.

15 Dias A, Patel V (2009) Closing the treatment gap for dementia in India. Indian J Psychiatry, 51(1):S93–97.

16 Zhang Z, Chen X, Liu X, Tang M, Zhao H, Jue Q, et al. (2004) A caregiver survey in Beijing, Xi'an, Shanghai and Chengdu: health services status for the elderly with dementia. Zhongguo Yi Xue Ke Xue Yuan Xue Bao, 26:116–21.

17 Prince MJ (2009) The 10/66 Dementia Research Group—10 years on. Indian J Psychiatry, 51(1):S8–S15.

18 Brodaty H, Green A, Koschera A (2003) Meta-analysis of psychosocial interventions for caregivers of people with dementia. J Am Geriatr Soc, 51:657–64.

19 Dua T, Barbui C, Clark N, Fleischmann A, Poznyak V, van Ommeren M, et al. (2011) Evidence-based guidelines for mental, neurological, and substance use disorders in low- and middle-income countries: summary of WHO recommendations. PLoS Med, 8:e1001122.

20 World Health Organization (2010) mhGAP intervention guide. Geneva: WHO.

21 Birks J (2006) Cholinesterase inhibitors for Alzheimer's disease. Cochrane Database Syst Rev, (1):CD005593.

22 Bruckner TA, Scheffler RM, Shen G, Yoon J, Chisholm D, Morris J, et al. (2011) The mental health workforce gap in low- and middle-income countries: a needs-based approach. Bull World Health Organ, 89:184–94.

23 Schneider LS, Tariot PN, Dagerman KS, Davis SM, Hsiao JK, Ismail MS, et al. (2006) Effectiveness of atypical antipsychotic drugs in patients with Alzheimer's disease. N Engl J Med, 355:1525–38.

24 Bottino CM, Carvalho IA, Alvarez AM, Avila R, Zukauskas PR, Bustamante SE, et al. (2005) Cognitive rehabilitation combined with drug treatment in Alzheimer's disease patients: a pilot study. Clin Rehabil, 19:861–9.

25 Shaji KS, Arun Kishore NR, Lal KP, Prince M (2002) Revealing a hidden problem. An evaluation of a community dementia case-finding program from the Indian 10/66 Dementia Research Network. Int J Geriatr Psychiatry, 17:222–5.

26 Ramos-Cerqueira ATA, Torres AR, Crepaldi AL, Oliveira NIL, Scazufca M, Menezes PR, et al. (2005) Identification of dementia cases in the community: a Brazilian experience. J Am Geriatr Soc, 53:1738–42.

27 Dias A, Dewey ME, D'Souza J, Dhume R, Motghare DD, Shaji KS, et al. (2008) The effectiveness of a home care program for supporting caregivers of persons with dementia in developing countries: a randomised controlled trial from Goa, India. PLoS One, 3(6):7.

28 Guerra M, Ferri CP, Fonseca M, Banerjee S, Prince M (1999) Helping carers to care: the 10/66 Dementia Research Group's randomized control trial of a caregiver intervention in Peru. Rev Bras Psiq, 33(1):47–54.

29 Gavrilova SI, Ferri CP, Mikhaylova N, Sokolova O, Banerjee S, Prince M (2009) Helping carers to care—the 10/66 Dementia Research Group' s randomized control trial of a caregiver intervention in Russia. Int J Geriatr Psychiatry, 24:347–54.

30 Bhan A (2012) Clinical trial ethics in India: one step forward, two steps back. J Pharmacol Pharmacother, 3(2):95–7.

31 Tharyan P (2006) Whose trial is it anyway? Reflections on morality, double standards, uncertainty and criticism in international collaborative health research. Monash Bioeth Rev, 24:53–68.

32 Tharyan P (2007) The role of prospective trials registration and trials registers in improving the design, conduct and reporting of randomized clinical trials from developing countries. XV Cochrane Colloquium, 23–7 October 2007, Sao Paulo, Brazil, pp. 78–9.

33 **Rafii MS** (2010) The pulse of drug development for Alzheimer's disease. Rev. Recent Clin Trials, **5**:57–62.

34 **Mittelman MS, Ferris SH, Shulman E, Steinberg G, Levin BA** (1996) Family intervention to delay nursing home placement of patients with Alzheimer disease. JAMA, **276**:1725–31.

35 **Alzheimer's and Related Disorders Society of India** (2010) The Dementia India Report 2010: prevalence, impact, costs and services for dementia. New Delhi: ARDSI.

36 **Maestre GE** (2012) Assessing dementia in resource-poor regions. Curr Neurol Neurosci Rep, **12**(5):511–19.

37 **Patel V, Prince M** (2001 Ageing and mental health in a developing country: who cares? Qualitative studies from Goa, India. Psychol Med, **31**:29–38.

38 **Prince M, Acosta D, Chiu H, Scazufca M, Varghese M** (2003) Dementia diagnosis in developing countries: a cross-cultural validation study. Lancet, **361**:909–17.

39 **American Psychiatric Association** (1994) DSM-IV-TR. Diagnostic and statistical manual of mental disorders, fourth edition. Arlington: American Psychiatric Association.

40 **Morris JC** (1993) The Clinical Dementia Rating (CDR): current version and scoring rules. Neurology, **43**:2412–14.

41 **Zarit SH, Reever KE, Bach-Peterson J** (1980) Relatives of the impaired elderly: correlates of feelings of burden. Gerontologist, **20**(6):649–55.

42 **Cummings JL, Mega M, Gray K, Rosenberg-Thompson S, Carusi DA, Gornbein J** (1994) The Neuropsychiatric inventory: comprehensive assessment of psychopathology in dementia. Neurology, **44**(12):2308–14.

43 **Fillenbaum G, Chandra V, Ganguli M** (1999) Development of an activities of daily living scale to screen for dementia in an illiterate rural older population in India. Age Ageing, **28**(2): 161–8.

44 **Prince M, Ferri CP, Acosta D, Albanese E, Arizaga R, Dewey M, et al.** (2007) The protocols for the 10/66 Dementia Research Group population-based research programme. BMC Public Health, **7**:165.

45 **Black JS** (1995) Telling the truth: should persons with Alzheimer's disease be told their diagnosis? Alzheimers Dis Int Global Perspective, **6**:10–11.

46 **Pinheiro JC, Bates DM** (2000) Mixed-effects models in S and S-PLUS. New York: Springer.

Chapter 13

Trials for people with mental disorders and conditions associated with stress

Wietse A. Tol, Mark J.D. Jordans,
Dessy Susanty, and Joop T.V.M. de Jong

The cluster randomized trials described in this chapter were made possible through funding from Plan Netherlands and Save the Children.

Introduction

In this chapter, we provide a brief overview of the knowledge on the effectiveness of interventions for mental disorders and conditions specifically related to exposure to stressors, including exposure to potentially traumatic events and bereavement. As an illustration of an intervention approach to address this wide range of mental conditions, we focus on the mental health of children in areas affected by armed conflicts. We discuss the factors that influence child mental health in conflict-affected settings, describing risk, protective, and promotive factors at different levels of the child's social environment. We summarize a series of studies that evaluated the effectiveness of a preventive school-based intervention in Burundi, Indonesia, Nepal, and Sri Lanka, focusing particularly on the study in Indonesia.

Mental disorders and conditions associated with stress

Exposure to negative life events, such as exposure to potentially traumatic events and bereavement, is common across the globe. The term traumatic events may refer to a range of adverse experiences, such as accidents, injuries, adverse childhood experiences (e.g. child maltreatment), exposure to violence, including sexual- and other forms of gender-based violence, and humanitarian crises such as natural disasters and armed conflicts. There is a large body of research that links exposure to potentially traumatic events to worse mental health outcomes. For example, in the World Mental Health Surveys, conducted with large representative samples of adults in 21 countries, childhood adversities were highly prevalent and interrelated. They accounted for 29.8% of all disorders across countries. Of the 12 childhood adversities included in the surveys, adversities related to maladaptive family functioning (parental mental illness, child abuse, neglect) were the strongest predictors of mental disorders (1). Another multi-country study examined the prevalence of intimate partner violence, i.e. psychological, physical, and sexual violence perpetrated by current or former partners, in 15 sites across ten countries. Seven of the sites had prevalence rates between 25% and 50%, and six sites had prevalence rates between 50% and 75% (2). Systematic reviews have found that intimate partner violence is strongly associated with worse mental health outcomes (3, 4). Similarly, armed conflicts and natural disasters are widespread and detrimental to mental health (5, 6).

Exposure to potentially traumatic events is linked with a wide range of mental health conditions and disorders. Some of these may also occur in the absence of exposure to potentially traumatic events, and are described in other chapters in this book (e.g. depression, substance use disorders, and suicide). Here, we describe mental conditions specifically related to exposure to stress, that is: symptoms of acute stress in the first month after exposure to a potentially traumatic event (acute traumatic stress symptoms, dissociative symptoms, sleeping problems, hyperventilation); PTSD; and bereavement. This terminology is consistent with the proposed classification in ICD-11 (7).

The proposed ICD-11 classification entails a new separate grouping of 'disorders specifically associated with stress', rather than the combination with anxiety disorders as in the DSM -IV or ICD-10. This grouping includes disorders related to stressful experiences within the normal range of experience (e.g. adjustment disorder, prolonged grief disorder), as well as negative life events outside the normal range (e.g. PTSD, complex PTSD) (7). Regarding symptoms of acute stress, the ICD-10 included acute stress reaction, described as emotional, cognitive, and behavioural reactions that disappear within days after experience of highly stressful events. For ICD-11, it is proposed that this set of symptoms be incorporated in the Z chapter, which includes categories representing reasons for clinical concern that are not in themselves disorders or diseases. This placement is preferred, as inclusion in the disorder section may inadvertently medicalize normal reactions to abnormal events, while still facilitating an intervention response to such symptoms (7). Also, ICD-11 prefers to describe this group of symptoms as a loosely related set of symptoms, rather than a specific diagnosis with set criteria, as the diverse symptoms of acute stress do not fit neatly into one diagnostic construct (8).

With regard to PTSD, the relevant working group wished to circumvent two key challenges: (1) the application of a diagnosis in people who are exposed to continuous stressors (e.g. ongoing intimate partner violence or armed conflict), for whom fear-related behaviours may be appropriate responses to actual threat, and (2) the risk that the existence of a traumatic stressor in a person's history necessarily leads to framing *all* symptomatology as PTSD-related, thereby risking underidentification of other common mental disorders, for example, depression. This resulted in a refocus on a smaller set of core PTSD symptoms, and the removal of non-specific symptoms that are also part of other disorders. The proposed diagnostic guidelines require the following symptoms for the diagnosis of PTSD: (1) re-experiencing of the traumatic event (e.g. flashbacks, nightmares), in which the event is not only remembered but also experienced as occurring again; (2) avoidance of reminders associated with re-experiencing of the traumatic event(s) (e.g. avoiding places or people that may be reminders of the event); and (3) a perception of heightened current threat, as indicated by arousal symptoms (e.g. hypervigilance, enhanced startle response). In addition, (4) symptoms must have started after experience of 'an event of an extremely threatening or horrific nature' and (5) must be associated with impaired functioning (7).

In addition to reworking PTSD, the ICD-11 proposals contain two new disorders: complex PTSD and prolonged grief disorder. Complex PTSD is intended to capture reactions to exposure to particularly severe and prolonged stressors, e.g. through several or repeated events. In addition to the three symptom components mentioned (re-experiencing, avoidance, hyperarousal), complex PTSD requires lasting problems in the domains of affect, self, and interpersonal relations. Prolonged grief disorder consists of 'intensely painful, disabling, and persistent responses to bereavement with specific symptoms such as pervasive yearning, or preoccupation with the deceased and associated emotional pain'. A key feature that distinguishes prolonged grief disorder from normative grief reactions is the longer duration of emotional difficulties. The ICD-11 proposal also includes adjustment disorder, which is one of the most frequently applied diagnoses by psychiatrists and psychologists globally. It describes this disorder as a maladaptive reaction to an identifiable stressor, including intrusive preoccupation with the stressor and an inability to adapt. These symptoms are noted to usually be transient in nature, emerging within a month of the onset of the stressor and resolving in 6 months (7).

Evidence for interventions

Recently, the WHO published guidelines for management of conditions specifically related to stress as part of the mhGAP (Box 13.1) (9, 10). The mhGAP is aimed at reducing the large treatment gap for mental disorders in LAMIC through building the capacity of non-specialized (e.g. primary health care) providers to deliver existing evidence-based treatments for a number of priority mental, neurological, and substance use disorders (11). The recent expansion for conditions specifically associated with stress focused on: (1) symptoms of acute stress in the first month after exposure to potentially traumatic events; (2) PTSD; and (3) bereavement (in the absence of a mental disorder such as depression or prolonged grief disorder). Development of the guidelines entailed the identification of recent systematic reviews of studies that evaluated psychological and pharmacological interventions, for children and adolescents, as well as adult populations. In searching for systematic reviews of controlled studies, the authors concluded that there is a great paucity of rigorous high-quality evidence for interventions for these three mental health conditions, particularly for children and adolescents, and most evidence has been collected with populations in HIC and in specialized health settings, so feasibility and acceptability of interventions is uncertain (8). Recommendations were based on existing evidence of intervention effectiveness and an appraisal of benefits vs harms; values and preferences; and feasibility.

In addition to the recommendations for the acute stress symptoms listed in Box 13.1, earlier guidelines have recommended psychological first aid (PFA) for this range of symptoms (12). PFA was intended as an alternative to psychological debriefing. Psychological debriefing entails the promotion of ventilation through recounting perceptions, thoughts, and emotional reactions experienced during a recent stressful event. A summary of rigorous studies that evaluated psychological debriefing showed that

Box 13.1 mhGAP recommendations for conditions specifically associated with stress in children, adolescents, and adults (8–10)

1. Symptoms in the first month after exposure to potentially traumatic events:

1A. Acute traumatic stress symptoms

- CBT with a trauma focus should be considered in adults (standard*)
- Benzodiazepines should *not* be offered to adults (strong)
- Antidepressants should *not* be offered to adults (standard)
- Benzodiazepines and antidepressants should *not* be offered to children and adolescents (strong)

1B. Sleeping problems (secondary acute insomnia)

- Relaxation techniques and advice about sleep hygiene should be considered for adults (standard)
- Benzodiazepines should *not* be offered to adults (standard)
- Benzodiazepines should *not* be offered to children and adolescents (strong)

1C. Bedwetting (secondary non-organic enuresis)

- Education about the negative effects of punitive responses should be given to caregivers of children (strong)
- Parenting skills training and the use of simple behavioural interventions should be considered.
  Where resources permit, alarms should be considered (standard)

1D. Hyperventilation

- Rebreathing into a paper bag should *not* be considered for children (standard)

2. PTSD

- Individual or group CBT with a trauma focus (CBT-T), eye movement desensitization and reprocessing (EMDR), or stress management should be considered for adults (standard)
- Individual or group CBT-T or EMDR should be considered for children and adolescents (standard)
- SSRIs and tricyclic antidepressants should *not* be offered as the first line of treatment in adults. SSRIs and tricyclic antidepressants should be considered if (a) stress management, CBT-T, and/or EMDR have failed or are not available, or (b) if there is concurrent moderate to severe depression (standard)
- Antidepressants should *not* be used in children and adolescents (strong)

Box 13.1 mhGAP recommendations for conditions specifically associated with stress in children, adolescents, and adults (8–10) (continued)

3. Bereavement, in absence of a mental disorder

- Structured psychological interventions should *not* be offered universally to bereaved children, adolescents, and adults who do not meet criteria for a mental disorder (strong)

- Benzodiazepines should *not* be offered to bereaved children, adolescents, and adults who do not meet criteria for a mental disorder (strong)

  Because of a lack of studies on these topics, it was not possible to make specific recommendations for the following questions of interest to the guideline developers: psychological interventions with children and adolescents for acute traumatic stress symptoms, insomnia, dissociative symptoms; psychological interventions with adults for dissociative symptoms; rebreathing into a bag for adults and adolescents for hyperventilation

* A *strong* recommendation indicates that the recommendation should be followed in all or almost all circumstances; a *standard* recommendation indicates that there may be circumstances in which the recommendation does not apply.

---

the intervention did not prevent PTSD symptoms, and in some cases even contributed to deteriorated mental health (13). In contrast to psychological debriefing, PFA is not aimed at encouraging emotional ventilation, but entails provision of practical and non-intrusive support; assessment of needs and concerns; helping people to address basic needs (e.g. health; food and non-food relief items; water, sanitation, and hygiene services); listening to people, but not pressuring them to talk; comforting people and helping them to feel calm; helping people connect to information, services, and social supports; and protecting people from further harm. PFA is evidence-*informed* but not evidence-based; in other words, it builds on existing expert consensus (14) and knowledge about what promotes long-term recovery after exposure to severely stressful events (15–17). The provision of social support, for example, is a well-known protective factor for the development of mental health problems in the longer term (18, 19). However, there is currently no rigorous evidence that directly supports the use of PFA in humanitarian settings.

Evidence in humanitarian settings

As part of the second *Lancet Series on Global Mental Health in 2011*, a systematic review and meta-analysis examined the evidence base for mental health and psychosocial support (MHPSS) interventions in humanitarian settings (i.e. armed conflicts and disasters) in LAMIC. For adults, the systematic review identified 13 controlled trials. Of these 13 studies, seven could be included in a meta-analysis (Fig. 13.1). These seven studies compared nine different interventions ($n = 486$) with a control arm ($n = 285$). Evaluated interventions included: control-focused behavioural therapy for survivors

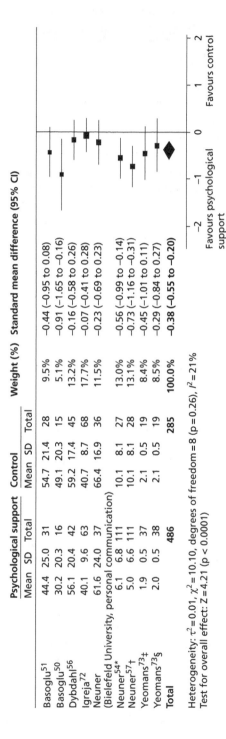

	Psychological support			Control			Weight (%)	Standard mean difference (95% CI)
	Mean	SD	Total	Mean	SD	Total		
Basoglu[51]	44.4	25.0	31	54.7	21.4	28	9.5%	−0.44 (−0.95 to 0.08)
Basoglu[50]	30.2	20.3	16	49.1	20.3	15	5.1%	−0.91 (−1.65 to −0.16)
Dybdahl[56]	56.1	20.4	42	59.2	17.4	45	13.2%	−0.16 (−0.58 to 0.26)
Igreja[72]	40.1	9.6	63	40.7	8.7	68	17.7%	−0.07 (−0.41 to 0.28)
Neuner	61.6	24.0	37	66.4	16.9	36	11.5%	−0.23 (−0.69 to 0.23)
(Bielefeld University, personal communication)								
Neuner[54*]	6.1	6.8	111	10.1	8.1	27	13.0%	−0.56 (−0.99 to −0.14)
Neuner[57†]	5.0	6.6	111	10.1	8.1	28	13.1%	−0.73 (−1.16 to −0.31)
Yeomans[73‡]	1.9	0.5	37	2.1	0.5	19	8.4%	−0.45 (−1.01 to 0.11)
Yeomans[73§]	2.0	0.5	38	2.1	0.5	19	8.5%	−0.29 (−0.84 to 0.27)
Total			486			285	100.0%	−0.38 (−0.55 to −0.20)

Heterogeneity: $\tau^2 = 0.01$, $\chi^2 = 10.10$, degrees of freedom = 8 (p = 0.26), $I^2 = 21\%$
Test for overall effect: Z = 4.21 (p < 0.0001)

Fig. 13.1 Meta-analysis of adult mental health interventions in LAMIC humanitarian settings. The figure shows random-effects meta-analysis with PTSD symptoms as outcome.

of an earthquake in Turkey; support groups for displaced mothers in Bosnia and Herzegovina; testimony therapy with war-affected people in Mozambique; narrative exposure therapy with refugees in Uganda and war-affected populations in Rwanda; trauma counselling with refugees in Uganda; and trauma healing and reconciliation workshops in Burundi, with and without psychoeducation sessions. Overall, these interventions showed a statistically significant benefit on PTSD symptoms, with limited statistical heterogeneity of intervention benefits between studies ($I^2 = 21\%$) (20).

For children and adolescents in LAMIC humanitarian settings, the review identified 19 controlled studies: 13 RCTs and six controlled trials. Six of these studies could be included in two meta-analyses: one focused on PTSD symptoms, and one analysed changes in internalizing (depressive/anxiety) symptoms (20). The first meta-analysis of PTSD symptoms (Fig. 13.2a) included five comparisons of school-based interventions, one in tsunami-affected areas in Sri Lanka (9–14 year olds, implemented by trained teachers) (21), and the others in conflict-affected areas in Indonesia (7–15 year olds) (22), Nepal (11–14 year olds) (23), and the occupied Palestinian territories (oPt) (two age groups: 6–11 and 12–16 year olds) (24). The interventions in the oPt and Sri Lanka were implemented by trained school counsellors or social workers and teachers, respectively, and did not involve screening (i.e. universal preventive intervention), whereas the interventions in Indonesia and Nepal were implemented by trained community members without a mental health background and were implemented with children identified as having psychological distress (i.e. they were selective preventive interventions). High statistical heterogeneity ($I^2 = 95\%$) was found in this meta-analysis, indicating large differences in the intervention effects observed across these studies. In two of the five comparisons (Sri Lanka, Indonesia) the study results clearly favoured the intervention, whereas no difference was found between the intervention and control arms in three of five comparisons (oPt both age groups, Nepal). Overall, no statistically significant effect of school-based universal and selective preventive interventions on reducing PTSD symptoms was identified (20).

The second meta-analysis of internalizing symptoms (Fig. 13.2b) lumped different types of interventions (eight comparisons), including the school-based preventive interventions already cited, as well as a study evaluating group IPT and creative play with war-affected adolescents in Uganda (14–17 year olds) (25), and an evaluation of weekly supportive group meetings with displaced mothers of preschool children (5–6 year olds) in Bosnia and Herzegovina (26). In the study in Uganda, group IPT was implemented by locally trained and supervised humanitarian workers, and creative play—consisting of creative activities aimed at strengthening resilience—was implemented by two staff from a humanitarian agency. Both interventions were implemented with adolescents screened for depression and function impairment (25). The mothers' groups in Bosnia and Herzegovina were aimed at promoting child development and wellbeing through parent involvement, support, and education, and focused on the importance of the mother–child interaction for child development and wellbeing. These groups were facilitated by trained preschool teachers, and all parents of children in the age group in the target area were invited to participate (26). Results of the meta-analysis of all the eight comparisons in this second meta-analysis showed high statistical heterogeneity ($I^2 = 63\%$), with four comparisons showing clear effects of

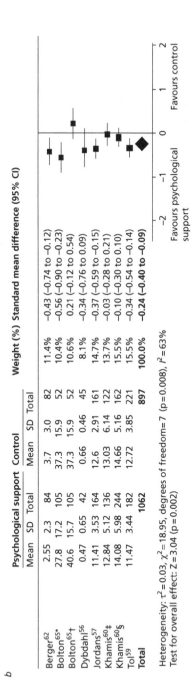

a

	Psychological support			Control			Weight (%)	Standard mean difference (95% CI)
	Mean	SD	Total	Mean	SD	Total		
Berger[62]	36.21	7.4	84	45.71	7.5	82	19.1%	−1.27 (−1.60 to −0.94)
Jordans[57]	17.71	4.83	164	18.62	5.26	161	20.2%	−0.18 (−0.40 to 0.04)
Khamis[60]*	30.69	12.37	136	29.85	13.01	122	20.0%	0.07 (−0.18 to 0.31)
Khamis[60]†	31.21	11.04	244	28.96	10.87	162	20.4%	0.20 (0.01 to 0.40)
Tol[59]	10.57	7.13	182	16.15	8.7	221	20.3%	−0.69 (−0.90 to −0.49)
Total			**810**			**748**	**100.0%**	**−0.36 (−0.83 to 0.10)**

Heterogeneity: $\tau^2 = 0.27$, $\chi^2 = 80.99$, degrees of freedom = 4 (p<0.0001), $I^2 = 95\%$
Test for overall effect: Z = 1.54 (p=0.12)

Note: random-effects meta-analysis with PTSD symptoms as outcome, Khamis * concerns a school-based intervention with 12–16 year olds, †
with 6–11 year olds

b

	Psychological support			Control			Weight (%)	Standard mean difference (95% CI)
	Mean	SD	Total	Mean	SD	Total		
Berger[62]	2.55	2.3	84	3.7	3.0	82	11.4%	−0.43 (−0.74 to −0.12)
Bolton[65]*	27.8	17.2	105	37.3	15.9	52	10.4%	−0.56 (−0.90 to −0.23)
Bolton[65]†	40.6	15.7	105	37.3	15.9	52	10.6%	0.21 (−0.12 to 0.54)
Dybdahl[56]	0.47	0.65	42	0.66	0.46	45	8.1%	−0.34 (−0.76 to 0.09)
Jordans[57]	11.41	3.53	164	12.6	2.91	161	14.7%	−0.37 (−0.59 to −0.15)
Khamis[60]‡	12.84	5.12	136	13.03	6.14	122	13.7%	−0.03 (−0.28 to 0.21)
Khamis[60]§	14.08	5.98	244	14.66	5.16	162	15.5%	−0.10 (−0.30 to 0.10)
Tol[59]	11.47	3.44	182	12.72	3.85	221	15.5%	−0.34 (−0.54 to −0.14)
Total			**1062**			**897**	**100.0%**	**−0.24 (−0.40 to −0.09)**

Heterogeneity: $\tau^2 = 0.03$, $\chi^2 = 18.95$, degrees of freedom= 7 (p=0.008), $I^2 = 63\%$
Test for overall effect: Z = 3.04 (p=0.002)

Note: random-effects meta-analysis with internalizing symptoms as outcome, Bolton * is group Interpersonal Psychotherapy, Bolton † is creative
play, Khamis ‡ concerns a school-based intervention with 6–11 year olds, Khamis § with 12–16 year olds

Fig. 13.2 Meta-analysis of child mental health interventions in LAMIC humanitarian settings.

the intervention, and no difference between study arms in the other four comparisons. Effects were found for the universal school-based intervention in Sri Lanka, group IPT in Uganda, and the selective school-based intervention in Indonesia and Nepal. Across studies, a statistically significant effect in favour of the intervention was found for internalizing symptoms (20).

Given these varied results of mental health interventions with children and adolescents, an important research direction concerns teasing apart the *moderators* (i.e. sub-groups for whom interventions may be effective, and conditions under which interventions may be effective) and *mediators* of interventions (processes through which the intervention may be effective). Studies in Burundi (27), Indonesia (28), and Sri Lanka (29) have started to address this question with regard to the selective preventive school-based intervention evaluated in Indonesia and Nepal. We will now discuss these results, after a discussion of risk, protective, and promotive factors for child mental health in areas of armed conflict, and a more detailed description of the RCT in Indonesia.

Case study: cluster randomized trial of a school-based intervention in Indonesia

Child mental health in areas of armed conflict

Estimates place the number of children living in areas affected by armed conflict at over 1 billion, almost one-sixth of the world population (30). In 2012 alone, 32 armed conflicts were recorded, the majority in Africa (13 armed conflicts) and Asia (ten armed conflicts) (31). Armed conflicts have far-reaching implications for the lives of children—through direct experiences of conflict-related violence, deterioration in access to basic needs including health care and education, and the disruption of supportive family and community contexts. We use the term 'mental health' here in line with the definition of the WHO as 'a state of well-being in which every individual realizes his or her own potential, can cope with the normal stresses of life, can work productively and fruitfully, and is able to make a contribution to her or his community'. The term mental health may thus refer to both psychological symptoms and positive aspects of functioning. Armed conflicts may have diverse impacts on children's mental health, spanning from improvements in functioning (e.g. post-traumatic growth) (32) and no change in mental health status, to transient psychological distress and major mental disorders. In addition, research has highlighted how armed conflicts impact the family, peer, and community and wider social conditions that lay the foundation for optimal child development and mental health (33, 34).

In terms of epidemiology, much of the literature has focused on establishing prevalence rates for PTSD, depressive, and anxiety symptoms. A meta-analysis of the child literature found pooled prevalence rates of 47% for PTSD (17 studies), 43% for depression (four studies), and 27% for anxiety (three studies). There was high heterogeneity in these prevalence rates, which was partially explained by study location (higher rates in the Middle East), by the type of symptom checklist used, or by the duration since exposure to war (higher rates in more recently affected areas) (35). Meta-analysis of epidemiological research with conflict-affected adults has shown that higher prevalence rates are more commonly found in smaller studies that do not use random samples or diagnostic interviews. In a sub-set of rigorous studies that applied representative sampling and diagnostic interviews, prevalence rates in conflict-affected adults were 15.4% for PTSD (30 studies) and 17.3% for depression (26 studies) (6).

In addition, epidemiologists have looked into risk, protective, and promotive factors. Risk, protective, and promotive factors for mental health exist at multiple levels of the environment in which children grow up (36). Reed and colleagues reviewed studies examining risk and protective factors for children displaced due to conflict in LAMIC. At the individual level, exposure to potentially traumatic events is the most well-established risk factor. In addition, girls commonly report higher levels of internalizing (e.g. depressive) symptoms, whereas boys generally have higher levels of externalizing symptoms (such as acting out behaviour). Much less research has focused on risk and protective factors of the family (e.g. parental mental health, family composition, parenting styles) and community levels (deterioration of supportive networks, socioeconomic situation, neighbourhood violence) (37).

With regard to protective and promotive factors, a recent systematic review focused on resilience in children affected by armed conflict (38), i.e. good mental health despite exposure to adversity (39). Even though it is not possible to draw robust conclusions on the basis of the current literature due to methodological limitations, the 53 studies included in this review pointed to a highly complex pattern of relations. Although some research has been conducted on protective factors, particularly factors associated with lower levels of PTSD and depressive symptoms, very little research has been conducted on promotive factors—i.e. factors associated with positive indicators of mental health. Overall, a relatively consistent finding was the protective effect of parental support and monitoring. However, factors that were protective in a period of active armed conflict could be risk factors in post-conflict settings, and protective factors in one place might be risk factors in other settings. For example, in a longitudinal study with children and adolescents in the oPt, political activity was protective for mental health problems during a period of relative stability, but not in a subsequent period of active conflict (40). Furthermore, the effect of protective factors varied according to gender and developmental stage. For example, in a large cross-sectional study with 14 year olds in oPt, parental monitoring (i.e. perceived level of parent's knowledge of after-school activities, friends, spending money) was associated with lower levels of depressive symptoms and antisocial behaviour in girls, but not in boys (41). Similarly, the qualitative studies identified by this review reported diverse ways in which populations across sociocultural settings described positive mental health outcomes, as well as differences in the processes that may lead to such outcomes. For example, two separate qualitative studies in Afghanistan (42, 43) described the importance of *tarbia* (a strong sense of morality, correct behaviour) and *wahdad* (family unity and honour) as indicators of wellbeing. The complexity suggested by these studies on resilience has an important implication for preventive interventions with children in areas of armed conflict. That is, they point to the need to carefully tailor interventions to sociocultural context, rather than assume that risk and protective factors will have similar impacts across different contexts (38).

From a research perspective, there is an urgent need to broaden our knowledge of child and adolescent mental health in areas of armed conflict through methodologically rigorous studies. To inform preventive interventions, there is a particular need for further mixed methods and longitudinal research that studies a wider range of predictors (risk, protective, promotive factors) and outcomes. With regard to risk factors specifically, it is important that researchers study the negative impact of factors beyond specific exposure to discrete conflict-related violence (e.g. exposure to bomb blasts, cross-fires, killings), to examine the structural violence, socioeconomic adversity and influence of deteriorated family and community contexts associated with armed conflicts (44). For example, research with adult refugees in LAMIC has found that ongoing stressors (e.g. intimate partner violence in refugee camps) and a lack of access to basic needs are key factors for psychological distress (45, 46). In these studies, ongoing stressors mediated the relationship between past exposure to violence and psychological distress. Although treatment of violence-related mental disorders will remain important, the possibility to prevent mental health problems through alleviating ongoing stressors warrants further study.

Despite these gaps in knowledge, there is overall agreement that children's mental health in areas of armed conflict is an important concern that needs to be addressed in humanitarian programmes. After a period of poorly coordinated programmes and heated ideological debate between humanitarian actors, much of it centring on whether therapeutic ('mental health' or PTSD-focused programmes) or preventive and promotion ('psychosocial') approaches would best meet existing mental health needs, there is now seemingly more consensus on best practices. In 2007, the Inter-Agency Standing Committee published guidelines developed by a group of 27 agencies. The guidelines refer to MHPSS interventions as 'any type of local or outside support that aims to protect or promote psychosocial wellbeing and/or prevent or treat mental disorder' (p.1) (47). Rather than the implementation of stand-alone services for specific disorders or target groups, the guidelines advocate a multilayered system of care that includes diverse levels of services for the variety of mental health needs in emergency settings. These levels are described as: social considerations in basic services and security (e.g. ensuring human rights protection for groups vulnerable to further violence); strengthening community and family supports (e.g. supporting community initiatives aimed at reconciliation); focused non-specialized supports (e.g. organizing support groups with family members of people who 'disappeared' during armed conflict; PFA); and specialized supports (e.g. psychotherapy for specific mental disorders).

Intervention approach

The Indonesia trial described in this section was part of a larger project with children affected by armed conflict in Burundi, Indonesia, Nepal, Sri Lanka, and South Sudan. The project ran from 2004 to 2009 and was coordinated by HealthNet TPO (<http://www.healthnettpo.org>) with funding from Plan Netherlands (Burundi, Indonesia, Sri Lanka, South Sudan) and Save the Children US (Nepal) (48, 49). This combined research and intervention project was aimed at implementing and evaluating a multilayered system of mental health and psychosocial care (50). The care package included school-based screening (51, 52), universal preventive activities (i.e. activities offered to children regardless of status on risk factors), the selective preventive intervention that is the focus of this case study (i.e. activities offered to children screened into intervention on the basis of risk), as well as more focused psychosocial counselling for children with higher levels of distress (53, 54). The structure of the care systems was the same across settings, but the content was adapted and adjusted based on local needs and sociocultural differences between sites. While the research into the efficacy of the school-based intervention was done in four countries, we will take the Indonesia study as an example.

Setting and conflict background

In Indonesia, project activities were implemented in Poso, a district in the province of Central Sulawesi on the island of Sulawesi. The project was implemented by Church World Service Indonesia, an NGO implementing humanitarian relief and development programmes in various areas in Indonesia. Central Sulawesi is one of the poorer provinces on the island, with around a quarter of the population living below the poverty line. Multiple ethnic groups live in the region, including the Pamona, Bugis, Makassarese, Togian, Balinese, Javanese, and Chinese (55). Traditionally, indigenous groups in the interior areas are Protestant. These groups were converted by Dutch colonizers who were interested in countering Muslim influence in coastal areas. Coastal areas were influenced through Muslim trade prior to Dutch rule (56). Although the large-scale communal violence in Central Sulawesi has largely played out along religious lines, the causes of violence between Protestant and Muslim groups are complex. Violence was rooted in changed economic relations (e.g. loss of the comparative economic advantage of Protestant groups due to limited profit for Protestant group from the new timber industry and cash-crop farming and increased economic pressure due to the Asian crisis on all ethnic groups); national political developments (e.g. state-sponsored migration changing ethnic population composition in the region, and a policy of decentralization that raised the stakes for local political control); indigenous groups' decreased access to ancestral land; and weak rule of law, allowing groups to stoke conflict for political gains, and causing rival groups to resort to vigilantism for retribution and self-protection (55, 56). Communal violence started in 1998 and moved through several cycles. Violence that started with small brawls turned into larger riots and escalated into more organized and larger scale killings and the arrival of radical Muslim militant groups (e.g. Jemaah Islamiyah). Reconciliation attempts resulted in the Malino Accords of December 2001, which were able to halt large-scale community rioting and reduce the level of violence. In the period of project implementation, violence was less overt but continued through mysterious shootings and killings, rumours, and occasional bombings (55–58). We chose to work in the Poso district, as this area had seen some of the worst violence, but appeared to have received less assistance from humanitarian agencies.

Unit of randomization and sample size considerations

A key consideration in the design of the trial concerned the unit of randomization. We were interested in implementing a school-based intervention and, from a design perspective, were worried about contamination. A risk of individual or classroom randomization was that children in the intervention arm of the trial would share learned skills or experiences with classmates or school friends in the control arm of the trial or try to get in the intervention arm, thus leading to potential underestimation of intervention benefits. To avoid contamination, we chose to randomize schools rather than individual children or classrooms (schools approximately 30–40 km apart). Cluster randomization has important implications for sample size, as children within clusters (i.e. schools in our case) are likely to be more similar than children between clusters—so-called intracluster correlation. Sample sizes in cluster randomized trials generally need to be considerably larger to obtain similar statistical power, and such trials require more advanced multilevel statistical analysis to account for intracluster correlation (59).

Our sample size calculation was based on the primary outcome measures for PTSD and depressive symptoms: the Child PTSD Symptom Scale (60) and Depression Self-Rating Scale (61), respectively. Based on two previous studies that applied these symptom checklists (62, 63), we calculated effect sizes of 1.10 for PTSD and 0.78 for depressive symptoms. To detect similar effect sizes with an α of 0.02 and β of 0.95, we calculated a minimum required sample size of 18 children (PTSD) and 35 children (depression) per study arm. To account for intracluster correlation we multiplied the sample size of 35 by $1 + (m-1)\rho$, with estimated average cluster size m at 30 children and intracluster correlation ρ at 0.1, resulting in a required sample size of 137 children per study arm (59). To allow for attrition, we aimed to recruit around 200 participants per study arm. As we expected to enrol approximately 30 children per school, we estimated that including seven schools per study arm would lead to sufficient sample size. To randomize schools we used a government list of schools in the Poso district (79 schools). From this list we included only schools in sub-districts that had been exposed to violence and that consisted of generally mixed fishing and farming communities. The list for these areas included 24 schools. Of these 24 schools we excluded three private and single-religious schools to ensure a homogeneous sample. Randomization of 14 schools to either arm was conducted with statistical software (SPSS) by the first author, after which implementing staff in Indonesia were notified of which schools were part of which study arm.

Screening and participants

Prior to the intervention we conducted a screening procedure to distinguish (1) children who did *not* experience traumatic events or who were doing comparatively well, from (2) children exposed to traumatic events and experiencing psychological distress. This was done to avoid a possible negative effect of processing traumatic experiences during the intervention on a group that is not having any such problems to start with, and also to maximally match resources with needs. Children screened out of the intervention were invited to participate in recreational group activities to avoid creating potential envy or stigma between the different groups. Screening occurred in schools subsequent to randomization, using symptom checklists for exposure to potentially traumatic events and symptom checklists for PTSD and anxiety. The nine-item exposure checklist was developed through free listing with staff of the implementing partner, in order to identify potentially traumatic events that were salient in the Poso context. Children were screened into the intervention if they had experienced one or more potentially traumatic events or if they scored above cut-off points on either the PTSD or anxiety symptom checklist (64). Criterion validation of these checklists indicated a need for higher scores than standard cut-off scores in western populations to identify probable disorder, but given our interest in including children with broader psychological distress in a selective preventive intervention, we retained the original cut-off scores for an inclusive screening process (22).

We screened 495 children, and included 403 children. Participants included 207 boys and 196 girls (48.6%) between 7 and 15 years old. The majority (79.8%) of children were between 9 and 11 years old (mean 9.9, SD 1.21). Around a third of the children reported their religion as Muslim (31.1%), almost half as Protestant (46.9%), and others as Hindu (12.9%), Catholic (7.1%), and other religions (5.2%). There were no differences at baseline between the study arms on exposure to traumatic events or any of the outcome measures, but 4% more children in the intervention arm were girls, the children in the intervention arm were on average 4 months older, and there were fewer children living in their original villages in the control arm.

Intervention and control arms

The classroom-based intervention (CBI) was developed in Boston by the Center for Trauma Psychology, and had been implemented in the US, the oPt, and Turkey (65). An RCT in the oPt had shown promising effects with 6–11 year olds (24). The intervention was implemented by people selected from local communities. These CBI facilitators had to be at least 18 years old and have at least a high-school education. They were selected through a selection procedure that assessed affinity and capacity to work with children through an interview and role-play selection process. Selected facilitators were trained in a 2-week practice-based and skills-oriented training programme, which included knowledge on mental health, basic intervention, and communication skills, the CBI protocol, ethics, and service provision. Most facilitators had no formal mental health background but had worked as volunteers in local organizations, or had teaching experience. They implemented the intervention for a year before research was initiated.

The manualized intervention consisted of 15 sessions with groups of about 15 children over 5 weeks. CBI combines cognitive behavioural techniques (e.g. psychoeducation, addressing coping skills, trauma processing) with cooperative play and creative-expressive exercises such as drama, dance, and music. The intervention has dual aims in reducing psychological distress and building resilience through improving positive coping skills and social support. CBI is phased and structured along/with the following themes: sessions 1–3 (week 1)—information, safety, and control (including psychoeducation); sessions 4–6 (week 2)—stabilization, awareness, and self-esteem; sessions 7–12 (weeks 3 and 4)—the trauma narrative; and sessions 13–15 (week 5)—reconnecting the child and group to his/her social context using resiliency-based themes and activities (manual available upon request). Trauma-focused elements in weeks 3 and 4 include non-forced sharing of trauma stories through drawing and drama games. Drawing consisted of 'silent storytelling', i.e. drawings related to traumatic events experienced by children, for example a drawing about what had happened during a particularly upsetting event, or a drawing of the people who supported the child right after this event. Children were invited, but not forced, to share these drawings with the other members in the group. Fidelity to the intervention manual was assessed through scoring 14 videotapes of randomly selected CBI groups using a structured checklist containing dichotomous items on presence or absence of prescribed activities for that session. Average adherence to the intervention manual was 89.7%. We opted for a waitlist-control design as we did not want to withhold a potentially effective intervention from other schools in the region. After the final measurements were concluded, the intervention team implemented CBI in the control arm.

Both the delivery mechanisms and the content were adapted to the local cultural setting in each of the sites. In practice, this meant that all country teams went through the manual and identified parts that were not compatible within the local culture (e.g. mixed gender groups, certain theatre games that were found too abstract, making a body outline on a large sheet of paper, some of the activities focused on strengthening self-esteem). Also, other parts of the intervention were changed to include favoured activities, for example the introduction of local dance moves, games, and music. During a 1-year period of adaptation and piloting the intervention, we learned the need to spend significant time in introducing the rationale and activities of the intervention For example, the use of pieces of white cloth as objects that children could colour and bring home with them (to provide a reminder and sense of continuity between sessions) raised questions in some Protestant communities, where this was perceived to be a Muslim headscarf (48).

Outcome measures

Assessments were conducted 1 week before the intervention, 1 week after the intervention, and 6 months after the intervention. Outcome measures were selected and developed after a qualitative study that was completed before the start of the trial. The aim of this qualitative study was to identify mental health and psychosocial consequences of the communal violence from the perspective of affected people, and to identify ways in which these consequences were dealt with. The qualitative study consisted of: focus groups with children ($n = 9$), parents ($n = 11$), and teachers ($n = 8$); semistructured interviews with families affected by communal violence ($n = 42$); and key informant interviews ($n = 33$). Participants were sampled through purposive and snowball sampling. Participants in the qualitative study highly prioritized socioeconomic adversity due to the violence, as well as emotional difficulties in children that were described as *trauma* (a broad range of fears, including realistic and generalized fears, and somatically phrased symptoms), morally inappropriate behaviour, and interreligious tensions. Based on these findings, we decided to use PTSD and anxiety symptom checklists as screeners for psychological distress, but we also included a standardized measure for depressive symptoms. In addition, we developed a somatic symptom checklist by selecting the somatic symptoms most commonly mentioned in the context of exposure to adversity. Given the dual aims of the study (i.e. decreasing psychological distress and enhancing strengths), we also chose to include measures for hope (66), coping behaviour (67), and social support (68). Existing standardized measures were translated using a previously advocated approach that included: translation by an indigenous group of experts; conceptual review by an independent bilingual professional; review by people similar to target research participants through focus groups; blind back translation; and piloting (69).

Finally, we developed a function impairment scale to identify potential benefits of intervention for locally salient daily activities through adapting qualitative methods proposed by Bolton and Tang with adults for children (70). This method entailed three steps: (1) brief participatory observation to identify important categories of daily activities and approximate time spent doing these activities; (2) diaries to collect specific activities; and (3) focus groups that explored children's own perspectives on important daily activities. This resulted in a scale with items covering individual, peer, family, and community activities that had satisfactory psychometric properties, including the hypothesized factor structure (71).

Ethical issues

Before starting research in the trial we introduced our research interests through community and school meetings, where we asked permission of principals, teachers, and other community leaders to conduct the study. Permission was also sought with the political leadership at the district level. We obtained written informed consent from children themselves (providing a highly simplified consent form, with reminders throughout), as well as from adults during parent meetings at schools and further follow-up visits, and collected data anonymously. The ethical review board of the VU University Amsterdam provided ethical clearance for the research activities. A key ethical challenge, both in the qualitative study and the cluster randomized trial, concerned provoking psychological distress in children through the discussion of psychologically sensitive topics, in a context where children appeared to not commonly discuss their emotional life with adults. Moreover, given the lack of mental health research resources, we relied on graduate-level research assistants without formal training in mental health research. We tried as much as possible to address this challenge through: (1) emphasizing in the informed consent procedure that children were free to not answer any questions they did not feel like answering, to ask for a break when they needed one, or to stop the interview at any time—without any negative consequences for participation in treatment, their school work, or anything else; (2) detailed attention to this in training of interviewers (e.g. role-plays on how to respond to children becoming upset); (3) the arrangement of a safety net (in Indonesia, research teams were joined by a psychosocial counsellor); and (4) a longer period of training research assistants than is commonly reported. Research assistants were trained in a 4-week period for the qualitative study and a 5-week training for the cluster randomized trial. Training materials avoided technical research jargon as much as possible, and training was strongly focused on practising skills through classroom role-plays and supervised practice. With regard to ethical concerns, even though intended for a different target group, we found the WHO Ethical and Safety Recommendations For Interviewing Trafficked Women useful in the design of training of research assistants (72).

Strengths and limitations

An important limitation of this cluster randomized trial is that, first, the study arm could not be masked. Research assistants conducted interviews at schools, and we could not control children or others disclosing whether CBI had been implemented in that school. We emphasized in the training of research assistants that an objective evaluation would be most beneficial to all stakeholders, but we cannot rule out that lack of masking had an impact on study results. Second, internal reliability of some of the measures was less than desirable, particularly of the five-item anxiety symptom checklist. Third, we selected standardized measures for both psychological symptoms and the strength-focused measures (hope, coping, social support). Although the symptom measures were selected based on the identification of relevant symptoms in the qualitative study, we feel that more intense research efforts are required to investigate the contextual validity of the strength-focused measures. Fourth, randomization of a limited number of schools likely resulted in the minimal, albeit statistically significant, differences at baseline.

Strengths of the study include its design according to rigorous CONSORT standards for cluster randomized trials, including sample size correction and a statistical analytic approach which aims to adjust for the cluster effect (59); the measurement of psychological symptoms, as well as strengths and (contextualized) function impairment to provide a more comprehensive picture of intervention benefits; the mixed methods approach with a preceding qualitative study that aimed to ensure relevance of measures to the study population; and the inclusion of three time points, allowing for longitudinal statistical analyses and the examination of sustained intervention effects at 6-month follow-up.

Trial results

Intervention benefits for children regardless of gender, age, or other variables (main effects) were found for a number of strength-focused outcomes: hope, positive coping methods, social support received from peers, and social support received through play. With regard to symptom outcomes, intervention effects for PTSD and function impairment were identified for girls only. No differences were found for depressive and anxiety symptoms, the trauma-related somatic symptoms, negative coping, and received emotional social support (22, 28).

As described, we were interested in potential moderators and mediators of intervention effects observed in this trial, which were analysed through parallel process latent growth curve modelling (28). Our hypothesis was based on the theoretical notion of ecological resilience, i.e. the assumption that strengthening protective factors at various levels of the child's social environment (e.g. the intervention benefits seen on hope, coping, and social support) would in turn be associated with a reduction in psychological symptoms (i.e. the improvements identified for PTSD symptoms and function impairment). However, contrary to our expectations, we found that social support received from peers mediated PTSD symptoms in the opposite direction. That is, increases in social support through play were associated with smaller reductions in PTSD symptoms. It is possible that for children with post-traumatic stress symptoms, the peer-support aspect of the intervention provided a means of distraction that was beneficial for aspects of wellbeing, but that took attention away from processing trauma symptoms. Although the improvements on the indicators of positive mental health (hope, positive coping, and social support) were encouraging, the association of play social support with reduced intervention benefits may point to the need for a sharper delineation between interventions aimed at promoting wellbeing and interventions with symptomatic children aimed at reducing psychological distress.

No other mediation effects were found, but we did identify several moderators of intervention effects. At the individual level, we found that girls showed larger intervention benefits for PTSD and function impairment. Furthermore, at the household level, children in smaller households and children relying more on social support from outside of their household reported larger intervention benefits for function impairment. We interpreted these moderation effects in terms of social vulnerability. Children living in situations where they received less support from within their households were able to benefit more from an intervention that was partially aimed at providing a more supportive social environment. As mentioned, the CBI has a strong focus on strengthening supportive relations between peers. In Indonesia, this focus on peer-level support seemed most beneficial for children who were lacking such support in their household. In that sense, the CBI appeared to fill a gap by complementing a child's social support system at a different socioecological level.

Comparison with findings in Burundi, Nepal, and Sri Lanka

Similar cluster randomized trials of this school-based intervention were conducted in Burundi, Nepal, and Sri Lanka (summarized in Table 13.1). These studies were not designed to be identical across countries, as we pragmatically wanted to allow for flexibility to accommodate to local circumstances and include contextually salient problems and strengths. However, they are similar enough in design to allow for cross-national comparisons. In Nepal, in a slightly adapted design with baseline and one post-intervention assessment with 325 children aged 11–14 years, no main effects of intervention were identified. However, sub-group analyses showed intervention benefits with regard to general psychological difficulties (a combined measure of hyperactivity, peer-, emotional-, and conduct-related complaints) and aggression for boys; increased prosocial behaviour for girls; and an increased sense of hope for older children (23).

In Sri Lanka, in a study with 399 children aged 9–12 years, a main effect on a locally developed symptom checklist for contextually salient conduct problems was found, which was stronger for younger children. These conduct problems included expressed worries by participants in the qualitative study that children had started viewing violence as an acceptable means of solving conflict, imitated the behaviour of soldiers, were becoming rude with family members and teachers, and were involved in violence and early sexual relations. In addition, intervention benefits for specific sub-groups were identified: boys showed benefits with regard to PTSD and anxiety symptoms; younger children showed benefits for prosocial behaviour; and children experiencing lower levels of current war-related stressors showed benefits on PTSD, anxiety, and

Table 13.1 Summary of findings of cluster randomized trials of a school-based intervention

	Burundi	Indonesia	Nepal	Sri Lanka
Included outcome measures: psychological symptoms	PTSD Anxiety Depression Function impairment**	PTSD Anxiety Depression Trauma-related somatic symptoms* Function impairment**	PTSD Anxiety Depression Psychological difficulties Aggression Function impairment**	PTSD Anxiety Depression Psychological difficulties Conduct problems* Supernatural complaints* Function impairment**
Included outcome measures: strengths	Hope Coping Social support	Hope Coping Social support	Hope Prosocial behaviour	Hope Coping Prosocial behaviour
Main effects	–	Hope Positive coping Peer social support Play social support	–	Conduct problems
Sub-group intervention effects/ moderators	**Larger households**: depression, function impairment **Living with both parents**: PTSD, function impairment **Younger age**: hope **Less past trauma exposure**: hope	**Girls**: PTSD, function impairment **Smaller households, social support outside of household**: function impairment **Younger age**: hope	**Girls**: prosocial behaviour **Boys**: general psychological difficulties, aggression **Older age**: hope	**Boys**: PTSD, anxiety **Younger age**: prosocial behaviour **Less ongoing war-related stressors**: PTSD, anxiety, function impairment
Negative findings	**Displaced children**: hope, function impairment	–	–	**Girls**: PTSD

* Locally constructed symptom checklists based on qualitative research; ** constructed locally through a mixed methods procedure

function impairment. However, an unexpected finding in this study was that girls in the wait-list arm showed stronger improvements in PTSD symptoms than girls in the intervention arm (29).

Similar to Nepal, no main effects were identified in a cluster randomized trial with 329 children aged 8–17 years in Burundi. Again, several sub-group effects were found. Children in larger households showed intervention effects for depressive symptoms and function impairment. Also, children living with both parents reported intervention benefits on PTSD and function impairment. Intervention benefits for a sense of hope were found in younger children and in children who reported lower levels of past conflict-related trauma exposure. However, a negative effect was observed for displaced children, i.e. wait-listed children who were not displaced showed more favourable trajectories on hope and function impairment (27).

Conclusion

In this chapter, we aimed to provide an overview of mental conditions and disorder associated with stress and the evidence for interventions targeting these conditions—both in general and in humanitarian settings specifically. We reviewed knowledge on child mental health in settings of armed conflict, and described the results of cluster randomized trials that were aimed at evaluating a school-based mental health intervention. We provided a more detailed summary of a trial in Indonesia. The summary of the emerging literature on risk, protective, and mental health promotion factors for children affected by armed conflict showed a complex set of relations. Risk, protective, and promotive factors have shown different relations to mental health according to gender, development stage, phase of conflict, and sociocultural setting. In the intervention trials, we found that the school-based intervention generally had modest beneficial effect on participants in each of the settings, but with variation in terms of types of effects and the factors that influenced these effects.

From an intervention perspective, overall, results of these trials confirm the usefulness of a socioecological intervention framework by highlighting the important role of individual-level, household-level, and wider contextual moderators, particularly in preventive interventions. Building on the qualitative studies conducted in these settings, we interpreted the findings in terms of the necessity for stability at other levels of children's socioecological environment in order for them to benefit from a school-level intervention. In Indonesia, where qualitative data suggested relatively intact family functioning in the context of low-intensity continuation of political violence, a school-based intervention seemed most effective for children in more socially vulnerable households (i.e. those in smaller households, relying more on social support from outside of the household). On the other side of the coin, in both Burundi and Sri Lanka, qualitative data seemed to suggest a more profound impact of armed conflict on family and community functioning, and these were settings where armed conflict was ongoing. In these settings, intervention seemed to only be beneficial for children in more socially stable settings. That is, in Burundi there were intervention benefits for children living with both parents, in larger households, and with less trauma exposure. In Sri Lanka, there were intervention benefits for boys and children with fewer ongoing war-related stressors. Interpreted from a socioecological perspective, the results of the studies suggest that a school-level intervention may be expected to be helpful when there is sufficient support and stability at other levels of the child's social environment (e.g. at family and community levels), but that one needs to proceed carefully—especially in settings where armed conflict is ongoing—when family and community functioning has deteriorated.

These findings are in need of further replication, but they seem to suggest a 'tipping point' of required stability in children's social environments. On the more stable side of that tipping point, school-based interventions may be beneficial—albeit still with differential effects for different sub-groups. On the more volatile side of that tipping point, intervention may be associated with unintended consequences for more socially vulnerable children. In such situations, it is advisable to conduct an analysis of the strengths and weaknesses in children's social support systems, and proceed with more carefully selected and homogenous groups of participants. If treatment of PTSD symptoms specifically is the main goal, there are interventions with a more consistent evidence base, such as CBT-T and EMDR (8–10). Feasibility of these interventions in humanitarian settings remains an important research question (8). Furthermore, findings across the countries show a consistent set of improvements on positive mental health outcomes (hope, prosocial behaviour, social support). Although important in themselves, it is yet unknown if these improvements translate over time in reductions in psychological symptoms.

In Burundi, we proceeded with the development of a family-based intervention for families in particularly vulnerable situations (73, 74). Collectively, the diverse findings emphasize the conclusions from epidemiological studies on protective factors (38) with regard to the vital importance of designing preventive interventions on knowledge of protective processes.

Another important intervention lesson that can be drawn from the collective studies is that the intervention may be overly relying on two paradigms, a preventive resilience-focused and a curative trauma-focused one. In Indonesia, we found that a resilience-focused element (i.e. the improvement in social support through play) was actually associated with smaller reductions of PTSD symptoms. While both are important, hence our development of a multilayered care package, the efficacy of CBI might be enhanced if there was a stronger separation between these aims. For example, a universal resilience-promotion intervention (without a focus on trauma symptoms) could be the entry point to intervention. As part of this intervention, systematic screening could refer children to an evidence-based cognitive behavioural intervention with a trauma focus, or other intervention depending on which types of symptoms were a priority.

In addition to these cluster randomized trials, we looked into the beneficiaries' perspectives on intervention benefits through analysis of routine monitoring and evaluation data of over 26,000 children, which demonstrated positive results across the board. The only point of concern was the high perceived level of burden among the CBI facilitators, something that was addressed as the programme evolved (50). The difference between conclusions based on these different data sets raises an important question. On the one hand, if the data from the trials are given prior weight, one might warn against hastily concluding that an intervention is beneficial based on monitoring and evaluation data, and infer that more rigorous quantitative evaluation is vital to truly understand intervention effects. On the other hand, we believe the monitoring and evaluation data, by collecting experiences with the intervention in stakeholders' own words, provide an important complementary perspective on the data from the trials. In this sense, we argue for the integration of more open-ended process evaluation with controlled trial methodology.

From a research perspective, three lessons may in our opinion be distilled from these four cluster randomized trials. First, we feel the trials support the benefits of mixed methods approaches to developing outcome measures in evaluations of mental health interventions in socioculturally diverse settings. The function impairment measure, developed through qualitative methods (71), successfully detected change in two out of the four trials, and in Sri Lanka we found main effects only for the symptom checklist developed through qualitative research. Second, the trials provide further arguments for debate on Bronfenbrenner's statement, 'If you want to know how it works, try to change it' (75), i.e. the possibility for intervention studies to address more basic science questions on protective and risk processes for mental health in children affected by adversity. On the one hand, the trials in Indonesia and Nepal generated important information on the differential effects of interventions by gender, age, and household size. On the other hand, the trials in Burundi and Sri Lanka also show the risks involved in intervening without detailed knowledge of how contextual variables may shape intervention effects, with the risk of doing harm in some sub-groups. Given this complexity, the four trials thereby strengthen the urgency for practitioners and researchers to debate what type of knowledge is required before initiating external intervention—a particularly burning question in an area of practice where needs and situational assessments are commonly skipped altogether (76).

Collectively, these four trials provide a more cautious note on what may be expected in terms of intervention benefits from relatively brief school-based psychosocial interventions implemented by trained non-specialists in challenging environments. There is room for optimism, in that moderate and sustained effects were identified in volatile settings with a relatively low-intensity intervention. From a public health perspective, a smaller intervention benefit that can be replicated at scale is at least as valuable as a resource-intensive clinical intervention with larger effect sizes. However, the research results emphasize that preventive psychosocial interventions with children in adversity could benefit from further advances in knowledge. Advances are required in the field of epidemiology, to further clarify and confirm risk, protective, and promotive factors on a broader range of symptoms with conflict-affected children. Further advances are also required in the more applied field of intervention development and evaluation, in order to more accurately capture the complex processes occurring during preventive interventions. Taken together, the trials reaffirm the critical need in this emerging field to combine interventions with dedicated efforts to rigorously evaluate outcomes.

References

1 Kessler RC, McLaughlin KA, Green JG, Gruber MJ, Sampson NA, Zaslavsky AM, et al. (2010) Childhood adversities and adult psychopathology in the WHO World Mental Health Surveys. B J Psychiatry, 197(5):378–85.

2 Garcia-Moreno C, Jansen HA, Ellsberg M, Heise L, Watts CH, WHO Multi-country Study on Women's Health and Domestic Violence against Women Study Team, et al. (2006) Prevalence of intimate partner violence: findings from the WHO multi-country study on women's health and domestic violence. Lancet, 368(9543):1260–9.

3 Trevillion K, Oram S, Feder G, Howard LM, et al. (2012) Experiences of domestic violence and mental disorders: a systematic review and meta-analysis. PLoS ONE, 7(12):e51740.

4 Howard LM, Oram S, Galley H, Trevillion K, Feder G, et al. (2013) Domestic violence and perinatal mental disorders: a systematic review and meta-analysis. PLos Med, 10(5):e1001452.

5 Satcher D, Friel S, Bell R (2007) Natural and manmade disasters and mental health. JAMA, **298**(21):2540–2.

6 Steel Z, Chey T, Silove D, Marnane C, Bryant RA, van Ommeren M (2009) Association of torture and other potentially traumatic events with mental health outcomes among populations exposed to mass conflict and displacement. JAMA, **302**(5):537–49.

7 Maercker A, Brewin CR, Bryant RA, Cloitre M, Reed GM, van Ommeren M, et al. (2013) Proposals for mental disorders specifically associated with stress in the ICD-11. Lancet, **381**(9878):1683–5.

8 Tol WA, Barbui C, van Ommeren M (2013) Management of acute stress, PTSD, and bereavement: WHO recommendations. JAMA, **310**(5):477–8.

9 World Health Organization and United Nations High Commissioner for Refugees (2013) Assessment and management of conditions specifically related to stress: mhGAP intervention guide module (version 1.0). Geneva: WHO.

10 World Health Organization (2013) Guidelines for the management of conditions specifically related to stress. Geneva: WHO.

11 World Health Organization (2010) mhGAP intervention guide for mental, neurological and substance use disorders in non-specialized health settings: mental health gap action programme (mhGAP). Geneva: WHO.

12 World Health Organization, War Trauma Foundation, and World Vision International (2011) Psychological first aid: guide for field workers 2011. Geneva: WHO.

13 Rose S, Bisson J, Churchill R, Wessely S, et al. (2009) Psychological debriefing for preventing post traumatic stress disorder (PTSD). Cochrane Database System Rev, (2):CD000560.

14 Bisson JI, Tavakoly B, Witteveen AB, Ajdukovic D, Jehel L, Johansen VJ, et al. (2010) TENTS guidelines: development of post-disaster psychosocial care guidelines through a Delphi process. B J Psychiatry, **196**(1):69–74.

15 Hobfoll SE, Watson P, Bell CC, Bryant RA, Brymer MJ, Friedman MJ, et al. (2007) Five elements of immediate and mid-term mass trauma intervention: empirical evidence. Psychiatry Interpers Biol Process, **70**(4):283–315.

16 Fox JH, Burkle FM Jr, Bass J, Pia FA, Epstein JL, Markenson D (2012) The effectiveness of psychological first aid as a disaster intervention tool: research analysis of peer-reviewed literature from 1990–2010. Disaster Med Public Health Preparedness, **6**(3):247–52.

17 Bisson JI, Lewis C (2009) Systematic review of psychological first aid. Geneva: WHO.

18 Trickey D, Siddaway AP, Meiser-Stedman R, Serpell L, Field AP (2012) A meta-analysis of risk factors for post-traumatic stress disorder in children and adolescents. Clin Psychol Rev, **32**(2):122–38.

19 Ozer EJ, Best SR, Lipsey TL, Weiss DS (2003) Predictors of posttraumatic stress disorder and symptoms in adults: a meta-analysis. Psychol Bull, **129**(1):52–73.

20 Tol WA, Barbui C, Galappatti A, Silove D, Betancourt TS, Souza R, et al. (2011) Mental health and psychosocial support in humanitarian settings: linking practice and research. Lancet, **378**(9802):1581–91.

21 Berger R, Gelkopf M (2009) School-based intervention for the treatment of tsunami-related distress in children: a quasi-randomized controlled trial. Psychother Psychosom, **78**(6):364–71.

22 Tol WA, Komproe IH, Susanty D, Jordans MJ, Macy RD, De Jong JT (2008) School-based mental health intervention for children affected by political violence in Indonesia: a cluster randomized trial. JAMA, **300**(6):655–62.

23 Jordans MJ, Komproe IH, Tol WA, Kohrt BA, Luitel NP, Macy RD, et al. (2010) Evaluation of a classroom-based psychosocial intervention in conflict-affected Nepal: a cluster randomized controlled trial. J Child Psychol Psychiatry, 51(7):818–26.

24 Khamis V, Macy R, Coignez V (2004) The impact of the classroom/community/camp-based intervention (CBI) program on Palestinian children. New York: Save the Children US.

25 Bolton P, Bass J, Betancourt T, Speelman L, Onyango G, Clougherty K, et al. (2007) Interventions for depression symptoms among adolescent survivors of war and displacement in northern Uganda: a randomized controlled trial. JAMA, 298(5):519–27.

26 Dybdahl R (2001) Children and mothers in war: an outcome study of a psychosocial intervention program. Child Dev, 72(4):1214–30.

27 Tol WA, et al. (2014) School-based mental health intervention for children in war-affected Burundi: a cluster randomized trial. In press, BMC Medicine.

28 Tol WA, Komproe IH, Jordans MJ, Gross AL, Susanty D, Macy RD, et al. (2010) Mediators and moderators of a psychosocial intervention for children affected by political violence. J Consult Clin Psychol, 78(6):818–28.

29 Tol WA, Komproe IH, Jordans MJ, Vallipuram A, Sipsma H, Sivayokan S, et al. (2012) Outcomes and moderators of a preventive school-based mental health intervention for children affected by war in Sri Lanka: a cluster randomized trial. World Psychiatry, 11(2):114–22.

30 Machel G (2009) Children and conflict in a changing world: Machel study 10-year review. New York: UNICEF.

31 Themner L, Wallensteen P (2013) Armed conflicts, 1946–2012. J Peace Res, 50(4):509–21.

32 Kimhi S, Eshel Y, Zysberg L, Hantman S (2010) Postwar winners and losers in the long run: determinants of war related stress symptoms and posttraumatic growth. Community Ment Health J, 46(1):10–19.

33 Tol WA, Reis R, Susanty D, de Jong JT (2010) Communal violence and child psychosocial well-being: qualitative findings from Poso, Indonesia. Transcult Psychiatry, 47(1):112–35.

34 Batniji R, van Ommeren M, Saraceno B (2006) Mental and social health in disasters: relating qualitative social science research and the Sphere standard. Soc Sci Med, 62:1853–64.

35 Attanayake V, McKay R, Joffres M, Singh S, Burkle F Jr, Mills E (2009) Prevalence of mental disorders among children exposed to war: a systematic review of 7,920 children. Med Conflict Survival, 25(1):4–19.

36 Betancourt TS, Kahn KT (2008) The mental health of children affected by armed conflict: protective processes and pathways to resilience. Int Rev Psychiatry, 20(3):317–28.

37 Reed RV, Fazel M, Jones L, Panter-Brick C, Stein A (2012) Mental health of displaced and refugee children resettled in low-income and middle-income countries: risk and protective factors. Lancet, 379(9812):250–65.

38 Tol WA, Song S, Jordans MJD (2013) Annual research review: resilience in children and adolescents living in areas of armed conflict: a systematic review of findings in low- and middle-income countries. J Child Psychol Psychiatry, 54(4):445–60.

39 Tol WA, Jordans MJD, Kohrt BA, Betancourt TS, Komproe IH (2013) Promoting mental health and psychosocial well-being in children affected by political violence: part I—current evidence for an ecological resilience approach. In: Fernando C, Ferrari M (eds) Handbook of resilience in children of war. New York: Springer.

40 Punamäki RL, Qouta S, El Sarraj E (1997) Models of traumatic experience and children's psychological adjustment: the roles of perceived parenting and the children's own resources and activity. Child Dev, 64(4):718–28.

41 Barber BK (2001) Political violence, social integration, and youth functioning: Palestinian youth from the Intifada. J Commun Psychol, **29**(3):259–80.

42 de Berry J, Fazili A, Farhad S, et al. (2003) The children of Kabul: discussions with Afghan families. New York: Save the Children US.

43 Eggerman M, Panter-Brick C (2010) Suffering, hope, and entrapment: resilience and cultural values in Afghanistan. Soc Sci Med, **71**(1–2):71–83.

44 Tol WA, Rees SJ, Silove D (2013) Broadening the scope of epidemiology in conflict-affected settings: opportunities for mental health prevention and promotion. Epidemiol Psychiatr Sci, **22**(3):197–203.

45 Rasmussen A, Nguyen L, Wilkinson J, Vundla S, Raghavan S, Miller KE, et al. (2010) Rates and impact of trauma and current stressors among Darfuri refugees in eastern Chad. Am J Orthopsychiatry, **80**(2):227–36.

46 Jordans MJ, Semrau M, Thornicroft G, van Ommeren M, et al. (2012) Role of current perceived needs in explaining the association between past trauma exposure and distress in humanitarian settings in Jordan and Nepal. Br J Psychiatry, **201**(4):276–81.

47 Inter-Agency Standing Committee (IASC) (2007) IASC guidelines on mental health and psychosocial support in emergency settings. Geneva: IASC.

48 Jordans MJ, Tol WA, Komproe IH, Susanty D, Vallipuram A, Ntamatumba P, et al. (2010) Development of a multi-layered psychosocial care system for children in areas of political violence. Int J Mental Health Syst, **16**:4–15.

49 Jordans MJ, Tol WA, Susanty D, Ntamatumba P, Luitel NP, Komproe IH, et al. (2013) Implementation of a mental health care package for children in areas of armed conflict: a case study from Burundi, Indonesia, Nepal, Sri Lanka, and Sudan. PLos Med, **10**(1):e1001371.

50 Jordans MJ, Komproe IH, Tol WA, Susanty D, Vallipuram A, Ntamatumba P, et al. (2011) Practice-driven evaluation of a multi-layered psychosocial care package for children in areas of armed conflict. Community Ment Health J, **47**(3):267–77.

51 Jordans MJ, Komproe IH, Ventevogel P, Tol WA, de Jong JT (2008) Development and validation of the child psychosocial distress screener in Burundi. Am J Orthopsychiatry, **78**(3):290–9.

52 Jordans MJ, Komproe IH, Tol WA, De Jong JT (2009) Screening for psychosocial distress amongst war-affected children: cross-cultural construct validity of the CPDS. J Child Psychol Psychiatry Allied Discipline, **50**(4):514–23.

53 Jordans MJ, Komproe IH, Smallegange E, Ntamatumba P, Tol WA, De Jong JT (2012) Potential treatment mechanisms of counseling for children in Burundi: a series of n = 1 studies. Am J Orthopsychiatry, **82**:338–48.

54 Jordans MJ, Komproe IH, Tol WA, Nsereko J, de Jong JT (2013) Treatment processes of counseling for children in South Sudan: a multiple n = 1 design. Community Ment Health J, **49**(3):354–67.

55 Brown G, Tajima Y, Hadi S (2005) Overcoming violent conflict, vol. 3: peace and development analysis in Central Sulawesi. Jakarta: UNDP.

56 Aragon LV (2001) Communal violence in Poso, Central Sulawesi: where people eat fish and fish eat people. Indonesia, **72**:45–79.

57 International Crisis Group (2004) Indonesia backgrounder: jihad in Central Sulawesi. Jakarta/Brussels: International Crisis Group.

58 Human Rights Watch (2002) Breakdown: four years of communal violence in Central Sulawesi. Washington, DC: Human Rights Watch.

59 Campbell MK, Elbourne DR, Altman DG (2004) CONSORT statement: extension to cluster randomised trials. BMJ, **328**:702–8.

60 Foa EB, Johnson KM, Feeny NC, Treadwell KR (2001) The Child PTSD symptom scale: a preliminary examination of its psychometric properties. J Clin Child Psychol, **30**(3):376–84.

61 Birleson P (1981) The validity of depressive disorder in childhood and the development of a self-rating scale—a research report. J Child Psychol Psychiatry Allied Discipline, **22**(1):73–88.

62 Cohen JA, Deblinger E, Mannarino AP, Steer R (2004) A multisite, randomized controlled trial for children with sexual abuse-related PTSD symptoms. J Am Acad Child Adolesc Psychiatry, **43**(4):393–402.

63 Layne CM, Pynoos RS, Saltzman WR, Arslanagić B, Black M, Savjak N, (2001) Trauma/grief-focused group psychotherapy: school-based postwar intervention with traumatized Bosnian adolescents. Group Dynamics Theor Res Practice, **5**(4):277–90.

64 Birmaher B, Khetarpal S, Brent D, Cully M, Balach L, Kaufman J, et al. (1997) The screen for child anxiety related emotional disorders (SCARED): scale construction and psychometric characteristics. J Am Acad Child Adolesc Psychiatry, **36**(4):545–53.

65 Macy RD, Macy DJ, Gross SI, Brighton P (2003) Healing in familiar settings: support for children and youth in the classroom and community. New Direction Youth Dev, Summer(98):51–79.

66 Snyder CR, Hoza B, Pelham WE, Rapoff M, Ware L, Danovsky M, et al. (1997) The development and validation of the Children's Hope Scale. J Pediatr Psychiatry, **22**:399–421.

67 Spirito A, Stark LJ, Williams C (1988) Development of a brief coping checklist for use with pediatric populations. J Pediatr Psychol, **13**(4):555–74.

68 Paardekooper B, de Jong JT, Hermanns JM (1999) The psychological impact of war and the refugee situation on South Sudanese children in refugee camps in northern Uganda: an exploratory study. J Child Psychol Psychiatry, **40**(4):529–36.

69 van Ommeren M, Sharma B, Thapa S, Makaju R, Prasain D, Bhattara R, et al. (1999) Preparing instruments for transcultural research: use of the Translation Monitoring Form with Nepali-speaking Bhutanese refugees. Transcult Psychiatry, **36**(3):285–301.

70 Bolton P, Tang AM (2002) An alternative approach to cross-cultural function assessment. Social Psychiatry Psychiatr Epidemiol, **37**(11):537–43.

71 Tol WA, Komproe IH, Jordans MJ, Susanty D, de Jong JT (2011) Developing a function impairment measure for children affected by political violence: a mixed methods approach in Indonesia. Int J Qual Health Care, **23**(4):375–83.

72 World Health Organization (2003) WHO ethical and safety recommendations for interviewing trafficked women. Geneva: WHO.

73 Jordans MJD, Tol WA, Komproe IH (2011) Mental health interventions for children in adversity: pilot-testing a research strategy for treatment selection in low-income settings. Soc Sci Med, **73**(3):456–66.

74 Jordans MJ, Tol WA, Ndayisaba A, Komproe IH (2012) A controlled evaluation of a brief parenting psychoeducation intervention in Burundi. Social Psychiatry Psychiatr Epidemiol, **48**(11):1851–9.

75 Bronfenbrenner U (1979) The ecology of human development: experiments by nature and design. Cambridge: Harvard University Press.

76 Tol WA, van Ommeren M (2012) Evidence-based mental health and psychosocial support in humanitarian settings: gaps and opportunities. Evidence-based Mental Health, **15**(2):25–6.

Chapter 14

Suicide prevention trials

Lakshmi Vijayakumar, Melissa Pearson, and Shuba Kumar

Introduction

Suicide is the tragic and untimely loss of human life which is all the more devastating and perplexing because it is a conscious act. It is a complex behaviour which is best understood as multidetermined and the result of the interactions between basic causal factors which render the individual susceptible and those that interact with this susceptibility to cause suicide. Suicidal behaviours tend to share common traits but not all are alike. The whole spectrum of suicidal behaviour includes suicides, non-fatal attempts, gestures, ideations, and indirect self-destructive behaviour. To call such diverse behaviour suicidal is vague and gives rise to a host of operational and measurement problems.

Every year around one million people die by suicide around the world. Suicide is one of three leading causes of death among those in the most economically productive age group (15–44 years) and the second leading cause of death in the 15–19 years of age group (1). In the Global Burden of Disease Study 2010, suicide accounted for 4.8% of female deaths and 5.7% of male deaths between 15 and 49 years (2). Patel and colleagues (3), in a nationally representative study in India, have shown that at ages 15–29 years, suicide accounted for nearly as many deaths as transport accidents in men and maternal deaths in women. About 3% of deaths at ages 15 and over were due to suicide. The majority of suicides (85%) in the world occur in LAMIC (4). It is also these countries that are relatively less equipped to prevent suicide as they are hindered by inadequate infrastructure and scarce economic and human resources. As a result, there are few sustained efforts and activities that focus on suicide prevention on a scale necessary to reduce the number of lives lost to suicide (5).

As part of its mhGAP programme, the WHO identified three evidence-based population-level strategies to prevent suicides:

1 restricting access to means of suicide, such as access to pesticides, firearms, and charcoal

2 developing policies to reduce harmful use of alcohol as a component of suicide prevention;

3 assisting and encouraging the media to follow responsible reporting practices of suicide.

In addition, a range of individual strategies have been recommended which include identifying and treating mental disorder at the primary health care level, providing

Table 14.1 Selected intervention trials in LAMIC for suicide prevention

	Charcoal restriction in Hong Kong (11)	Postcards from Persia, Iran (12)	Mobile phone psychotherapy, Sri Lanka (13)	Multicentre trial treatment of schizophrenia to reduce suicidal behaviours InterSePT, 2003 (14) (US, UK, Czech Republic, Hungary, Croatia, South Africa, Argentina, Chile)
Journal/authors	*British Journal of Psychiatry*, 2010 Yip et al.	*British Journal of Psychiatry*, 2011 Hassanian-Moghaddam et al.	*Journal of Telemedicine and Telehealth*, 2012 Marasinghe et al.	*Archives of General Psychiatry*, 2003 Meltzer et al.
Study design	Exploratory controlled trial	RCT	RCT	Randomized (open-label) trial
Sample size	Population of intervention arm 502,000 Population of control arm 534,000	Estimated sample size was 1100 per group. 2113 individuals were enrolled: intervention group (n = 1043); control group (n = 1070)	68 participants were recruited from patients admitted with episode of self-harm and randomized to immediate or delayed brief mobile treatment (I-BMT or D-BMT)	Men and women aged 18–65 with a diagnosis of schizophrenia or schizoaffective disorder and a high risk of suicide. 980 patients enrolled: olanzapine 477, clozapine 479
Intervention	Access to charcoal was limited by removing all barbecue charcoal packs from the open shelves of stores and storing in a locked container accessed by staff only. Follow-up was for a period of 12 months	A modified 'Postcards from the Edge' intervention (15). Eight postcards were mailed to suicide attempters at 1, 2, 3, 4, 6, 8, 10, and 12 months after discharge. A ninth postcard was sent at participant's birthday. The intervention group also received TAU	The I-DBT included face-to-face training in problem-solving therapy, meditation, a brief intervention to increase social support, as well as advice on alcohol and other drugs, and ten telephone calls of 10–15 minutes duration at days 2 and 4, and at 1, 2, 4, 6, 10, 12, 18, and 24 weeks post discharge, access to continuous access to audio messages, and SMS reminders.	Patients were randomly allocated to treatment of either olanzapine or clozapine. Weekly and biweekly clinical visits were matched in the groups. Other clinically necessary interventions were allowed

Table 14.1 (continued) Selected intervention trials in LAMIC for suicide prevention

	Charcoal restriction in Hong Kong (11)	Postcards from Persia, Iran (12)	Mobile phone psychotherapy, Sri Lanka (13)	Multicentre trial treatment of schizophrenia to reduce suicidal behaviours InterSePT, 2003 (14) (US, UK, Czech Republic, Hungary, Croatia, South Africa, Argentina, Chile)
Results	At 12 months the observed changes in the suicide rate showed a reduction in suicides by 31.8% in the intervention arm and 1.6% in the control arm (intervention arm from 17.9 to 12.2 per 100,000 and control arm from 12.7 to 12.5 per 100,000). The suicide rate from charcoal burning was reduced by a statistically significant margin in the intervention region ($p < 0.05$) but not in the control region	At 12 months there was a significant reduction in suicidal ideation (RRR = 0.31, NNT = 7.9), suicide attempt (RRR = 0.42, NNT = 46.1), and number of suicide attempt events per person (IRR = 0.64). There was no significant reduction in any self-cutting (RRR = 0.14) or self-cutting events (IRR = 1.03)	Participants who received the intervention had significant improvements in reducing suicidal ideation and depression compared to TAU. The intervention group also experienced a significant improvement in social support. However, the intervention group did not demonstrate a significant effect in reducing actual self-harm and most substance use, and differential effects on alcohol use were restricted to men	Suicidal behaviour was significantly less in patients treated with clozapine compared to olanzapine. Fewer clozapine-treated patients attempted suicide, required hospitalizations or rescue interventions to prevent suicide, or required concomitant treatment with antidepressants or anxiolytics or soporifics

IRR incidence rate ratio; NNR number needed to treat; RRR relative risk reduction and activating psychosocial support, and maintaining regular contact and follow-up for those who have attempted suicide (<http://www.who.int/mental_health/mhgap>) (see Table 14.1).

There are a number of studies in LAMIC where the focus has been on the treatment of depression. While treatment for mental disorders and specifically for depression is strongly recommended for the prevention of suicide in HIC the evidence in LAMIC is more debated (1–4). However, regardless of the importance of the role of mental illness and depression in suicide in LAMIC, it can still be assumed to be an important component of any suicide intervention strategy. A recent review of effective interventions for the treatment of depression (5) identified studies in Uganda (6), India (7), Chile (8), Pakistan (9), and Mexico (10). In four of these studies there was no discussion of suicide, suicidal behaviours, or suicidal ideation, and only the Indian study reported suicide, but not as an outcome measure. This highlights the difficulties in incorporating suicide outcome measure into studies even in high-incidence countries such as India.

Case studies

Interventions for suicidal acts are aimed at different target groups, such as the general population, suicidal attempters, and suicidal completers. The following section addresses different intervention strategies, wherein using the case study approach two interventions are described. The first is an intervention for those who have attempted suicide and the second is an intervention that seeks to limit access to means of suicide.

Case study 1: SUPRE-MISS

Research has established that persons who attempt suicide are at a high risk of committing suicide. An important strategy to reduce suicide mortality is to provide effective interventions for those who have attempted suicide. There is very limited knowledge about the burden of attempted suicide and effective intervention for suicide attempters in LAMIC. To address this issue, the WHO initiated the Suicide Prevention Multisite Intervention Study for suicidal behaviour (SUPRE-MISS) in five culturally diverse settings (Campinas—Brazil, Chennai—India, Colombo—Sri Lanka, Karaj—Iran, and Yuncheng—China). The objective of the RCT was to assess the effectiveness of brief intervention and contact as an intervention strategy for suicide attempters.

Rationale

Long-term contact with high suicide risk psychiatric patients is known to be associated with a significant reduction in suicide. The contact comprised regular short letters expressing concern for the persons well-being and inviting them to contact (20–22). Carter and colleagues (19) have also shown in a randomized trial that intervention using postcards reduced repetition of hospital-treated deliberate self-harm poisoning. These studies suggested that regular contact with high suicide risk population had the potential to reduce suicidal behaviour. Brief interventions, for example for alcohol problems, which include information, feedback, health education, and practical advice, were found to be effective in reducing alcohol-related problems (23, 24) and were also found to be as effective as more extensive treatment. Repeated follow-up visits were recognized as a factor favouring behaviour change and maintenance. Taking into consideration the human and economic resource limitation in LAMIC, brief intervention and contact (BIC) was selected as the intervention for suicide attempters.

Intervention

The brief intervention module included a 1-hour individual information session as close to the time of discharge as possible. A standard protocol was adhered to by all sites and included information about suicidal behaviour as a sign of psychological and/or social distress, risk and protective factors, basic epidemiology, alternatives to suicidal behaviour, and referral options. There were nine follow-up contacts (visit or phone calls) at 1, 2, 4, 5, and 11 weeks and 4, 6, 12, and 18 months by a nurse, psychologist, or doctor. The treatment as usual (TAU) condition was according to the norms prevailing in the respective emergency departments (ED). Typically only medical treatment was given and no routine psychological assessment or referral system was in place in all the sites.

Instruments

The questionnaire, based on the European Para-suicide Study Interview Schedule (EPSIS) of the WHO/EURO multicentre study on suicidal behaviour, was used (25). It covered detailed sociodemographic information, the history of suicidal behaviour and family data, physical health, contact with health services, mental health, questions related to social support, substance use, hopelessness, traumatic events, legal problems, and antisocial behaviour, and modified Becks suicide intent scale (26), the Beck depression inventory (27), Spielberger trait anger scale (28), WHO well-being index (29), WHO psychiatric disability assessment schedule (30), and Eysenk impulsiveness scale (31). The SUPRE-MISS questionnaire was translated, back translated, and field tested in the regional language and the interviewers were trained in the administration of the questionnaire (32).

Results

All the sites used the same protocol and recruited 1867 suicide attempters identified by medical staff in the emergency care department of the hospitals. All participants ($n = 1867$) were randomly assigned to BIC ($n = 922$) or TAU ($n = 945$) based on a random number table. Completed suicide was the primary outcome measure. For a significance level of 95% (two sided) and power of 80% assuming 3% suicides in the TAU and 1% in the BIC group at 18 months follow-up, a total of 1730 subjects were required. The overall dropout rate was 9% (BIC 5.4% and TAU 12.5%). At the end of 18 months, 18 (2.2%) in the TAU had died by suicide compared to 2 (0.2%) in the BIC group ($x2 = 13.83; p < 0.001$) (33).

The study had several limitations. Several eligible cases were not enrolled due to inadequate recording, intentional misreporting, and rapid departure from the ED. The sample size was different in different sites. The ascertainment of mortality was from the informants and not substantiated by official mortality statistics. As attempted suicide is a punishable offence in India, recruiting the participants was a challenge in itself, as many patients absconded as soon as they were reasonably medically stable. Hence unlike other countries, only 40% of eligible patients were recruited in India.

The dropout at follow-up was highest (15%) in Chennai, India. The follow-up of subjects proved to be a major challenge due to the complex setting and high mobility. A substantial number of persons who lived in rental dwellings moved to a different house after the suicide attempt, due to cultural beliefs and stigma. Sometimes even people who owned their house moved to a rental dwelling elsewhere. To address this issue, the contact sheet had provision for a minimum of two addresses, the nearest bus stop, the nearest temple, mobile phone number, if available, etc. In spite of these methods, it was time-consuming to trace the subjects and identify their whereabouts. It was also necessary to be careful when male psychologists were assigned to follow-up young female suicide attempters.

The major advantage of BIC is that it required little training as opposed to more sophisticated psychological interventions. Considering the low availability of human and economic resources, it is suitable for extensive use in LAMIC.

Case study 2: restricting access to pesticides to reduce suicides

Background

The WHO considers that the single most important means of suicide worldwide is by ingestion of pesticides and accounts for one-third of all suicides (34). Gunnell and colleagues (35) surmised that at least 275,000–370,000 suicides per year are by pesticide poisoning. Mortality data on international suicide patterns revealed that in Asia, rural Latin American countries, and Portugal, pesticide suicide was a major problem, notably among women (36). There is enough evidence now that ingestion of pesticides is the most common method of suicide in the world. Studies from rural India reveal that pesticide is the commonest method of suicide (37). More recently, Patel and colleagues (3), in a nationally representative study from India, reported that suicides in 49% of men and 44% of women were primarily through pesticide poisoning, which is much higher than the data provided by the Government of India (38).

Studies from Asia have found that pesticide suicides are impulsive acts, undertaken during stressful life events, and the majority of people involved do not suffer from mental disorders (39, 40). Case fatalities from pesticide poisoning are estimated to be between 10 and 20% in Asian countries (41). Restricting easy access to pesticides in rural households, to prevent their use in impulsive self-harm, has become a popular recommendation (42–44) for suicide prevention strategies. There is convincing evidence that restricting access to commonly used, highly lethal methods of suicide not only reduces method-specific suicide rates, but also can significantly reduce overall suicide rates (35, 41, 45). Gunnell and colleagues (46) have shown that restricting sales of highly toxic pesticides has coincided with a reduction in suicides in Sri Lanka. Hawton and colleagues (47) discovered that the introduction of individual lockable boxes for storing pesticides in farming households in Sri Lanka was acceptable. Konradsen and colleagues (40, 48) reported that lockable boxes were beneficial for safe-keeping, but they also raised some concerns. The introduction of these storage boxes (see Fig. 14.1) had resulted in the farmers shifting from storing the pesticides in the fields to the home. The authors believed that keeping the storage boxes in the home could

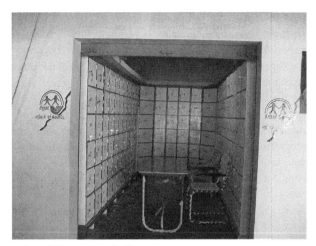

Fig. 14.1 Central pesticide storage facility.

increase the risk of impulsive self-poisoning as the pesticides were now more easily accessible. The pesticide industry has long argued for secure storage and the use of locked boxes to prevent pesticide poisoning, and has started projects testing and scaling up the use of safe storage boxes (49).

What follows is a description of a community controlled trial from South India illustrating the restricting access to means of suicide strategy suggested by the WHO.

The setting

The study was carried out in Kattumannarkoil taluk, Cuddalore district, Tamil Nadu state, in southern India. There is a high utilization of pesticides in this area. While the majority of the villages cultivate paddy, teak, etc., a few of them are primarily engaged in floriculture (e.g. Jasmine, Kanakambaram, and Mullai). The Ministry of Health and Family Welfare at the state level and the Police Department had both shown interest in testing out the effectiveness of a central storage facility for storing pesticides as a means of reducing/preventing suicide and suicidal behaviour. Given this, we decided to undertake the study in Kattumannarkoil taluk, where, besides high utilization of pesticides, we also had governmental support. We visited the District Revenue Office (DRO) from whom we obtained information on the villages governed by this taluk. We learnt that the taluk administers 161 villages. The number of households in each village ranges from a minimum of about 500 to around 1000.

Design and unit of randomization

This was a community controlled trial with two arms (intervention and control). To randomize intervention and control villages we needed to ensure that all selected villages were demographically similar. During the initial field visit made by the research team in May 2008, villages engaging in floriculture (information obtained from the taluk office) were identified from which to randomize the intervention and control sites. (A *taluk* is an *administrative division* and consists of an area of land with a city or town that serves as its headquarters, with possible additional towns, and usually a number of villages. As an entity of local government, the taluk office exercises certain fiscal and administrative power over the villages and municipalities within its jurisdiction.) However, when the study team revisited the sites almost a year later in April 2009, some changes were noted. Several villages in the study area had stopped engaging in floriculture. We therefore had to revisit the taluk office and once again map out potential villages, following which the randomization was done.

Eight villages were identified as predominantly engaging in floriculture which requires spraying of pesticides twice a month, resulting in higher and frequent pesticide usage. The lottery method was used to select four villages. The first two villages were allocated for intervention and the second two became the controls. The villages of Kandamangalam and Kurungudi with 935 and 693 households, respectively (total 1628 households), were the intervention site, and the villages of Pazhanjanallur and Karunagaranallur with 835 and 541 households, respectively (total 1376 households), served as the control sites, following the randomization exercise.

The sample

For the study, pesticide suicides included attempted and completed pesticide suicides, and all suicides included attempted and completed pesticide suicide and attempted and completed suicides by other methods. Suicide attempts are usually 10–40 times more frequent than completed suicides (50). This fact, coupled with data from previous epidemiological studies (37, 51) in rural Tamil Nadu, helped us arrive at an estimate of nearly 10/1000. Factoring in a power of 80, α error at 0.05, one-sided test, and expecting a 50% reduction, the sample size required was estimated at 3578 persons in each arm.

Method

Six trained research assistants (RAs) carried out a baseline door-to-door survey of all households in the study sites using a structured interview schedule which was administered to one adult member in the household. This survey was done before the construction of the storage facilities. In addition to documenting sociodemographic characteristics of the household, information on types of pesticides used, pesticide storage and disposal, and knowledge about health risks of pesticides was obtained. Histories of alcoholism and mental disorder in the family were noted. Information on attempted or completed suicides and/or accidental deaths occurring in the family over the previous 18 months was also obtained. The survey was repeated at the end of 18 months in both sites. Verbal autopsies were conducted for all deaths occurring during the intervention period. This information was cross-checked with the death certificate which is issued by the district taluk office and which confirms cause of death. In case of suicide, psychological autopsy was carried out. A surveillance system involving monthly visits to physicians, health workers, teachers, hospitals, and police stations located in the study area was carried out to document reports of attempted or completed suicides occurring during the study period.

The intervention arm

The idea that reducing access to pesticides can have the potential to reduce pesticide suicides has been endorsed by the WHO and demonstrated by studies carried out in

Sri Lanka. We decided to test this idea in India, with one change. Instead of having individual pesticide storage boxes, we decided on setting up a central storage facility wherein farmers residing in a particular village could keep their pesticides under lock and key in individual lockers (Fig. 14.1). The rationale behind a central storage facility was to avoid the lacunae reported in the Sri Lankan study, namely, that these boxes which were kept at home were often not locked and provided relatively easy access to the pesticide. Storing pesticides in a central facility located at some central point in the village thus deterred easy access. It also had the added advantage of having two supervisors who took turns to be present at the facility throughout the day. These supervisors acted as gatekeepers, and kept a record of farmers who accessed their lockers and the quantum of pesticides taken. Thus, a farmer had to go through these gatekeepers to access the pesticide.

The other important aspect of our intervention was the manner in which it was introduced to the villagers. We realized that for the intervention—indeed for any community-based intervention—to work efficiently, the need for community acceptance of the programme was critical. Thus, well before the commencement of the study, we involved the local panchayat (village council) leaders and other decision-makers in the selected villages in a series of meetings wherein issues concerning pesticide-related suicides and ways in which this could be handled were discussed at length. It was obvious at that time that such suicides were common and were a matter of concern among the village folk. The idea of setting up a central pesticide storage facility was presented and discussed at these meetings and welcomed by most. The only concerns a few expressed related to the location of the facility and how convenient it would be for farmers to access it. These meetings and the discussions that ensued played an important role in not only enhancing acceptance of the intervention, but also infusing a sense of ownership amongst the farmers. Thus, it was the village leaders who decided the location of the facility, the supervision of its construction, and finally the selection of two local persons charged with the responsibility of managing the facility. In the process, the facility received adequate publicity among the households in the villages to the extent that people from neighbouring villages came over and asked us when we would be setting up a similar facility in their village.

Two centralized storage facilities (one in each village) were identified with the help of the panchayat. Within these buildings and based on available space, 167 and 132 storage boxes, respectively (similar to a bank locker) were constructed. These boxes, 2 ft by 2 ft in size and made of wood, were fixed to the wall and could not be removed from the facility. Each box could be locked (Fig. 14.1). With the help of the panchayat and other key persons in the villages, public meetings were organized to create awareness among residents about the storage facilities, their purpose and benefits. Farmers had access to their pesticide storage boxes at any time during the day from about 7 a.m. in the morning until about 7 p.m. in the evening. They had a key to their own locker and a duplicate key was kept with the manager of the central storage facility. Four managers (two for each facility) were identified by the local community and were in charge of managing the facility. They were given training on the importance of safe storage and disposal of pesticides and orientation regarding the purpose of the storage facility and their role in managing it in terms of regular attendance so as not to cause hardship to the farmers. They also maintained a register where they recorded frequency of usage.

The control arm

Control villages were those where floriculture was being practised and therefore pesticides were being used regularly. The aim was to ensure maximum demographic similarity between control and intervention villages. All the baseline and follow-up assessments carried out in the intervention villages were done here too; however, no central storage facility was provided for farmers here.

The outcomes

Our primary study outcome was suicidal behaviour, i.e. attempted or completed suicides, and/or accidental deaths in the family over the last 18 months. As the study was based on the premise that the central storage facility would reduce easy access to pesticides and thereby pesticide-related suicides, assessing the incidence of pesticide-related suicides during the study period was both logical and necessary. In addition to the household survey, we gathered data on suicides through surveillance which involved making monthly visits to physicians, health workers, teachers, hospitals, and police stations located in the study area to document reports of attempted or completed suicides occurring during the study period.

Ethical issues

Our proposal was approved by the ethics committee of the Voluntary Health Society, a 500-bed hospital in Chennai which caters to both urban and semi-urban populations. Consent forms were developed and translated into Tamil. Administering the consent form is always a challenge, particularly among populations with poor literacy. Our RAs were trained to read out the consent form, stopping to explain its contents, and checking to determine if the respondent had understood the contents. Some of the respondents were wary of affixing their signature/thumb imprint to the document and, in such cases, the RAs sought the help of the panchayat leaders to help convince and assure the respondents that no harm would befall them by signing the consent form. This process of obtaining consent took up a considerable amount of time, and therefore reduced the number of households that could be surveyed in a day. As we had the support of the panchayat, cooperation from the village residents was, by and large, good. In some cases, respondents even asked the RAs to skip the consent process, stating that they understood and wanted the RAs to simply begin administering the questionnaire. In such cases our RAs explained to the respondents that, since this was a research study, the consent process still needed to be adhered to.

Another problem that we encountered was that nothing could remain a secret in these villages. Neighbours were well aware of suicide attempts that had occurred, which was particularly awkward and embarrassing for the attempter, more so if it happened to be a young woman. In one such case, the woman who had attempted suicide refused to talk to us and her family members denied that she had even attempted suicide and glossed it over as an accident. It was only after one of our senior researchers met with and spoke to the family and the girl that she finally agreed to participate in an interview.

Key findings

Attempted pesticide suicides With respect to attempted pesticide suicides at baseline, there were 16 cases in the intervention sites and five in the control sites. At follow-up there were three in the intervention and two in the control sites. The rate of change from baseline to follow-up in the intervention sites was nearly 292/100,000 individuals. In the control sites this was nearly 91/100,000 individuals. The difference in change from intervention to control site for a year was 135/100,000 individuals (95% CI 8.5–260.5; $p < 0.05$).

Completed pesticide suicides With regard to completed pesticide suicides, at baseline there were ten cases in the intervention sites while there were none in the control sites. At follow-up there were two cases in the intervention and two in the control sites. The rates of change from baseline to follow-up in the intervention and control sites were nearly 180/100,000 and −60/100,000 individuals, respectively. The reduction in completed pesticide suicides per year was 160/100,000 individuals (95% CI 98.9–221.7; $p < 0.001$).

Combined attempted and completed pesticide suicides We also analysed attempted and completed pesticide suicides as a combined variable. There were 26 cases in the intervention sites at baseline and five in the control sites. At follow-up there were five in the intervention sites and four in the control sites. The rates of change from baseline to follow-up in the intervention and control sites were 472/100,000 and 30/100,000, respectively. The difference in change when calculated for a year was 295/100,000 individuals (95% CI 154.7–434.8; $p < 0.001$).

All suicides Finally we analysed all suicides which included all means of attempting and completing suicides inclusive of pesticides. There were 33 cases of all suicides in the intervention sites at baseline and ten in the control sites. At follow-up there were five cases of all suicides in the intervention sites and six in the control sites. The rates of change from baseline to follow-up in the intervention and control sites were 630/100,000 and 121/100,000, respectively. The difference in change when calculated for a year was 339/100,000 individuals (95% CI 165.3–513.2; $p < 0.001$) (52).

The rates of change were also calculated based on per protocol analysis. For pesticide suicides the difference in change was 300/100,000 individuals (95% CI 153.0–447.1; $p < 0.01$), while for all suicides it was 334/100,000 individuals (95% CI 146.1–521.0; $p < 0.01$), similar to the rates emerging from the intention to treat (ITT) analyses. The findings emerging from this study may provide useful insights into the effectiveness of these storage boxes in preventing pesticide suicides. The storage facility may have had a role in minimizing suicides in the intervention sites. Important to note was the fact that in all those cases of attempted ($n = 3$) and completed ($n = 2$) suicides that took place in the intervention sites at follow-up, the pesticides had not been stored in the storage facility but had been kept at home.

Strengths and limitations

A key strength of the study was the participatory process of developing the intervention. We conducted focus group discussions (FGDs) before commencement of the community-based intervention. These FGDs provided deep insights into the phenomena of suicides and suicidal behaviour, use of pesticides and peoples awareness of the health risks associated with it, and their attitude towards the idea of a centralized pesticide storage facility. It became evident that in cases where an individual had swallowed pesticides, care was sought from a private medical practitioner and not from a government health care facility. The bureaucratic hassles and delays in care provision, associated with bringing a person who had attempted suicide to a government health facility, acted as a major deterrent. People feared that bringing the victim to a government health facility was as good as signing his/her death warrant. Despite the fact that it involved spending a lot of money, the private doctor was perceived as the only one who could resuscitate the patient. What was equally striking were the reasons that forced individuals to resort to suicide. These ranged from petty quarrels between husbands and wives, parents reprimanding their teenage children, to failure in love and examinations. It was also evident that people had poor understanding of first-aid steps that needed to be taken to help a victim and also had poor knowledge of the health risks associated with pesticide use. Therefore the need to build awareness about safe use of pesticide was perceived to be very important. These findings provided valuable information that informed the development of our intervention and assessments.

A major limitation in our study was, first, that the intervention was only carried out in two villages. A larger number of villages followed up over a longer period of time would be necessary to prove effectiveness. Second, the baseline differences in the incidence of suicides between the intervention and control sites precluded our ability to establish the effectiveness of the storage facility as a pesticide suicide prevention strategy. Third, the follow-up duration of 18 months may not have been adequate to assess the sustainability of the storage facility. Fourth, we observed a 19% loss to follow-up in the control villages due to migration of an entire community who had been residing in those villages. Despite these limitations, our study has provided preliminary findings on the feasibility and acceptability of the storage facility as a probable pesticide suicide prevention strategy. The major strength of the central storage facility lies in its simplicity and cultural acceptability and the fact that it was designed and built through involvement and participation of the community, thereby contributing to its sustainability. Future studies involving larger populations are necessary to assess the effectiveness of such storage facilities in a variety of settings.

Challenges in the field

There were other challenges that the field team faced during the survey. With the villages spread out and with poor transportation facilities, getting from one place to another was both time-consuming and difficult. This became worse during the monsoon when heavy rains rendered many roads unusable. The other problem they faced was getting an eligible adult household member to participate in the interview. The farmers, quite often both the husband and wife, would usually leave for the agricultural fields in the early hours of the morning and return only in the evening. On several occasions the researchers had to travel to these agricultural fields and either schedule a time for the interview in the evening when they returned home or else carry out the interview in the field itself.

Floriculture is both expensive and labour intensive and because of the susceptibility to infestation by pests, major losses can affect farmers engaged in floriculture. Consequently, many farmers had given up flower cultivation in favour of teak. Not engaging in floriculture meant that pesticide use was minimal and therefore these villages could not be included in the randomization process. This posed a major challenge for us and highlights genuine problems such community-based studies face. Often, by the time the study gets all the necessary approvals a substantial period of time lapses, during which many changes tend to occur, which was the case in this study.

Conclusion

There has been an upsurge of knowledge about suicidal behaviour in the last three decades. However, the complexity, variability, and multi-dimensionality of suicide has practical consequences in reducing the burden of suicide. A universally accepted nomenclature for suicidal behaviour which is necessary to further research and interventions remains elusive. Although knowledge about risk factors in the longer term (previous 12 months) is clear, factors or markers for acute risk of suicide (hours to days) is unclear. There is an urgent need to address this gap as it has the potential to reduce suicides. There is also insufficient understanding of the pathway from despair, to suicidal ideation, to impulse, to behaviour.

Although RCTs are recognized as a gold standard, it is difficult to mount a sufficiently powered study on the subject of suicides. The low base rate or incidence of suicide together with a large number of false positives that are predicted on the basis of conventional risk factors imposes clinical and research limitations, particularly in demonstrating the effectiveness of treatment (53). For example, to demonstrate a 15% reduction in suicide among those discharged from psychiatric hospitals where there is a 0.9% suicide in the subsequent year, over 140,000 patients would be required to be studied (54). The sample size required to detect a significant change is thus so large that RCTs with suicide as the outcome tend to become both uneconomical and unfeasible. This is apart from the ethical question of placebo treatment for those who are suicidal and exclusion of high-risk suicidal persons from clinical studies.

Addressing high-risk groups, as in the case of the SUPRE-MISS, nesting suicide prevention strategies in other large-scale prevention efforts such as injury control and violence prevention and primary health care could possibly answer the effectiveness question. Large-scale interventions at the community level and involving collaborators from different settings using the same protocol are other possibilities. The heterogeneity of suicide in different contexts highlights the need for an effective surveillance system to understand the patterns and risk factors in different countries. Routine surveillance systems are required, although challenges exist in their implementation. Underreporting of suicide is common in LAMIC because of cultural norms and at times due to legal barriers surrounding the reporting of suicides. In addition, cultural issues in diagnostic criteria complicate the recoding of suicide.

Suicide in India is a punishable offence under the Indian Penal Code and families fear disclosing information for fear of social stigma and harassment. There is also the fear of protracted legal battles if such cases are reported to the authorities. Consequently, many cases go unreported. Interestingly, none of the suicidal attempts or deaths that had been recorded in the case study from south India had been reflected in the police and official records. Therefore, the need to bring in surveillance strategies as a means of detecting suicide cases has immense value. Not only does it afford a means of identifying attempters, thereby enabling interventions that could perhaps help to save lives, but also it brings us closer to better understanding this complex phenomenon. Policy makers, health care providers, and the public at large have to learn to look upon suicidal behaviour as an emotional and mental health problem, rather than as a criminal offence, as a first and important step towards decriminalizing it.

Another factor to be highlighted is that much of suicide research today has predominantly focused on suicidal attempts and ideation and less on completed suicides. There is thus a need to study the latter phenomenon more closely in large populations from varied cultures, thereby aiding us in developing more effective interventions.

Suicide, being a personal tragedy and a sensitive issue, needs to be dealt with tactfully. Any intervention needs to take into account the local cultural belief systems and work towards acceptability of the interventions. Engagement with local and national level policy makers is critical to the success of these programmes, enabling as it does translation of research into policy and practice. Reducing alcohol availability and consumption, unemployment, poverty, domestic violence, and social inequities, increasing mental health awareness, and improving mental health services are other important issues that need to be addressed in order to reduce suicides. While a multipronged approach addressing these factors would be a necessary long-term strategy, the central storage facility as described in the study from south India, as a medium-term strategy, is likely to be a feasible step for reducing pesticide suicides in developing countries.

Acknowledgements

We acknowledge with grateful thanks the efforts of the study teams from India whose diligent hard work enabled the efficient conduct of the study. We are also deeply grateful to Dr R Thara, Director of the Schizophrenia Research Foundation, who critically reviewed this chapter and provided insightful comments. The valuable funding support provided by the WHO enabled us to carry out these studies, for which we are most grateful. Lastly, we would like to convey our heartfelt thanks to all the men and women from the study areas, whose cooperation and involvement made it possible for us to execute the study.

References

1 Patton GC, Coffey C, Sawyer SM, Viner RM, Haller DM, Bose K, (2009) Global patterns of mortality in young people: a systematic analysis of population health data. Lancet, **374**:881–92.

2 Lozano R, Naghavi M, Foreman K, Lim S, Shibuya K, Aboyans V, et al. (2012) Global and regional mortality from 235 causes of death for 20 year age groups in 1990 and 2010, a systematic analysis for the Global Burden of Disease Study 2010. Lancet, **380**:2095–128.

3 Patel V, Ramasundarahettige C, Vijayakumar L, Thakur JS, Gajalakshmi V, Gururaj G, et al. (2012) Suicide mortality in India; a nationally representative survey. Lancet, **379**(9834):2343–51.

4 Krug EG, Mercy JA, Dahlberg LL, Zwi AB (2002) World report on violence and health. Geneva: WHO.

5 Vijayakumar L, Pirkis J, Whiteford H (2005) Suicide in developing countries: prevention efforts. Crisis, **26**(3):120–4.

6 Chen Y-Y, Wu KC-C, Yousuf S, Yip PS (2012) Suicide in Asia: opportunities and challenges. Epidemiol Rev, **34**:129–44.

7 Eddleston M, Karalliedde L, Buckley N, Fernando R, Hutchinson G, Isbister G, et al. (2002) Pesticide poisoning in the developing worlda minimum pesticides list. Lancet, **360**:1163–7.

8 Hendin H, Phillips MR, Vijayakumar L, Pirkis J, Wang H, Yip P, et al. (2008) Suicide and suicide prevention in Asia. Mental health and substance abuse. Geneva: WHO.

9 Patel V, Araya R, Chatterjee S, Chisholm D, Cohen A, De Silva M, et al. (2007) Treatment and prevention of mental disorders in low-income and middle-income countries. Lancet, **370**:991–1005.

10 Bolton P, Bass J, Neugebauer R, Verdeli H, Clougherty KF, Wickramaratne P, et al. (2003) Group interpersonal psychotherapy for depression in rural Uganda. JAMA, **289**: 3117–24.

11 Patel V, Chisholm D, Rabe-Hesketh S, Dias-Saxena F, Andrew G, Mann A (2003) Efficacy and cost-effectiveness of drug and psychological treatments for common mental disorders in general health care in Goa, India: a randomised controlled trial. Lancet, **361**:33–9.

12 Araya R, Rojas G, Fritsch R, Gaete J, Rojas M, Simon G, et al. (2003) Treating depression in primary care in low-income women in Santiago, Chile: a randomised controlled trial. Lancet, **361**:995–1000.

13 Ali BS, Rahbar MH, Naeem S, Gul A, Mubein S, Iqbal A (2003) The effectiveness of counseling on anxiety and depression by minimally trained counselors: a randomized controlled trial. Am J Psychother, **57**:324–36.

14 Lara M, Navarro C, Rubí N, Mondragón L (2003) Outcome results of two levels of intervention in low-income women with depressive symptoms. Am J Orthopsychiatry, **73**:35–43.

15 Yip PS, Law C-K, Fu K-W, Law Y, Wong PW, Xu Y (2010) Restricting the means of suicide by charcoal burning. Br J Psychiatry, **196**:241–2.

16 Hassanian-Moghaddam H, Sarjami S, Kolahi A-A, Carter GL (2011) Postcards in Persia: randomised controlled trial to reduce suicidal behaviours 12 months after hospital-treated self-poisoning. Br J Psychiatry, **198**:309–16.

17 Marasinghe RB, Edirippulige S, Kavanagh D, Smith A, Jiffry MT (2012) Effect of mobile phone-based psychotherapy in suicide prevention: a randomized controlled trial in Sri Lanka. J Telemed Telecare, **18**:151–5.

18 Meltzer HY, Alphs L, Green AI, Altamura AC, Anand R, Bertoldi A, et al. (2003) Clozapine treatment for suicidality in schizophrenia: international suicide prevention trial (InterSePT). Arch Gen Psychiatry, **60**:82–91.

19 Carter GL, Clover K, Whyte IM, Dawson AH, DEste C (2005) Postcards from the edge project: randomised controlled trial of an intervention using postcards to reduce repetition of hospital treated deliberate self poisoning. BMJ, **331**(7520):805.

20 Motto JA (1976) Suicide prevention for high-risk persons who refuse treatment. Suicide Life Threat Behav, **6**:223–30.

21 Motto JA, Hellbron DC, Juster RP, Bostrom AG (1981) Communication as a suicide prevention program. In: Soubrier JP, Vedrienne J (eds) Depression and suicide. Pergamon, Paris, pp. 143–66.

22 Motto JA, Bostrom AG (2001) A randomized controlled trial of post-crisis suicide prevention. Psychiatr Serv, **52**:828–33.

23 Babor TF, Higgins-Biddle JC (2000) Alcohol screening and brief intervention; dissemination strategies for medical practice and public health. Addiction, **95**:677–86.

24 Babor TF, Higgins-Biddle JC (2001) Brief intervention for hazardous and harmful drinking; a manual for use in primary care. Geneva: WHO.

25 Kerkhof A, Bernasco W, Bille-Brahe U, Platt S, Schmidtke A (1999) European Parasuicide Study Interview Schedule (EPSIS). In: Bille-Brahe U (ed.) Facts and figures: WHO/EURO. Copenhagen: WHO Regional Office for Europe.

26 Beck AT, Schuyler D, Herman I (1974) Development of suicidal intent scales. In: Beck AT, Resnik HLP, Lettieri DJ (eds) The prediction of suicide, pp. 45–56. Bowie: Charles Press.

27 Bec, AT, Steer RA Brown GK (1996) BDI-II, Beck depression inventory: manual, 2nd edn. Boston: Harcourt Brace.

28 Spielberger CD (1988) Professional manual for state trait anger expression inventory. Odessa: Psychological Assessment Resources.

29 WHO (1998) WHO (five) well-being index (1998 version). Geneva: WHO.

30 WHO (1988) WHO psychiatric disability assessment schedule. <http://whqlibdoc.who.int/publications/1988/9241561114.pdf>.

31 Eysenck SBG, Pearson PR, Easting G, Allsopp JF (1985) Age norms for impulsiveness, venturesomeness and empathy in adults. Personality Individual Difference, **6**(5):613–19.

32 Bertolote JM, Fleischmann A, DeLeo D, Phillips M, Botega N, Desilva D, et al. (2005) Characteristics of attempted suicides seen in emergency care settings of general hospitals in eight low and middle income countries. Psychol Med, **35**:1467–74.

33 Fleischmann A, Bertolote JM, Wasserman D, De Leo D, Bolhari J, Botega NJ, et al. (2008) Effectiveness of brief intervention and contact for suicide attempters: a randomized controlled trial in five countries. Bull World Health Organ, **86**(9):703–9.

34 Bertolote JM, Fleischhmann A, Eddelston M, Gunnell D (2006) Death from pesticides poisoning: a global response. Br J Psychiatry, **189**:201–3.

35 Gunnell D, Eddleston M, Phillips MR, Konradsen F (2007) The global distribution of fatal pesticide self-poisoning: systematic review. BMC Public Health, **7**:357.

36 Gross VA, Weiss MG, Ring M, Hepp U, Bopp M, Gutzwiller F, et al. (2008) Methods of suicide: international suicide patterns derived from the WHO mortality database. Bull World Health Organ, **86**:657–736.

37 Gajalakshmi V, Peto R (2007) Suicide rates in rural Tamil Nadu, south India. Verbal autopsy of 39,000 deaths in 1997–8. Int J Epidemiol, **36**:203–7.

38 National Crimes Records Bureau (2011) Suicides in India. In: Accidental death and suicides in India. Ministry of Home Affairs. <http://ncrb.nic.in/CD-ADSI2009/suicides-09.pdf>.

39 Phillips MR, Yang G, Zhang Y, Wang L, Ji, H, Zhou M (2002) Risk factors for suicide in China: a national case-control psychological autopsy study. Lancet, **360**:1728–36.

40 Konradsen F, Van der Hoek W, Peiris P (2006) Reaching for the bottle of pesticidea cry for help. Self-inflicted poisonings in Sri Lanka. Soc Sci Med, **62**:1710–19.

41 Eddleston M, Karalliedde L, Buckley N, Fernando R, Hutchinson G, Isbister G, et al. (2002) Pesticide poisoning in the developing worlda minimum pesticides list. Lancet, **360**:1163–7.

42 Mishara BL (2007) Prevention of deaths from intentional pesticide poisoning. Crisis, **28**(1):10–202.

43 Mann JJ, Apter A, Bertolote J, Beautrais A, Currier D, Haas A, et al. (2005) Suicide prevention strategies: a systematic review. JAMA, **294**(16):2064–74.

44 Manoranjitham S, Abraham S, Jacob KS (2005) Towards a national strategy to reduce suicide in India. Natl Med J India, **18**(3):118–22.

45 Hawton K (2007) Restricting access to methods of suicide: rationale and evaluation of this approach to suicide prevention. Crisis, **28**(1): 4–9.

46 Gunnell D, Fernando R, Hewagama M, Priyangika WD, Konradsen F, Eddleston M (2007) The impact of pesticide regulations on suicide in Sri Lanka. Int J Epidemiol, **36**:1235–42.

47 Hawton K, Ratnayeke L, Simkin S, Harriss L, Scott V (2009) Evaluation of acceptability and use of lockable storage devices for pesticides in Sri Lanka that might assist prevention of self-poisoning. BMC Public Health, **9**:69.

48 Konradsen F, van der Hoek W, Cole DC, Hutchinson G, Daisley H, Singh S, et al. (2003) Reducing acute poisoning in developing countries—options for restricting the availability of pesticides. Toxicology, **192**(23):249–61.

49 Pearson M, Konradsen F, Gunnell D, Dawson AH, Pieris R, Weerasinghe M, et al. A community-based cluster randomised trial of safe storage to reduce pesticide self-poisoning in rural Sri Lankastudy protocol. BMC Public Health, **11**:879.

50 Schmidtke A, Bille-Brahe U, DeLeo D, Kerkhof A, Bjerke T, Crepet P, et al. (1996) Attempted suicide in Europe: rates, trends and sociodemographic characteristics of suicide attempters 1989–92. Results of the WHO/EURO multicentre study on parasuicide. Acta Psychiatr Scand, **93**:327–38.

51 Aaron R, Joseph A, Abraham S, Muliyil J, George K, Prasad J, et al. (2004) Suicides in young people in rural southern India. Lancet, **363**:1117–18.

52 Vijayakumar L, Jeyaseelan L, Kumar S, Mohanraj R, Devika S, Manikandan S (2013) A central storage facility to reduce pesticide suicides—a feasibility study from India. BMC Public Health, **13**:850.

53 Goldney RD (2005) Suicide prevention: a pragmatic review of recent studies. Crisis, **26**(3):128–40.

54 Gunnell D, Frankel S (1994) Prevention of suicide: aspirations and evidence. BMJ, **308**:1227–33.

Part 3

Beyond trials: reducing the mental health treatment gap

Chapter 15

Economic modelling for global mental health

David McDaid

Introduction

A good level of physical and mental health is a key goal in most societies. It must be balanced alongside other priorities such as boosting economic growth, providing high levels of education and good-quality housing, tackling crime, and ensuring good levels of security. Even in the world's wealthiest countries, decision-makers will have to consider how best to make use of the resources that they have to best achieve their intended goals. Choosing how to allocate these resources is never easy. While decision-makers will be interested in receiving rigorous information on the effectiveness, quality, and appropriateness of potential interventions to promote health or any of these other goals, one of the most significant factors in any policy-making process is likely to be an assessment of the costs involved with different policy options and any future return on their investment. A lack of information on the economic benefits of investment is a key barrier to successfully making the case for investment in the development of mental health systems (1–3).

Economic evaluation methods, which synthesize information on the costs and effectiveness of two or more interventions, have long been used to inform policy deliberations in high-income settings (4). Chapter 6 of this book describes the principal types of economic evaluation that may be used. It also highlights the small but growing use of economic evaluation in LAMIC. While many of these studies are conducted alongside controlled trials, modelling studies can also be used to inform decision-making. These modelling techniques are the focus of this chapter.

Models essentially are mathematical frameworks that estimate the consequences of different policy and practice decisions (5). Modelling plays an important role in decision-making in health technology assessment (HTA) processes around the globe that assess the costs and benefits of different technologies (6). In resource-constrained LAMIC contexts, it may be the most practical way of assessing the effectiveness and economic case for investing in innovative packages of care and delivery systems for mental disorders. This information might otherwise be missing from the policy-making process, due to limited opportunities for local controlled trials.

This chapter sets out the case for making use of models, including an acknowledgement of some of the limitations in the evidence generated within clinical trials, before briefly describing the most common alternative types of model. Strengths and limitations of these models are discussed and examples of how they have been used to inform policy-making highlighted. Mechanisms to deal with uncertainty are briefly described. The chapter ends by setting out key steps that should be taken when planning a modelling study and in the presentation of findings.

Why make use of economic models?

There are many different reasons for making use of economic models (Box 15.1). Paramount is the need to reduce any uncertainty about the strength of evidence on the effectiveness and costs of different mental health interventions. Such uncertainty increases the likelihood of making a sub-optimal policy decision. Poor decisions are not without consequence; at best, opportunities to improve health are missed, but in the worst case there may be detrimental impacts. Poor decisions imply a waste of resources on expensive investment in strategies that are inferior to other policy options. Moreover, once these investment decisions are made they may be difficult to reverse. Disinvestment can be politically and practically difficult.

There will always be limitations in relying solely on findings from the results of a single trial—even one that is very well conducted. Issues of external and internal

---

Box 15.1 The role of economic modelling for mental health policy and practice

- Addressing uncertainty in the results of any one clinical trial.
- Synthesizing data from multiple trials on different costs and effects of interventions, often using different head-to-head comparators rather than relying on findings from one trial alone.
- Modelling the costs and effectiveness of different interventions for longer time periods than seen in most clinical trials.
- Modelling potential intervention pathways, and their effectiveness and costs in contexts and settings where local empirical evidence is unavailable.
- Modelling the costs and effectiveness of interventions for specific sub-population groups.
- Modelling the cost-effective implications of differing rates of coverage, uptake, and continued engagement with different interventions.
- Modelling the budgetary impacts of investing in changes to mental health system organization and infrastructure to implement cost-effective interventions.
- Complying with formal requirements for modelling as part of technology appraisal processes in some countries.
- In the absence of definitive empirical studies, helping to prioritize where scare research funds may be invested in empirical trials.

validity of trial findings have been discussed in Chapter 1; there will always be questions about the representativeness of trial populations to real-world settings, and how well results achieved within trial conditions really translate to every-day effectiveness. In HIC, these uncertainties mean that economic models can be a formal requirement in HTA decision-making processes, even when good data are available from economic evaluations conducted alongside clinical trials. While such formal requirements remain rare in LAMIC, examples can be identified in Latin America and Asia (7–9).

Models can help address uncertainty in the generalization of the findings of controlled trials. For instance, models can look at how different assumptions about population characteristics, levels of resource use, unit costs, or effectiveness may impact on cost-effectiveness. Another potential uncertainty concerns the comparator interventions used in clinical trial findings, particularly when the trial has been conducted in a different system or setting to that where an argument for investment is to be made. Are the comparators used in the trial appropriate to the local context? Have the usual alternative treatment options been included? Did the trial look at appropriate combinations of treatments or stepped-care approaches?

One single trial may not always include all relevant alternative approaches, although these may be available in different trials perhaps conducted in different settings. Economic modelling can be used to pool effectiveness estimates of a broader range of interventions from a number of different trials, with various statistical techniques used to adjust for the lack of head-to-head comparison between some of these alternative interventions and the potential new intervention under consideration (5).

Modelling is often the only way of estimating the impacts of an intervention over the mid- to long term. Most trials follow up participants for no more than a few years at best (10). The economic case for investing in a package of care for mental health based solely on the short-term outcomes of a 12-month controlled study may be very different from a study with the same package evaluated over a longer follow-up period (11). Models can extrapolate from trials and other sources of information to provide estimates of longer term cost-effectiveness. They can make different assumptions, for instance on the persistence of effectiveness of any intervention, as well as the need for ongoing or booster treatments. These longer term models can also be designed to take account of the risk of future negative events and patterns of disease progression. In the case of chronic mental disorders this may involve looking at the risk of a relapse or how past suicidal behaviour impacts on the risk of further suicidal events.

Models can also be used to look at the impacts of adapting the evidence on effective interventions for different contexts and settings. The cost and resource use data reported in a trial in one LIC setting may not be representative of current infrastructure, practice, and costs, even in a neighbouring country. The relevance of any estimates of quality of life elicited in a trial may not be easily transferable to other population groups. Existing models can be adapted or new models created, obtaining information on the resources required to deliver the intervention locally, taking account of differences in health care infrastructure and practice. These models could consider the potential health consequences of different service configurations, i.e. in settings where resources are more limited and different clinical pathways are likely to be used.

Models can also be used to estimate the potential cost-effectiveness of modifications to single interventions or packages of care to improve uptake in specific population groups. For instance, they could quantify additional costs required for the provision of peer-led support to encourage contact with mental health services, as well as the potential impact of this additional action on the total number of service contacts. Models might also be used to look at the minimum level of engagement and continued use of an intervention that would be needed for an intervention to be considered cost-effective in every day rather than ideal trial conditions.

In the absence of evidence from trials, models can also be used to help prioritize areas for evaluation or piloting of that intervention. For instance, modelling was used to argue in a UK context that antistigma campaigns, if effective, also had the potential to be cost-effective (12). This type of information can strengthen the merits of empirical studies, especially if findings indicate that only very modest levels of effectiveness need to be achieved in order for the intervention to be considered cost-effective. Modelling techniques can also be used to identify what has been termed the 'expected value of information'; that is, whether the costs of investing in additional research to reduce uncertainty over the effectiveness of an intervention itself represents value for money (13, 14).

What are the main approaches to decision modelling?

The starting point for any potential model is to carefully specify the question to be addressed and the information that will be needed by policy makers to reach a decision. This will usually involve defining the intervention, characteristics of the target population, nature of comparator intervention(s), timeframe to be covered, and the economic perspective to be adopted (typically at a minimum either that of the health system and/or intervention funder, plus in some instance costs to service users and their families, other sectors, including costs in the workplace, and perhaps overall impacts on the economic output of society). Outcome measures may be condition specific or cover all health problems, such as QALYs or DALYs. Outcomes other than health, such as impacts on education, might also be considered. This is followed by conceptual development of the model, ensuring that potential care pathways are appropriate and logical. This usually will be done in partnership with local health system experts. Alternatively, this may be about adapting the structures of an existing model for a different context.

At this stage a decision is then made on what type of modelling technique is best suited to the decision question. This chapter cannot provide detailed information on these modelling techniques, but instead provides an overview of the most common methods, together with some information on their strengths and weaknesses. Three approaches are described: simple decision tree models, cohort and individual level Markov models, and micro-simulation modelling. Most of these models can be built using spreadsheet software packages, but complex models may require high-cost specialist software and hardware. In a later section in this chapter, some of the factors to consider when choosing between modelling approaches are discussed.

Decision tree models

Decision tree models are the most commonly used method for assessing the cost-effectiveness of interventions in HIC (11, 15). However, despite the relatively modest levels of resources and time needed for these models, few examples from LIC settings related to mental health interventions can be identified (16–19).

Figure 15.1 shows a simple decision tree, looking at the merits of a hypothetical community group 'art on prescription' intervention delivered to a hypothetical cohort of 44 UK adults as a frontline intervention in people with mild to moderate depression. It is compared with referral to group-based psychotherapy. The model also assumes that where group art classes do not reduce depression, individuals are also then referred to psychotherapy. The time period covered by this model is very short, being 6 months in total. Costs to health and social care services, as well as the costs of lost employment, are included in the model.

A square decision node at the start of the tree indicates a decision point between two or more alternative options. Intervention pathways can then be developed and validated in consultation with appropriate local mental health professionals and service users, in order to ensure that these indeed represent local care processes. Circular chance nodes on the tree indicate the differing probabilities of following one of two or more alternative pathways.

Information on the probabilities of events occurring has to be estimated at every chance node point in the tree. For instance, in our illustrative model even if an individual is referred to a community group arts programme or psychotherapy, this does not mean that they will actually attend. Estimates for the probability of attendance are often drawn from previous large publications, pilot studies, or observed participation rates in similar types of health schemes. This tree also requires information on the probabilities of recovery from depression following each intervention option, as well as the underlying rate of recovery without use of either intervention. In a situation where no plausible probability estimates can be identified from previous studies, one option is to rely on expert opinion.

Each mutually exclusive pathway or branch of the tree ends with a triangle, which represents a terminal node. Payoffs are associated with each terminal node. In this case they consist of at least one effectiveness outcome, in this case a measure of QALYs gained, but outcomes will vary in models. This could have been DALYs or a measure of depression-free days, etc. Another payoff quantifies the total costs incurred for treatment, other health and social care use, and lost employment. Figure 15.2 shows the payoffs that would be achieved for each pathway when the model is run. If all participate in community group activities and subsequently recovered from moderate depression, then total costs would be £39,858 with 32.03 QALYs gained. Alternatively, if community group activities were not successful, with no-one going on to have psychotherapy and with no recovery, total costs would be £108,630 with 24.51 QALYs gained.

Using all this information on the likelihood of uptake, costs, effectiveness of interventions, impact on health status collated in the model, and expected costs and QALYs gained, expected values for each branch of the tree synthesize the costs and outcomes with the probabilities of following each pathway. For example, the expected costs

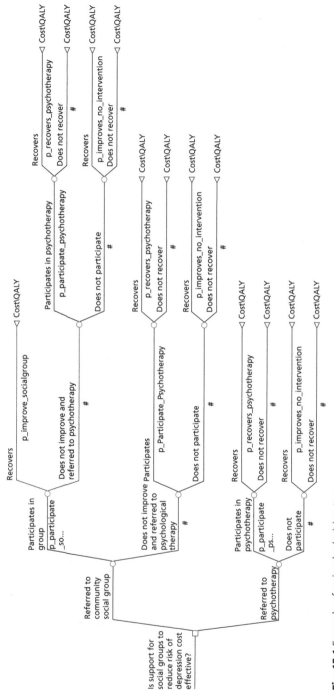

Fig. 15.1 Example of a simple decision tree.

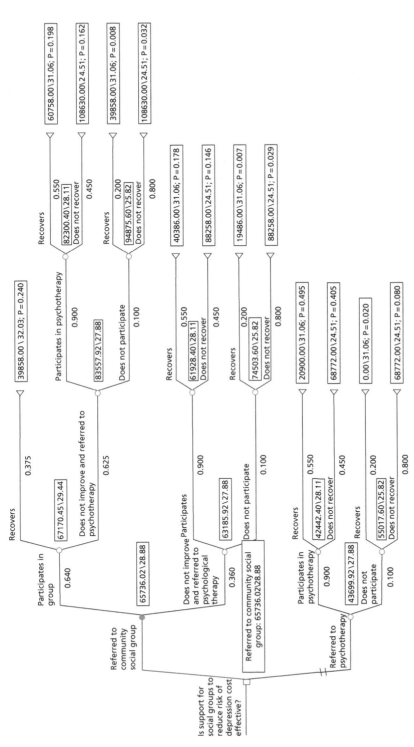

Fig. 15.2 Calculation of costs and health outcomes for a simple decision tree.

of participation in the group arts programme will be £67,170 for an expected 29.44 QALYs. Overall, the expected per person net costs of following the community arts pathway would be £22,000 (£65,700 vs £43,700) greater than those of the psychotherapy pathway for an additional gain of 1 QALY. In an HIC, where costs per QALY gained of around £30,000 are not controversial, this outcome would generally be considered cost-effective.

Cohort and individual level Markov models

Simple decision trees, while providing valuable information to policy makers, are limited in their flexibility. Our hypothetical model in Fig. 15.1 does not, for instance, say anything about the possibility of relapse after a period of recovery from depression. It also says nothing about the persistence of effect from either psychotherapy or group art sessions over the longer term. Markov (or state-transition) modelling can help deal with some of these complexities (20). The approach is common in health economic analysis and has been applied to some mental health interventions in LIC settings (21–23). These models can also be used to help predict patterns of service utilization (24) or to model the course of a disease (25).

Specified periods of time known as Markov cycles are defined, typically being periods of several months or perhaps 1 year. The total number of cycles in the model is also specified—e.g. to cover a 10-year period or the lifetime of the population in the model. Figure 15.3 shows an excerpt from a Markov model. In this excerpt all those

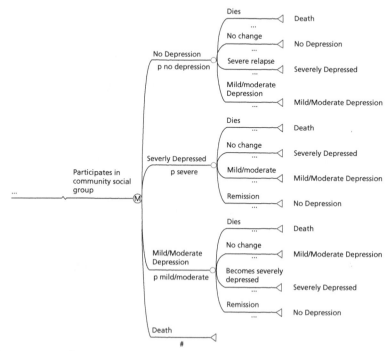

Fig. 15.3 Excerpt from the Markov Model.

who participate in the community group art classes initially are in a state of mild to moderate depression; they then have a probability of remaining in that state, developing severe depression, and moving to remission from depression or dying.

At the end of the next cycle individuals who have not died will again have a probability of remaining in the same state or transitioning to a different state within the next defined Markov cycle. The probability of moving between different states can also be varied as the number of cycles increases, e.g. to perhaps increase the risk of death with advancing age. This process is then repeated until all cycles have been completed or all of the population have entered a terminal state (often death). Overall expected costs and outcomes are calculated by summing up total costs and outcomes from the expected time spent in each health state in all model cycles.

The simplest versions of Markov models will have a hypothetical cohort representing a target population group. Each individual in the cohort is identical, with the same demographic and health characteristics. In many instances this will be fine for modelling purposes, but the 'lack of memory' in Markov models can be problematic. This is because in a cohort-level Markov model the probability of moving between health states at any point in time is not influenced by the past pattern of health states experienced by members of the cohort. For some health problems, including many mental disorders, the risk of relapse or adverse events, e.g. suicidal acts, may be influenced by both the total past number of acute episodes and the time since the last of these events.

One way to overcome this challenge is to construct individual-level (Monte Carlo simulation) Markov models. Literally, these models are run separately for each individual in the target population. This allows for different probabilities of transition between states, reflecting differences in individual characteristics and treatment histories. With this type of model the mean costs and health gains are then estimated after aggregating findings observed for each individual-level model. Expected costs and benefits from different options in the model are then calculated.

Micro-simulation models

Another approach to modelling is to use more complex micro-simulation models (26). Unlike a Markov model, there is no series of regular cycles where individuals have a probability of being in different health states. Instead, in these models individuals move along the model pathway, experiencing changes in health status, such as recurrence of depression, at varying points in time after the previous event. The simulation model then considers the likelihood of a further event and when this is likely to occur.

Variants on these simulation models can also be used to look at the economic challenges related to implementation and scale-up, as well as assess the case for packages of mental health-related interventions. Like previous models they can also be adjusted to take account of issues such as uptake, but have the advantage of being able to take account of structural issues in health systems, which may, for instance, impact on the level of coverage and/or access to services in a country.

These models need a great deal of data and can take a long time to build and run. They often make use of specific software programs or add-on to spread sheets. In the case of depression, in order to accurately model the probability of moving between different health states, information would be needed on the risk of recurrence of depression relative to the amount of time since an individual has been in remission from depression. Detailed information would also have to be collected on resources in terms of personnel, equipment, and buildings, etc. needed to deliver interventions. Even more sophisticated models might include transition probabilities for the onset/recurrence of illness linked to changes in socioeconomic circumstances, the presence of physical illness, and interactions between individuals, etc.

Simulation modelling has been used by the WHO as part of its CHOICE programme to look at the cost-effectiveness of different packages of interventions for different mental health problems for the 17 sub-regions or geographical clusters of countries that are members of the WHO (27). Because CHOICE has largely been conducted at a pan-national level, all interventions have been modelled against a do-nothing option, negating the need to identify available infrastructure and treatment pathways in any country, although budgetary constraints are used to determine the types of intervention that could be made available in different countries.

To date, WHO CHOICE has relied on information from the Global Burden of Disease Study on the incidence, prevalence, remission, and case-fatality of different mental disorders. The lack of published data on resource use in LIC settings led the CHOICE programme to initially obtain estimates through a Delphi process involving more than 60 mental health professionals in LIC settings (28). The impact of interventions on health status is modelled and compared with impacts on health status if the mental disorder in question follows its natural course without intervention. As with Markov models, the costs of treatment and the cost-consequences of being in different health states are aggregated over the lifetime of the model. In CHOICE models, outcomes are expressed in terms of DALYs, with costs (to the health care system only) adjusted to take account of differences in purchasing power and expressed in international dollars.

This use of simulation modelling in the CHOICE programme has certainly raised awareness across the globe that even in the most resource-poor region of the world, cost-effective packages of mental health care are available (29). The relative cost-effectiveness of interventions for different mental disorders can be compared—these can, for instance, highlight that for people with schizophrenia or bipolar disorder in sub-Saharan Africa, a package of community outpatient care, older generation psychotropics, and psychosocial care is far more cost-effective and less costly than relying on inpatient care using the latest antipsychotics (29).

While the economic information from CHOICE is powerful, it can be even more powerful if country-specific simulation models can be constructed. In Nigeria, for example, modelling was used to identify a package of interventions for a number of conditions: epilepsy, schizophrenia, depression, and hazardous alcohol use. (30). CHOICE model regional data were replaced, wherever possible, by Nigerian-specific parameters and assumptions. Using the model, a package of actions costing less than $320 per DALY avoided was identified. This would be cost-effective in a Nigerian context. The analysis also highlighted important differences in the cost-effectiveness of some interventions compared with the regional estimates, due to substantive difference in local unit costs for some drug therapies.

One challenge is that this process of adaptation requires some collaboration between the authors of the regional model and country partners; this may limit the number of country-specific models in development at any one time. The limits in expertise and resources for modelling in many LAMIC are another barrier to country-specific models.

How can models deal with uncertainty?

Sensitivity analysis can be conducted with all of these models to deal with uncertainty in the underlying evidence base from clinical trials and other studies, in model parameters, and in population characteristics. The simplest types of deterministic sensitivity analysis allow the values of one or more of the input parameters in these models to be varied independently or in combination. For instance, the probability of an intervention being effective, the level of change in quality of life scores, and the costs/incidence of adverse events might be changed between high and low values and the change in cost-effectiveness ratios presented. The lower the change in any cost-effectiveness findings in these sensitivity analyses, the more confidence decision-makers can have in the findings.

Threshold analysis can also be used to identify the minimum level of effectiveness or population uptake that would need to be achieved in order for the intervention to be considered cost-effective. For instance, this might be the minimum level of participation by the target population group or minimum level of recovery that must be achieved. If these threshold values are low, then even with uncertainty in the model this will mean that in the majority of scenarios the intervention is likely to be cost-effective, which may be helpful in policy-making deliberations.

Probabilistic sensitivity analysis should also be used (31). As well as uncertainty on model parameters, there can be uncertainty over the representativeness of populations, in both models and trials. This can be overcome by repeated random sampling (typically several thousand times) of members of the population and recording the impact on cost-effectiveness results observed (32). The values of input parameters used in models could also be randomly sampled within parameter distribution confidence intervals to similarly produce a distribution of cost-effectiveness results. These techniques can be combined to further explore the distribution of uncertainty around baseline cost-effectiveness results. These distributions can be visually plotted as cost-effectiveness acceptability curves, illustrating the likelihood that the intervention will be cost-effective at different societal levels of the willingness to pay for health shown (33).

In the interests of transparency when undertaking any sensitivity analysis, or looking at the results of a sensitivity analysis, a justification should be provided for any assumptions made over the distribution of variance in estimates of baseline parameter values—in some cases they may be normally distributed, but other distribution patterns may be more likely and should be reflected in sensitivity analysis. Justifications should also be provided for any change in model parameters when adapting a model to a different local context.

What should be considered when adapting existing models?

It may be the case that a model already exists and needs its structure and input parameters adapting to a different context. Example of this includes adaptation of a decision tree model looking at drug therapies for the treatment of major depression in Canada (34) to the Brazilian context (17), as well as tailoring mental health models in the CHOICE programme to country-specific contexts (30, 35). When adapting models it is important to discuss with service planners, service users, and others, whether interventions are appropriate and acceptable. Would the intervention need adaptation in order to help encourage the target population to make use of the service and what would the resource implications be of this adaptation? Is there any evidence on the effectiveness of the intervention from trials in a similar LIC setting rather than an HIC? What are the resource implications and unit costs in this setting? Is the comparator appropriate or should a different alternative treatment pathway be used? What about infrastructure? It may be the case that resources and skills are so scarce that no intervention is currently provided, in which case a 'do nothing' alternative might be modelled. The appropriate cost-effectiveness threshold will also need adaptation to local circumstances; for instance, using some ratio between GDP per capita per year and years of good-quality life gained (36).

What modelling approach should be used?

This chapter has demonstrated that economic models come in different formats, which involve different levels of complexity and time to develop. So which approach should be used to strengthen the evidence base? Well, this should be led very much by the decision problem under consideration, the ability of different models to address this problem, and the timeframe and resources available to undertake this work (37).

Decision tree or Markov models should be perfectly suitable for many decision problems. In fact, for many models comparing a few specific interventions, the difference in the conclusions of decision tree, Markov, and simulation models may be modest (26). Decision trees can be constructed relatively quickly or adapted from existing models, but still make use of sophisticated sensitivity analysis to deal with many aspects of uncertainty. They do not require investment in expensive computing equipment or in the development of bespoke software, but quickly become unwieldy when considering more than five or six different strategies or population groups.

Markov modelling, often embedded into a simple decision tree, can ensure that the long-term impacts of mental health interventions are assessed. Most Markov studies tend to use a hypothetical identical population cohort; if time allows, individual-level Markov modelling can be used to take account of how differences in personal characteristics and patterns of illness may impact on outcomes. Existing service user administrative data sets might be a source of individual characteristics in some settings. Running complex sensitivity analysis is more complex as ideally model parameters have to be varied for each individual-level model run. While cumbersome, this is becoming less of an issue as access to fast computer processors increases.

Well-conducted macro-simulation modelling can have additional value to policy makers. Complex simulations can take account of many more factors that influence outcomes compared to decision tree and Markov models. They can also more easily look at the impacts of changes in uptake in the use of multiple interventions or different packages of interventions by a population; the costs and time needed to scale up existing interventions can also be modelled.

However, macro-simulation models are unlikely to be suitable when there are time pressures on producing evidence to inform policy making. It can take a team of researchers many months to build and test these models from scratch. Sourcing the data for these models is also more time-consuming, as many individual probabilities on transitions between health states are needed. These models require a large amount of computational power; it is not untypical for some complex simulation models covering national populations, with many different possible health state transitions, to take many days to run, even when using powerful mainframe computers. From a practical point of view, debugging these models and making sure that they are error free can also become a frustrating and time-consuming process.

It is not surprising therefore that macro-simulation modelling remains uncommon, or restricted to relatively narrow decision problems. However, when it comes to global mental health it is possible to build on mental health simulation models that have already been constructed as part of the ongoing WHO CHOICE programme. These models have already been successfully adapted to better reflect the situation at country level for some mental disorders, e.g. in Chile, Nigeria, and Sri Lanka (30, 35); providing more country-specific recommendations on packages of care taking the CHOICE model as a starting point could be invaluable to facilitating more investment in mental health.

The importance of transparency

This chapter has indicated many ways in which models can be used to complement evidence from clinical trials and strengthen the evidence base for global mental health. Modelling can be very powerful; demonstrating that highly cost-effective interventions for mental health are available can play an important role in the planning of mental health services across the globe. With models, an economic case for action can be built rapidly, whereas evidence from a local trial may take several years to come to fruition. This is not always about developing new models, but also about adapting existing models to LAMIC settings. Furthermore, models can act as a catalyst for empirical studies to help reduce uncertainty and strengthen the local evidence base.

One recent review for depression reported a wide variety of model structures, modelling techniques, time horizons, and sources of data being used (11). Transparency in model structures, sources of evidence, limitations, and the reporting of results is therefore critical if they are to be seen as a credible source of information for the decision-making process (38, 39). It is important to provide a rationale for use of a model, crucially including the justification for the time horizon adopted. Given that many mental health problems may be chronic but episodic in nature, any model that focuses on short-term outcomes only may be questionable and lead to erroneous conclusions being reached. A highly effective treatment might appear cost-effective in the long term, but not in the short term (11).

Guidance and checklists are available to help promote better standards in model design and reporting (25, 40, 41). This, for instance, should indicate how relevant data taken from trials to the local context are, and to what extent they have been adjusted to take account of the likely difference in effectiveness seen in controlled trials and everyday practice. Where expert opinion has been used for the model, it should state any potential conflicts of interest. How, for instance, have models taken account of the risk of adverse events or relapse? These have been included and reported very inconsistently in economic evaluations (42). In the case of depression, for example, the cost-effectiveness of different interventions may be very different if models do or do not include risks of relapse or risk of suicidal events (11, 43).

It is much better to highlight caution and the level of uncertainty in model findings rather than gloss over limitations. Policy makers need to have confidence in the strengths and weaknesses of model findings when referring to model results in their deliberations. Take, for instance, one example from England where simple decision trees and Markov models have been used to rapidly model the economic case for investing in 15 mental health promotion and mental disorder prevention interventions to inform national mental health policy (44). Care was taken not to model interventions without reasonable evidence from trials of effectiveness; but short-, mid-, and long-term economic impacts were modelled where the data allowed. Limitations in modelling methods and assumptions used were highlighted. Assumptions about effectiveness and cost consequences were conservative and subject to a range of sensitivity analyses. Notwithstanding these caveats, the economic models were cited heavily in an official economic assessment of the new mental health strategy (45).

Conclusion

In summary, modelling should not be seen as an alternative to undertaking controlled trials; rather it is a complement. Information from RCTs will inform models, while information from models can be used to identify potentially attractive areas for further empirical research. There are clearly trade-offs between investing in highly complex models that more accurately reflect real-world situations against the need for time-critical, policy-relevant information and the level of resources available for modelling.

Ultimately in respect of global mental health, where evidence from RCTs conducted in low-income settings is still sparse, the advantages of producing economic models, erring on the side of caution in terms of their effectiveness and costs, undertaking a wide range of sensitivity analyses, and being transparent about their strengths and limitations, are likely to far outweigh any disadvantages of their simplicity.

References

1 McDaid D, Knapp M, Raja S (2008) Barriers in the mind: promoting an economic case for mental health in low- and middle-income countries. World Psychiatry, 7(2):79–86.

2 Saxena S, Thornicroft G, Knapp M, Whiteford H (2007) Resources for mental health: scarcity, inequity, and inefficiency. Lancet, 370(9590):878–89.

3 Jenkins R, Baingana F, Ahmad R, McDaid D, Atun R (2011) Social, economic, human rights and political challenges to global mental health. Mental Health Family Med, **8**(2):87–96.

4 Maynard A, McDaid D (2003) Evaluating health interventions: exploiting the potential. Health Policy, **63**(2):215–26.

5 Briggs A, Sculpher M, Claxton K (2006) Decision modelling for health economic evaluation. Oxford: Oxford University Press.

6 Buxton MJ, Drummond MF, Van Hout BA, Prince RL, Sheldon TA, Szucs T, et al. (1997) Modelling in economic evaluation: an unavoidable fact of life. Health Econ, **6**(3):217–27.

7 Attieh R, Gagnon MP (2012) Implementation of local/hospital-based health technology assessment initiatives in low- and middle-income countries. Int J Technol Assess Health Care, **28**(4):445–51.

8 Cruz L, Lima AF, Graeff-Martins A, Maia CR, Ziegelmann P, Miguel S, et al. (2013) Mental health economics: insights from Brazil. J Mental Health, **22**(2):111–21.

9 Oortwijn W, Mathijssen J, Banta D (2010) The role of health technology assessment on pharmaceutical reimbursement in selected middle-income countries. Health Policy, **95**(2–3):174–84.

10 Hodgson R, Bushe C, Hunter R (2007) Measurement of long-term outcomes in observational and randomised controlled trials. British J Psychiatry Suppl, **50**:s78–84.

11 Haji Ali Afzali H, Karnon J, Gray J (2012) A critical review of model-based economic studies of depression: modelling techniques, model structure and data sources. PharmacoEconomics, **30**(6):461–82.

12 McCrone P, Knapp M, Henri M, McDaid D (2010) The economic impact of initiatives to reduce stigma: demonstration of a modelling approach. Epidemiol Psichiatria Sociale, **19**(2):131–9.

13 Claxton KP, Sculpher MJ (2006) Using value of information analysis to prioritise health research: some lessons from recent UK experience. PharmacoEconomics, **24**(11):1055–68.

14 Fenwick E, Claxton K, Sculpher M (2008) The value of implementation and the value of information: combined and uneven development. Med Decis Making, **28**(1):21–32.

15 Zimovetz EA, Wolowacz SE, Classi PM, Birt J (2012) Methodologies used in cost-effectiveness models for evaluating treatments in major depressive disorder: a systematic review. Cost Effect Resource Alloc, **10**(1):1.

16 Kongsakon R, Bunchapattanasakda C (2008) The treatment of major depressive disorders (MDD) in Thailand using escitalopram compared to fluoxetine and venlafaxine: a pharmacoeconomic evaluation. Chotmaihet Thangphaet, **91**(7):1117–28.

17 Machado M, Iskedjian M, Ruiz IA, Einarson TR (2007) The economic impact of introducing serotonin-noradrenaline reuptake inhibitors into the Brazilian national drug formulary: cost-effectiveness and budget-impact analyses. PharmacoEconomics, **25**(11):979–90.

18 Machado M, Lopera MM, Diaz-Rojas J, Jaramillo LE, Einarson TR (2008) Pharmacoeconomics of antidepressants in moderate-to-severe depressive disorder in Colombia. Rev Panam Salud Publica, **24**(4):233–9.

19 Yang L, Li M, Tao LB, Zhang M, Nicholl MD, Dong P (2009) Cost-effectiveness of long-acting risperidone injection versus alternative atypical antipsychotic agents in patients with schizophrenia in China. Value Health, **12**(3):S66–9.

20 Sun X, Faunce T (2008) Decision-analytical modelling in health-care economic evaluations. Eur J Health Econ, **9**(4):313–23.

21 Siskind D, Araya R, Kim J (2010) Cost-effectiveness of improved primary care treatment of depression in women in Chile. British J Psychiatry, **197**(4):291–6.

22 Siskind D, Baingana F, Kim J (2008) Cost-effectiveness of group psychotherapy for depression in Uganda. Journal Mental Health Policy Econ, **11**(3):127–33.

23 Lindner LM, Marasciulo AC, Farias MR, Grohs GE (2009) Economic evaluation of antipsychotic drugs for schizophrenia treatment within the Brazilian Healthcare System. Rev Saude Publica, **43**(1):62–9.

24 Fisher DL, Knesper DJ (1983) Markov models and the utilization of mental health services: a study of endogenously depressed patients. Socio-econ Plan Sci, **17**(1):21–31.

25 Caro JJ, Briggs AH, Siebert U, Kuntz KM (2012) Modeling good research practices—overview: a report of the ISPOR-SMDM Modeling Good Research Practices Task Force-1. Med Decis Making, **32**(5):667–77.

26 Karnon J (2003) Alternative decision modelling techniques for the evaluation of health care technologies: Markov processes versus discrete event simulation. Health Econ, **12**(10):837–48.

27 Chisholm D (2005) Choosing cost-effective interventions in psychiatry: results from the CHOICE programme of the World Health Organization. World Psychiatry, **4**(1):37–44.

28 Ferri C, Chisholm D, Van Ommeren M, Prince M (2004) Resource utilisation for neuropsychiatric disorders in developing countries: a multinational Delphi consensus study. Soc Psychiatry Psychiatr Epidemiol, **39**(3):218–27.

29 Chisholm D, Saxena S (2012) Cost effectiveness of strategies to combat neuropsychiatric conditions in sub-Saharan Africa and South East Asia: mathematical modelling study. BMJ, **344**:e609.

30 Gureje O, Chisholm D, Kola L, Lasebikan V, Saxena S (2007) Cost-effectiveness of an essential mental health intervention package in Nigeria. World Psychiatry, **6**(1):42–8.

31 Briggs AH, Weinstein MC, Fenwick EA, Karnon J, Sculpher MJ, Paltiel AD (2012) Model parameter estimation and uncertainty analysis: a report of the ISPOR-SMDM Modeling Good Research Practices Task Force Working Group-6. Med Decis Making, **32**(5):722–32.

32 Hunink MG, Bult JR, de Vries J, Weinstein MC (1998) Uncertainty in decision models analyzing cost-effectiveness: the joint distribution of incremental costs and effectiveness evaluated with a nonparametric bootstrap method. Med Decis Making, **18**(3):337–46.

33 Barton GR, Briggs AH, Fenwick EA (2008) Optimal cost-effectiveness decisions: the role of the cost-effectiveness acceptability curve (CEAC), the cost-effectiveness acceptability frontier (CEAF), and the expected value of perfection information (EVPI). Value Health, **11**(5):886–97.

34 Einarson TR, Addis A, Iskedjian M (1997) Pharmacoeconomic analysis of venlafaxine in the treatment of major depressive disorder. PharmacoEconomics, **12**(2 Pt 2):286–96.

35 Chisholm D, Gureje O, Saldivia S, Calderon MV, Wickremasinghe R, Mendis N, et al. (2008) Schizophrenia treatment in the developing world: an interregional and multinational cost-effectiveness analysis. Bull World Health Organ, **86**(7):542–51.

36 Shillcutt SD, Walker DG, Goodman CA, Mills AJ (2009) Cost-effectiveness in low- and middle-income countries: a review of the debates surrounding decision rules. Pharmaco-Economics, **27**(11):903–17.

37 Barton P, Bryan S, Robinson S (2004) Modelling in the economic evaluation of health care: selecting the appropriate approach. J Health Services Research Policy, **9**(2):110–18.

38 Eddy DM, Hollingworth W, Caro JJ, Tsevat J, McDonald KM, Wong JB (2012) Model transparency and validation: a report of the ISPOR-SMDM Modeling Good Research Practices Task Force-7. Med Decis Making, **32**(5):733–43.

39 Watkins JB (2012) Creating models that meet decision makers' needs: a US payer perspective. Value Health, **15**(6):792–3.

40 Evers S, Goossens M, de Vet H, van Tulder M, Ament A (2005) Criteria list for assessment of methodological quality of economic evaluations: consensus on health economic criteria. Int J Technol Assess Health Care, **21**(2):240–5.

41 Husereau D, Drummond M, Petrou S, Carswell C, Moher D, Greenberg D, et al. (2013) Consolidated Health Economic Evaluation Reporting Standards (CHEERS) statement. BMJ, **346**:f1049.

42 Craig D, McDaid C, Fonseca T, Stock C, Duffy S, Woolacott N (2010) Are adverse effects incorporated in economic models? A survey of current practice. Int J Technol Assess Health Care, **26**(3):323–9.

43 Haji Ali Afzali H, Karnon J, Gray J (2012) A proposed model for economic evaluations of major depressive disorder. Eur J Health Econ, **13**(4):501–10.

44 Knapp M, McDaid D, Parsonage M (eds) (2011) Mental health promotion and mental illness prevention: the economic case. London: Department of Health.

45 Department of Health (2011) No health without mental health: a cross-government mental health outcomes strategy for people of all ages. Supporting document—the economic case for improving efficiency and quality in mental health. London: Department of Health.

Chapter 16

Evaluation of interventions in the real world

Mary J. De Silva, Alex Cohen, and Vikram Patel

Introduction

The preceding chapters in this book have described the conduct of RCTs to evaluate the efficacy and effectiveness of mental health interventions for specific mental disorders in a variety of settings. These trials generate evidence of what works in relatively controlled or ideal conditions. Nevertheless, the goal of these trials is to generate knowledge which can be implemented in the 'real world'. The 'real world', however, is a messier place in many ways: interventions are less well circumscribed, patient populations are more difficult to precisely define, co-morbidities between mental disorders and physical disorders are common, attention to delivery of the intervention is less well structured, and, perhaps most importantly, there may be practical and ethical concerns regarding randomization when the interventions proposed are already 'evidence-based'. Knowing that the effect of interventions in the real world may be different from, and most likely much smaller than, the effect sizes reported in trials, it is essential that we evaluate their implementation and effect when they are 'scaled-up' as real programmes. The evaluation of scaled-up health programmes typically involves the use of multiple methods which are triangulated to address the key questions of the programme leaders or investigators. This chapter aims to describe what outcomes we might be interested in evaluating and the methods we might use to assess these outcomes, and presents selected case studies which demonstrate these methods in action.

What to evaluate

The OECD's Health Care Quality Indicators Project (HCQI) framework (1) provides a useful framework to determine which aspects of a programme need to be evaluated to determine its impact. The HCQI framework identifies three core dimensions of health care system performance which can be assessed at the level of a health care programme: quality, access, and cost/expenditure. Evaluating these three domains will answer the following questions: what is the level of quality of care across the range of patient care needs, who uses the programme and does it cover those people in need in services, and what does this performance cost? We will cover each of these domains in turn. It should be noted that broader social, political, economic, and cultural factors may affect the outcome and impact of any given mental health programme. The most powerful programme evaluations include an assessment of these contextual factors in their methodology.

Quality of care

The HCQI framework defines three dimensions within quality of care: effectiveness, safety, and responsiveness/patient centredness (1).

- *Effectiveness* is perhaps the most important performance dimension. Effectiveness is defined as the extent to which attainable improvements in health are actually attained (2) and is most often measured by the change in patient clinical (and less often functioning, quality of life, and economic) outcomes as a result of being treated by the programme. The notion of effectiveness can be linked with that of access to services to evaluate effective coverage. In order to evaluate the effect of treatment on patient outcomes, the process of care must also be evaluated. This comprises collecting process indicators such as: which interventions were delivered to which types of patients, how well these interventions were administered, and the extent to which patients were willing and able to take advantage of the available interventions.

- *Safety* is the extent to which the programme prevents or avoids any potential adverse outcomes as a result of the interventions it provides. It is therefore closely linked to effectiveness, for to produce measurable improvements in patient outcomes, the programme must also be safe for patients and avoid adverse outcomes. For mental health programmes, serious adverse events include: deleterious side-effects from psychotropic medication, increased risk of suicide, and premature mortality from other causes.

- *Responsiveness*, or patient-centredness, refers to how well a programme meets the needs of patients by placing their needs at the centre of the delivery of health care (1). It is measured by patients' reports of their experience of the care provided by the programme, going beyond issues of general satisfaction with the service (1). Continuity of care can also be considered as another dimension of responsiveness, assessing the extent to which care is coordinated across time and across providers (for example, process indicators such as how well referral systems work, and the extent to which medication is continuously supplied). Patient-centredness can also encompass an assessment of timeliness, defined as the degree to which patients are able to obtain care promptly, and to move through the care pathway in a timely manner (3).

Access to care

The second broad domain listed in the HCQI framework is access to the programme. The evaluation of access can be conceptualized as the coverage of a programme, defined as the extent to which those in need of a health intervention get it. Individuals in need of a specific health service pass through a number of stages before they can receive the full therapeutic benefit of an intervention (4). Specifically, the intervention needs to be (1) physically available (services exist); (2) financially and geographically accessible (services are affordable and located where people can use them); (3) acceptable (people want to use, and are satisfied with the quality of, the services); (4) used (people actually use the services); and (5) delivered appropriately and effectively so that people are able to receive the expected health benefit from the services. Accessibility also includes notions of equity, in that services are equally accessible to those who could benefit from the service, irrespective of their age, gender, socioeconomic, or ethnic group, or other indicators of equity.

Even if physical availability or *potential* coverage is 100%, each of the subsequent filters could easily reduce the preceding ratio by a third, resulting in a final or *effective* coverage of only 20%. Such approaches have been used to assess the coverage of interventions in other areas of health care, for example the coverage of mosquito nets (5) and malaria treatment (6).

The five levels of service coverage developed by Tanahashi (4) provide a useful conceptual framework for understanding programme coverage (Fig. 16.1 lists the five levels of coverage and provides examples of how each level can be measured). The first three levels address the *potential* coverage of a programme, comprising the availability of a service, how accessible it is, and how acceptable the treatment provided is.

For *service availability* (level 1), a range of tools have been developed and applied in a number of different country contexts for the purpose of comparing the structure, range, and supply of specialist adult mental health services in a catchment area. Examples of these at a national level are the WHO Project ATLAS (7) and the WHO AIMS instrument which collects detailed information about the mental health system of a country (8). However, these methods have rarely been applied at a programme level.

Service accessibility (level 2) is also measured at the health system rather than the individual level and requires a separate set of evaluation methods, including national-level monitoring and evaluation (M&E) systems (e.g. (10)) and targeted surveys

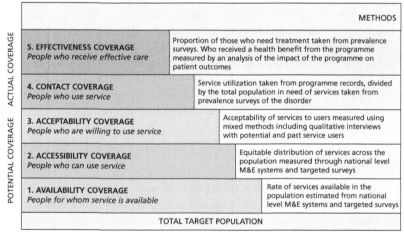

Fig. 16.1 Levels of programme coverage. (Reproduced from (9), originally adapted from (4). Figure reproduced with permission from De Silva M J, Lee L, Fuhr D, Rathod S, Chisholm D, Schellenberg J, et al. Estimating the coverage of mental health programmes: a systematic review. *International Journal of Epidemiology*. In press, originally adapted from Tanahashi T. Health service coverage and its evaluation. *Bulletin of the World Health Organization*, 1978; 56(2):295–303)

(e.g. using the WHO AIMS instrument (8)) to assess how accessible mental health services are to the population in domains such as geographical distribution of services and financial affordability. However, as these methods involve the collection of national level data rather than assessing individual programmes, they can only provide an overview of the geographical distribution of services. For more accurate programme level measures of accessibility, data need to be collected through situation analyses at the level of defined populations (e.g. a district).

Acceptability of the services to potential and actual services users (level 3) is most often measured through mixed methods, including qualitative interviews with service users.

These three types of coverage do not in themselves capture the concept of contact or effective coverage as they are preconditions of coverage rather than coverage itself. Levels 4 and 5 of the Tanahashi framework (4) measure *actual* rather than potential coverage, and are the critical domains for evaluating programme coverage.

Contact coverage: this corresponds to level 4 of the Tanahashi framework and captures the proportion of persons in need of a service (e.g. the number of cases with a diagnosable disorder such as schizophrenia or depression) who receive an intervention that is appropriate to their condition. It is calculated as the ratio between the numerator of those receiving services and the denominator of those estimated to need those services in the population. Contact coverage also includes equitable coverage which assesses whether the service covers different sociodemographic or other groups equitably.

Effective coverage: this corresponds to level 5 and has been defined as 'the probability that individuals will receive health gain from an intervention if they need it' (11). Effective coverage links the three concepts of need, utilization of services, and quality of care received, including issues of therapeutic response as well as provider and patient adherence (12). Effective coverage therefore places intervention-specific coverage within a health system constraints perspective. Effective coverage is calculated by assessing the proportion of those in need of a service who receive the intended health benefit from that service. It therefore combines measures of intervention effectiveness (also defined as quality of care), measured by tracking changes in patient clinical outcomes over the course of treatment, with measures of contact coverage.

A systematic review of all mental health programmes that had evaluated programme contact or effectiveness coverage found only seven studies globally (9). However, clear methods of how to measure programme coverage emerged from the review. Case study 1 presents an overview of the Increased Access to Psychological Therapies (IAPT) programme in England, an excellent example of how a programme can routinely evaluate the contact and effectiveness coverage of a national-level mental health programme. However, as shown by the systematic review (9), such evaluations are extremely rare.

This lack of evidence is partly due to the methodological difficulties of estimating contact coverage. To estimate the denominator of the population in need of services in a catchment area, estimates of the prevalence of the disorder in the catchment population are needed. Collecting this information is beyond the scope of individual programmes, so routine data need to be utilized. In HIC, prevalence data may be available through routine national surveys such as the Adult Psychiatric Morbidity Survey in England (13) and the national Survey of Mental Health and Wellbeing in Australia (14). In settings where national- or regional-level survey data are not available, reference can be made to the estimated prevalence of mental disorders in the scientific literature, for example in the World Mental Health Surveys (15) and the national prevalence rates for different disorders calculated as part of the Global Burden of Disease Study 2010 (16). However, prevalence data are patchy, with more complete prevalence data for North America and Australia, highly variable data from Europe, Latin America, and Asia Pacific, and poor levels of data in other regions of Africa and Asia (17).

In addition, the prevalence estimates that do exist are often for specific regions of a country, sub-groups of the population, or for specific disorders, and may not represent the population or disorders that a specific programme seeks to serve. If no such prevalence estimates exist, then the number treated can be compared to the total population size to provide a ratio of the number treated per 100,000, which remains an informative metric for planning services, tracking changes in service utilization over time, and comparing programme coverage to other non-mental health programmes, though they cannot provide an estimate of the proportion of those in need who are receiving services.

Better estimates of programme contact and effective coverage, the equity of that coverage, and the factors that affect coverage are needed to ensure that there is optimal investment of scarce resources into existing programmes, and that new mental health services are designed to optimize the effective and equitable programme coverage of those in greatest need.

Case study 1: evaluation of the IAPT programme in England

Evidence base

Since 2004, the National Institute of Clinical Excellence (NICE) in England reviews of the evidence base from trials evaluating the effectiveness of a variety of interventions for depression and anxiety disorders have led to clear guidelines for the recommended use of certain psychological therapies. This evidence base was cited by economists and researchers to argue that increasing access to psychological therapies would largely pay for itself through a reduction in public costs, including welfare benefits and costs to the UK National Health Service (NHS), and through an increase in revenues from people being able to return to work, resulting in increased productivity and tax revenue (18). In 2006 these developments resulted in a political commitment to increase access to evidence-based psychological therapies through the NHS across England (19).

Programme description

The IAPT programme is a large-scale national initiative that aims to greatly increase the availability of psychological treatments for depression and anxiety disorders within

NHS-commissioned services in England. After successful pilots during which many lessons for widespread implementation were learnt (19), a national phased roll-out started in 2008. Since then, the IAPT programme has trained over 3600 new therapists, with a further 2400 to be trained by 2014, and by 2012 had provided access to psychological therapies for more than 1.1 million people (20).

Evaluation methodology

A comprehensive M&E system is core to the IAPT model. The system collects session-by-session performance data on service access, treatment provision, and routine patient-reported outcomes recorded using validated symptom scales (the Patient Health Questionnaire-9 (PHQ-9) for depression (21) and Generalized Anxiety Disorder 7-item (GAD-7) for anxiety disorders (22)). These data are collated nationally and analysed as part of routine programme evaluation to provide critical data for service improvement and to advocate for further scaling up of the programme.

Results

Contact coverage is evaluated by taking the number of patients treated by the programme, taken from the M&E system, and dividing it by the national prevalence of depressive and anxiety disorders derived from the Adult Psychiatric Morbidity Survey (13). The IAPT programme has set a target of reaching 15% of the population with these disorders by 2015, based on assumptions relating to the number of people with depression and/or anxiety who will seek treatment, the number of those who will receive a diagnosis of depression/anxiety, and the number of those who will opt for psychological therapy. Since the programme started in 2008, average access rates have increased annually, treating over 1.1 million people by 2012. In 2012, IAPT services were commissioned by 150 of the 151 Primary Health Care Trusts in England, and they estimate that 60% of the population has access to these services. In 2012 the IAPT programme treated two-thirds (9.7% out of 15%) of the 900,000 cases that it aims to treat every year, a contact coverage of 64.5% (20).

Equitable coverage: some services do not have representative access from their local communities with regard to age, ethnicity, and other factors, but the biggest gains in access and recovery have been among groups who are traditionally excluded from health care (20).

Effective coverage: of the people who use the service, 60% complete the course of treatment and 45% of these recover. This is comparable to a target recovery of 50% estimated from clinical trials of psychological therapies, and reflects the need for a downward adjustment for the difference between efficacy demonstrated in clinical trials and the effectiveness of the treatment delivered in routine care. The effective coverage of the IAPT programme is therefore 35% of the total population that the programme aims to serve.

Effect on patient outcomes: as outlined, in 2012, 45% of those who were adherent to the treatment recovered. In addition, 45,000 people treated by the IAPT programme have moved off sick pay and benefits.

Programme costs

The IAPT programme has been allocated a total of £397 million between 2008 and 2015, increasing the percentage of the total NHS adult mental health spend on psychological therapies from 3.2% to 6.6% (20). Cost-benefit modelling conducted before the IAPT programme was rolled out estimates that as the cost per patient treated was relatively small (£750), the cost to the government would be fully covered by the savings in incapacity benefits and extra taxes (18). These projections have not been tested by real programme data.

Cost of care

Economic information about programmes is essential for determining whether investing in a particular programme is a sound financial investment. Moreover, it enables comparisons among programmes to determine which programmes produce the best results at the lowest cost.

There are two domains within the assessment of cost of care which provide different types of economic information. The first is the absolute cost of delivering a programme, which is often presented as a cost per patient treated or a cost per treatment session. Such information is collected by adding up the financial and other inputs to the programme (e.g. salary costs, medication supply and distribution costs, training costs, cost of maintaining the physical space needed to house the programme, administration costs).

The second domain is the efficiency of the programme, defined as the system's optimal use of available resources to yield maximum benefits or results (23). Programme efficiency is calculated by comparing the costs of a programme with the benefits or outcomes of that programme, to determine the cost of producing a desired outcome.

A full economic evaluation is a specific type of analysis which is rarely possible for evaluations of scaled-up programmes, as it requires the comparison of the programme against an alternative (normally usual care) to determine whether one programme type is more cost-effective (produces better outcomes for cheaper) than another. A cost-outcome description, whereby the costs of the programme are compared to the outcomes achieved without reference to a comparison group, is often the most pragmatic way to assess the efficiency with which a programme achieves the desired outcomes. If similar programmes also conduct cost-outcome descriptions, then the comparative efficiency of different programmes can be compared.

Information on costs can be used to estimate the costs of scaling up the programme to cover a wider population. Affordability and cost are critical for setting budgets, estimating resource gaps, and mobilizing resources. In order to address the overall question of how much it will cost to scale up a mental health care programme, it is necessary to: (1) define the programme and how much it costs to deliver; (2) estimate current versus target levels of intervention need and coverage; and (3) calculate the year-on-year resource costs required over a specified investment period in order to reach the desired coverage.

As an example, if there is a 20% prevalence rate of hazardous alcohol use in a total population of 1 million persons, the total *population in need* of services is 200,000 individuals. All these individuals could benefit each year from a brief intervention in primary care that is currently delivered to only 10% of the population in need at, say, a cost of $1 per treated case to deliver. The *annual total cost* of the current coverage of the programme is therefore $20,000 (200,000 × $1 × 10%). This information can be used to estimate the cost of covering a larger population. For example, if the desired level of coverage is 50% of the target population, then the total *cost of target coverage* is five times greater at $100,000 (200,000 × $1 × 50%). The *incremental cost* is the difference between the current and target level of coverage ($100,000 − $20,000 = $80,000). The *cost per capita* is calculated by dividing the total cost by the total number of people in the population (annual cost per person would rise from $20,000/1,000,000 people = $0.02 to $100,000/1,000,000 people = $0.10, an increment of $0.08) (Chisholm, personal communication).

Evaluation methods

Useful guidance has been produced on the steps needed to design an evaluation of a health care programme (24). Box 16.1 outlines these stages.

As explored in the chapter on intervention development (Chapter 3), developing a programme-level ToC during the design of an intervention provides a useful framework for its formal evaluation. As ToC was originally developed to design and evaluate

---

Box 16.1 Steps to design a programme evaluation. (Adapted from 'Ten steps to systems thinking: applying a systems perspective in the design and evaluation of interventions' (24), p. 54)

1 Determine indicators: decide on indicators that are important to track in the redesigned intervention (e.g. input, process, output, and outcome indicators) across the affected sub-systems.

2 Choose methods: decide on evaluation methods to best measure the indicators and track changes over time.

3 Select the evaluation design: opt for the evaluation design that best manages the methods and fits the nature of the intervention.

4 Develop plan and timeline: collaborate with relevant stakeholders from different disciplines (e.g. clinical staff, policy makers, and researchers) to develop an evaluation plan and timeline.

5 Set a budget: determine the budget and scale by considering implications for both the intervention and the evaluation partnership.

6 Source funding: assemble funding to support the evaluation before the intervention begins.

Adapted from 'Ten steps to systems thinking: applying a systems perspective in the design and evaluation of interventions' (24), p. 54.

real-life programmes (25), its use as an evaluation framework to guide the evaluation of scaled-up mental health programmes is recommended. If a ToC has not already been developed for the programme, one may be retrospectively generated by programme staff and other key stakeholders and used as the framework for an evaluation plan. Box 16.2 provides an example of how ToC has been used as a framework for the evaluation of district-level mental health care plans (MHCPs) as part of the PRIME project.

Evaluations designs

The three core domains to include in evaluations of mental health programmes can be measured though a variety of evaluation designs. These range from analysis of data collected by programmes as part of their routine M&E procedures, to in-depth evaluations of the programme by independent evaluators. A range of different study designs can be employed to evaluate programmes, with the choice of method dependent upon the resources available for the evaluation and the strength of the conclusions needed to be drawn from the analysis. Potential methods include the analysis of routinely collected programme data, repeat surveys, observational cohorts of patients followed over time to assess changes in patient outcomes, and randomized evaluations comparing the programme to a control group of patients receiving either no service or an alternative service. Often a combination of methods is required, for example combining a patient cohort with process data derived from routinely collected programme data to determine the strength of programme implementation or the costs of delivering care.

Analysis of routinely collected programme data

The most common method to evaluate real-life programmes is for the programmes to routinely collect M&E data though health information systems (HIS). Monitoring refers to the continuous collection of programme inputs and outputs which are continuously monitored to make decisions about the management of a programme (e.g. to determine the exact case load and patient profile of a programme, and to determine current programme costs). Evaluation refers to the periodic analysis of data routinely collected in order to measure changes in programme delivery and coverage, including changes in patient outcomes. Such data can be used to review and strengthen programme delivery.

If a core set of HIS indicators are used across similar programmes, or across the same programme implemented in a number of different areas, these data can be aggregated to provide information about not only individual service providers and programme beneficiaries, but also the impact of the programme as a whole.

Such evaluations can be simple and cover a brief set of process indicators to measure access, such as number of people referred to the programme, number treated, and number discharged, broken down by diagnosis and key equity indicators such as gender and age. Equally, they can be more complex and cover the whole spectrum of the HCQI framework domains including access, quality of care, and cost. Such evaluations may include routine assessments of patient outcomes collected by administering outcome assessment tools to all patients at key follow-up times. These data are used to evaluate the effectiveness of the programme on patient outcomes and to track any possible safety issues. Case study 1 presents a description of the IAPT programme in England as an excellent example of how a programme can routinely evaluate all the domains of health care quality, access, and costs, resulting in valuable information for programme planners and policy makers.

The key feature of programme M&E is that data are routinely collected by the programme staff on all patients treated by the programme (as opposed to a sub-set for research purposes). Mechanisms for data collection are built into the routine functioning of the programme and form part of the programme staff's roles and responsibilities. As such, data can be collected at relatively low cost, and can be continually monitored and fed back to staff to enable continuous quality improvement. The IMPACT programme is a powerful example of how such systematic collection and analysis of programme data can be fed back to produce demonstrable improvements in service quality (26). In this programme for late-life depression in primary care in the US, a web-based data management system was used as a clinical management tool and also to continuously monitor the effectiveness of the programme. Subsequent iterations of this system, combined with Pay for Performance incentives tracked by the M&E system, have been shown to improve timely follow-up and shorten recovery time for people with depression (27). The key limitation of routine data collected by programmes is concerns over the reliability and validity of the data collected. For example, as the data are not collected by independent evaluators, there may be an incentive for programme staff to show that the programme is successful, leading to potential reporting bias.

Case study methodology

As noted in the Introduction, the 'real worlds' in which mental health programmes function are always messier than the contexts in which clinical trials are conducted. This is especially true of programmes in low-resource settings as a result of, for example: shortages of health workers with the skills to diagnose and manage mental, neurological, and substance abuse disorders; lack of adequate and reliable supplies of medication; and lack of financial resources to support the full range of evidence-based interventions. Assessing how and how well programmes function under such constraints is critical to efforts to initiate, develop, and expand mental health services in low-resources settings. However, it is unlikely that it will be possible to employ the methods because programmes in low-resource settings lack the health information systems that provide the routine process and outcomes data that are usually considered the essential foundations of M&E.

Conducting case studies—which can be defined as detailed narrative accounts of real-life events, people, or institutions—is one strategy for evaluating *in situ* mental health programmes in low-resource settings (28). Case studies are well suited for this task for two reasons. First, rather than trying to isolate and measure the extent to which a given intervention is effective in the treatment of a given disorder—as is done in RCTs—the case study methodology is used to examine and understand how programmes function and the results that are achieved amidst the 'messiness' of local worlds. Second, case studies rely on multiple sources of quantitative and qualitative evidence—interviews, participant-observation, document reviews, data extraction from programme records, and surveys—that allows one to examine the programme from different perspectives.

Thus, case studies produce detailed and comprehensive accounts of the effectiveness of programmes. In addition, case studies may highlight a programme's success in a particular area or bring attention to a particular challenge or difficulty.

The Case Studies Project at the London School of Hygiene and Tropical Medicine was established in 2008 to develop a methodology that would facilitate conducting case studies of functioning mental health programmes in LIC (29). The methodology was developed during a series of site visits to programmes in Nigeria, Ghana, India, East Timor, the Philippines, and South Africa. These experiences suggested that a number of domains were of particular importance when assessing programme effectiveness (see Box 16.1). Case study 2 presents the results from a case study evaluation of three mental health programmes in low-resource settings.

Case study 2: three models of community mental health services in LIC (29)

Description of programmes

The three programmes that were the subjects of this case study were:

- Services for People with Disabilities, Abuja, Federal Capital Territory, Nigeria: mental health services were one component of a community-based rehabilitation project that was co-funded by CBM International and the Archdiocese of Abuja.

- Holy Face Rehabilitation Center for Mental Health, Tabaco City, Albay Province, the Philippines: provided inpatient and outpatient care, as well as outreach and livelihood activities; co-funded by CBM International and the Brothers of Charity.

- Asia Psychosocial Rehabilitation Programme, Karakonam, Kerala, India: provided inpatient and outpatient treatments at a hospital, as well as community clinics and outreach. Funded by CBM International but salaries for staff are paid, in part, by the Dr Somervell Memorial CSI Medical College and Hospital.

Evaluation methodology

Following the case study methodology, site visits were made to each of the programmes. Site visit activities included accompanying staff in the field and on home visits, observing community clinics, visiting with self-help groups, and interviewing staff. Whenever possible, documentary evidence was utilized to confirm and/or augment the information collected during site visits. Narrative accounts of site visits, transcripts of interviews, and documentary evidence were analysed using qualitative data analysis software.

Results

Although all three programmes were established, either directly or indirectly, in response to the Indian Ocean tsunami, during the period 2004–2006, and were considered to be providing community mental health services, the case study revealed significant differences in: the service models utilized, diagnostic profiles of clients, strategies for recruitment and follow-up, initial and ongoing training activities, size of

Box 16.2 Domains of interest for case study methodology

Context

Domain 1—Environment in which the programme functions: physical, sociocultural, socioeconomic, and political environments

Domain 2—Health system in which the programme functions: present general and mental health services, as well as alternative sources of care, available in catchment area

History

Domain 3—History: 'when, where, why, what, who, and how' the programme was established

Programme model

Domain 4—Conceptual framework: orientation of services and attitudes about evidence-based practice and evaluation

Domain 5—Engagement with broader systems: work in the political and international spheres

Programme organization

Domain 6—Resources: human, transportation, funding, other

Domain 7—Management: organizational structure, finances, safety; plans for improvement and/or scaling up

Client populations

Domain 8—Client characteristics: diagnostic categories, sociodemographics, treatment coverage

Domain 9—Pathways to care: patterns of help-seeking, case-finding, referral networks

Interventions

Domain 10—Clinical interventions: diagnostic procedures, treatments offered, operational processes, protocols and guidelines, outcomes, methods of evaluation

Domain 11—Medications

(a) Domain 12—Psychosocial interventions: treatment, prevention and promotion, protocols and guidelines, outcomes, methods of evaluation

(b) Domain 12a—Self-help groups and livelihood programmes

(c) Domain 13—Accessibility of services: location, provision of transportation, affordable fees, service hours, in-home services

(d) Information system

(e) Domain 14—Information system: relative availability of statistics on number of active clients, and their clinical and social characteristics, use of services, and clinical and functional outcomes catchment areas, and the extent to which each programme was able to provide a range of interventions. At the same time, the programmes faced two common challenges: lack of sustainability without funding from CBM International and comparative lack of human resources. It was also found that all of the programmes were in need of information systems that could routinely generate basic sociodemographic, diagnostic, and clinical data about clients. A major strength of undertaking this case study methodology was demonstrating how using a defined set of narrative topics and programme-level indicators makes it possible to compare and contrast the relative strengths and weaknesses of programmes that utilize similar or different models of care.

Repeated surveys

Repeated cross-sectional surveys can be used instead of or in addition to programme M&E data to assess specific aspects of the programme such as coverage or detection rates. If the survey is repeated over time, then changes in these key indicators can be tracked. Such surveys can be conducted by the programme itself, by independent evaluators, or by utilizing data collected by external surveys conducted for other purposes. An example of this is the assessment of the coverage of the National Depression Detection and Treatment Programme in Chile, outlined in case study 3.

Case study 3: evaluation of the coverage of the Chilean National Depression Detection and Treatment Programme (30)

Evidence base

As discussed in Chapter 10, a series of trials in Chile have demonstrated the effectiveness and cost-effectiveness of a collaborative stepped-care programme in primary care to treat depression (31). These results, supplemented with evidence from subsequent clinical trials (32–34), were then used to scale up a treatment for depression nationally (35).

Programme description

The National Depression Detection and Treatment Programme was launched in 2003 with a network of more than 500 primary care centres across Chile to provide universal access to treatment for depression. Each primary health centre has a general clinical team composed of primary care doctors, nurses, and auxiliary nurses delivering the programme. The programme offers improved case identification, timely and adequate treatment, and closely monitored follow-up for all enrolled cases.

Evaluation methodology

The evaluation compared independently collected, national-level, cross-sectional community survey data obtained before the programme was implemented in 2003 and again post-implementation in 2009–10. The national survey measured the population prevalence of depression (denominator of population in need) and the proportion of those with depression who had accessed services (numerator of those in contact with the service). As the national programme was the only service providing treatment for depression in primary care, positive responses to whether patients had seen a doctor in connection with a depressive episode in the past 12 months were taken as the numerator of service utilization for contact coverage. The study therefore estimated the increase in coverage that happened after the national programme was introduced, which may have been due to factors other than the programme itself.

Results

Contact coverage: the likelihood a depressed individual has access to treatment for depression increased significantly after the programme was introduced (OR 1.87; 95% CI 1.21–2.90).

Equitable coverage: depressed women (41.6% (33.0–50.2) vs 66.3% (58.9–73.7); $p < 0.0001$) and those with less education (40.3% (30.0–50.7) vs 66.5% (55.8–77.3); $p = 0.001$) were the primary beneficiaries of the introduction of this universal programme for depression.

Specific aspects of programmes, for example whether they increase contact coverage or improve rates of detection, correct diagnosis and initiation of evidence-based treatment over time, are also usefully evaluated through repeat cross-sectional surveys. Such surveys are likely to be undertaken as an independent research exercise, as the time and resource demands of such surveys may constrain programmes from conducting these evaluations without additional resources. The suite of methods used by the Programme for Improving Mental Health Care (PRIME) to evaluate district-level MHCPs in five LAMIC provide good examples of such repeat surveys, in the form of pre- and post-programme implementation community surveys to measure coverage, and repeat cross-sectional Facility Detection Surveys to assess changes in adequate diagnosis and initiation of appropriate initiation of evidence-based treatment over time (case study 4).

Cohort studies

Cohort studies are the most powerful methodology for tracking changes in patient outcomes over time when a comparison group is not feasible, as in most programme evaluations. Though analysis of M&E data collected from the same patients at repeated time points (as in the IAPT programme in case study 1) is also a cohort study, conducting a more detailed study on a sub-group of patients who receive treatment from a service produces a much more detailed set of data which can be used to answer a range of different research questions in addition to the impact on patient outcomes. The disease-specific cohorts which are part of the PRIME suite of evaluation methods are an excellent example of this methodology (case study 4).

The ASHAGRAM cohort study is a further excellent example. This cohort described the scaling up and impact of a community-based rehabilitation programme for people with psychotic disorders in a very low-resource setting in India (36). They followed up 256 people with psychotic disorders who had been ill for on average 8 years, for a median follow-up time of 46 months. The cohort demonstrated significant reductions in disability over time. It also provided valuable information on the predictors of good outcomes which included family engagement with the programme, medication adherence, and being a member of a self-help group. Such information can be used to refine the delivery of the programme to enhance its effectiveness, e.g. by more actively engaging with family members, and setting up self-help groups as part of the programme (36).

Case study 4: the PRIME evaluation of district-level MHCPs in five LAMIC

Background

As demonstrated by some of the case studies of RCTs in this book, there is an emerging evidence base from RCTs for cost-effective interventions to treat mental disorders in LAMIC. This evidence has been summarized into treatment guidelines for non-specialist health workers in primary care by the mhGAP project (37). However, very little is known about how to practically implement these guidelines as treatment programmes in routine care settings such as primary care and maternal health clinics.

The aim of the PRIME consortium is to generate evidence on the implementation and scaling up of integrated packages of care for priority mental disorders (depression, AUD, and psychosis) in primary and maternal health care contexts in Ethiopia, India, Nepal, South Africa, and Uganda (38). PRIME is working initially in one district or sub-district in each country. The project is developing and evaluating district-level MHCPs which integrate mental health into primary care at three levels of the health system: the health care organization, the health facility, and the community.

Overview of the evaluation

PRIME is using the MRC framework for complex interventions (39) combined with ToC to provide a robust evaluation framework for the project to measure common themes across countries and to ensure that both process and outcome evaluations are conducted. The overall research questions to be answered in the evaluation are to assess the implementation, coverage, detection rates, and effect on patient outcomes of the MHCPs.

A suite of four study designs have been developed to answer the cross-country research questions. The study designs, and the primary research question they seek to answer, are listed below.

Community survey

Primary research question: what is the coverage of treatment for any current episode of depression or AUD among adults living in the implementation district?

Methods: repeat cross-sectional population-based community surveys conducted before the MHCPs are implemented, repeated 2 years after, to assess changes in the treatment gap for depression and AUD. Treatment coverage was considered adequate for those who screen positive if they have seen a clinician with regard to the relevant symptoms, and have been provided with an adequate dose of appropriate medication and/or counselling.

Facility Detection Survey

Primary research question: what is the initiation of evidence-based care, including detection for those with depression and/or AUD?

Methods: repeat cross-sectional surveys conducted in primary health care facilities before the MHCPs are implemented and at regular intervals after it has been implemented to track changes in detection of depression and AUD over time. Information on diagnoses, treatments prescribed, and referrals from the clinical consultation is collected for all patients who screen positive, along with 10% of those who screen negative. The interim results will also be reported back to the clinicians to help them improve their detection and treatment strategies.

Cohort studies

Primary research question: what are the clinical, social, and economic effects of the MHCP on patients diagnosed with depression, AUD, and psychosis?

Methods: separate cohorts of patients with depression, AUD, and psychosis who have been diagnosed by clinicians in the implementation areas are followed up for 9–12 months to assess changes in patient clinical, social, and economic outcomes. A wide range of information from interviews with patients and caregivers of patients with psychosis at repeated time points enables a detailed analysis of the baseline moderators that affect programme effectiveness for individual patients (e.g. severity of symptoms, socioeconomic status, and gender) and the mediators that affect outcomes (e.g. which interventions were received and how adherent patients were to them). In-depth qualitative interviews are conducted with patients and their caregivers to assess the acceptability of the care provided, barriers to adhering to treatment, and their experience of stigma and discrimination.

Case studies

Primary research questions: how well are different aspects of the MHCP implemented, how much do they cost to implement, and how is the impact of each MHCP affected by their interaction with the districts' political, cultural, and social contexts?

Methods: a set of studies answering specific research questions related to the process of implementing the MHCPs. Community-, facility-, and district-level profiles measure process indicators to assess how well the MHCPs are implemented at each level of the health system, and how much the implementation costs. This includes the extent of engagement of district authorities with the MHCP, the adequacy of the psychotropic drug supply, and qualitative interviews with service delivery and district-level planners to explore the acceptability and feasibility of the MHCPs and barriers to their implementation. The district profile also includes an assessment of the broader social, political, economic, and cultural factors that may affect the effectiveness of the MHCP in each district. A separate study assesses the quality and fidelity of the training and supervision delivered as part of the MHCPs.

Challenges to evaluation

There are a number of challenges to conducting such a complex evaluation. Critical among these is the Hawthorn effect whereby the research evaluation becomes an intervention in its own right and may therefore alter the effect of the programme. For example, knowing that the content of patient sessions is being recorded in the Facility Detection Survey may directly affect the behaviour of clinicians, leading them to improve their diagnostic skills through a heightened awareness of mental health. In addition, the evaluation methods are complex, multilevel, and multidisciplinary. This creates challenges, including the overburdening of participants and staff at the health facilities, building clinical and research capacity in each site to deliver and evaluate the MHCPs, and measurement challenges involved with the selection of locally valid tools to assess adults for the presence of mental disorders—by both clinicians and researchers—in diverse cultural contexts.

Randomized designs

As emphasized throughout this book, RCTs of various designs are the only way in which the effect of an intervention (or in this case a programme) can be definitively determined. If the political will power and financial resources are available, and it is ethically and conceptually appropriate to randomize, it is possible to conduct a randomized evaluation of a real-world programme. However, largely due to these constraints, examples of such evaluations are rare.

One of the most feasible designs is randomizing patients to be referred to the new service or to an existing one with represents a treatment as usual control arm. A good example of such a trial is the Lambeth Early Onset (LEO) early intervention for psychosis programme in London, UK. All people referred to specialist mental health services with newly diagnosed psychosis were randomized to receive either community-based services from the LEO programme or treatment from standard services (40). Patient outcomes and costs were compared between the LEO group and standard care, and demonstrated that the early-intervention LEO service was cost-effective compared to standard care (40).

An alternative way in which randomization can be introduced into programme evaluation once a new programme has been approved is to randomize the roll-out of the programme into new clinics or populations, in a stepped wedge design. Clusters that have not yet set up the programme contribute data to the control arm of the trial, then move to contribute data to the intervention arm as soon as the programme has been implemented in that cluster. The order in which the programme will be rolled out into the clinics and communities is ascertained randomly.

Though randomized evaluations of real-life programmes can provide definitive evidence of a programme's impact, it must be noted that if the intervention has been adequately tested in a pragmatic RCT before being scaled up, continued intensive evaluation of its effectiveness may not be warranted. Indeed, there are many situations in which a non-randomized evaluation of a scaled-up programme using the methods outlined in this chapter are in fact the most appropriate methodology. Non-randomized evaluations are particularly convincing if the confounders are well understood and measured, and the causal pathways through which the intervention has its effect are well understood and measured (e.g. by using ToC), where the expected effect of the programme is large or where the evidence suggests that there is little chance of harm (41).

Conclusion

The 'messiness' of the real world in which mental health programmes are implemented and the resulting reduced impact they have compared to the results observed in RCTs, means that it is essential that we continue to evaluate the impact that programmes have after they are implemented. Three core dimensions of a health care programme should be evaluated: quality of care in terms of the impact on patient outcomes, how accessible the care is, and the cost of providing the care. These domains can be measured using a range of different evaluation methodologies, including routine programme monitoring and evaluation, a detailed case study of the programme, collating information from a range of different sources, surveys, and cohorts of patients tracked through care, and RCTs. The choice of method will be dependent upon the resources available, the purpose of the evaluation, the setting in which the programme is implemented, and political, ethical, or other constraints. Often, a combination of methods is most appropriate.

There is a huge lack of evaluation of mental health programmes globally. In a systematic review of evaluations of mental health programmes, we found only a hundred or so evaluations of any scaled-up mental health programme globally, only a handful of which were from low-resource settings (9). Without clear evidence as to which programmes provide equitable access to services, and prove the most cost-effective at improving patient outcomes, the policy imperative to scale up mental health services will remain weak, and the treatment gap will remain unacceptably large.

References

1 Kelley E, Hurst J (2006) Health care quality indicators project: conceptual framework paper. Paris: OCED.

2 Donabedian A (2003) An introduction to quality assurance in health care. Oxford: Oxford University Press.

3 Institute of Medicine (2001) Crossing the quality chasm: a new health system for the 21st century. Washington, DC: National Academy Press.

4 Tanahashi T (1978) Health service coverage and its evaluation. Bull World Health Organ, **56**(2):295–303.

5 Marchant T, Schellenberg D, Nathan R, Armstrong-Schellenberg J, Mponda H, Jones C, et al. (2010) Assessment of a national voucher scheme to deliver insecticide-treated mosquito nets to pregnant women. Can Med Assoc J, **182**(2):152–6.

6 Hetzel MW, Obrist B, Lengeler C, Msechu JJ, Nathan R, Dillip A, et al. (2008) Obstacles to prompt and effective malaria treatment lead to low community-coverage in two rural districts of Tanzania. BMC Public Health, **8**:317.

7 World Health Organization (2011) Mental health atlas. Geneva: WHO.

8 World Health Organization (2009) Mental health systems in selected low- and middle-income countries: a WHO-AIMS cross-national analysis. Geneva: WHO.

9 De Silva M, Lee L, Fuhr D, Rathod S, Chisholm D, Schellenberg J, et al. (2014) Estimating the coverage of mental health programmes: a systematic review. International Journal of Epidemiology. In press.

10 Rotondi NK, Rush B (2012) Monitoring utilization of a large scale addiction treatment system: the Drug and Alcohol Treatment Information System (DATIS). Subst Abuse, 6:73–84.

11 Shengelia B, Tandon A, Adams OB, Murray CJ (2005) Access, utilization, quality, and effective coverage: an integrated conceptual framework and measurement strategy. Soc Sci Med, 61(1):97–109.

12 Lozano R (2006) Benchmarking of performance of Mexican states with effective coverage. Lancet, 368:1729–41.

13 Jenkins R (1997) The National Psychiatric Morbidity Surveys of Great Britain—strategy and methods. Psychol Med, 27:765–74.

14 Parslow RA Jorm AF (2000) Who uses mental health services in Australia? An analysis of data from the National Survey of Mental Health and Wellbeing. Austr N Z J Psychiatry, 34(997–1008).

15 Wang PS, Aguilar-Gaxiola S, Alonso J, Angermeyer MC, Borges G, Bromet EJ, et al. (2007) Use of mental health services for anxiety, mood, and substance disorders in 17 countries in the WHO world mental health surveys. Lancet, 370(9590):841–50.

16 Wang H, Dwyer-Lindgren L, Lofgren KT, Rajaratnam JK, Marcus JR, Levin-Rector A, et al. (2012) Age-specific and sex-specific mortality in 187 countries, 1970–2010: a systematic analysis for the Global Burden of Disease Study 2010. Lancet, 380(9859):2071–94.

17 Baxter A, Patton G, Scott K, Degenhardt L, Whiteford H (2013) Global epidemiology of mental disorders: what are we missing? PLoS One, 8(6):e65514.

18 Layard R, Clark D, Knapp M, Mayraz G (2007) Cost-benefit analysis of psychological therapy. Natl Inst Econ Rev, 202(1):90–8.

19 Clark D (2011) Implementing NICE guidelines for the psychological treatment of depression and anxiety disorders: the IAPT experience. Int Rev Psychiatry, 23(4):318–27.

20 Department of Health (2012) IAPT three-year report: the first million patients. London: Department of Health.

21 Kroenke K, Spitzer RL, Williams JB (2001) The PHQ-9: validity of a brief depression severity measure. J Gen Intern Med, 16(9):606–13.

22 Löwe B, Decker O, Müller S, Brähler E, Schellberg D, Herzog W, et al. (2008) Validation and standardization of the Generalized Anxiety Disorder Screener (GAD-7) in the general population. Med Care, 46(3):266–74.

23 Joint Commission on Accreditation of Healthcare Organizations (1997) National Library of Healthcare Indicators. Health plan and network edition. Oakbrook Terrace, IL:The Joint Commission.

24 de Savigny D, Adam A (eds) (2009) Systems thinking for health systems strengthening. Geneva: WHO.

25 Anderson A (2005) The community builder's approach to Theory of Change. A practical guide to theory development. Washington, DC: The Aspen Institute.

26 Unützer J, Choi Y, Cook IA, Oishi S (2002) A web-based data management system to improve care for depression in a multicenter clinical trial. Psychiatr Serv, 53(6):671–3, 678.

27 Unützer J, Chan YF, Hafer E, Knaster J, Shields A, Powers D, et al. (2012) Quality improvement with pay-for-performance incentives in integrated behavioral health care. Am J Public Health, 102(6):e41–5.

28 Cohen A, Eaton J, Radtke B, de Menil V, Chatterjee S, De Silva M, et al. (2012) Case study methodology to monitor & evaluate community mental health programs in low-income countries. Bensheim: CBM International.

29 Cohen A, Eaton J, Radtke B, George C, Manuel BV, De Silva M, et al. (2011) Three models of community mental health services In low-income countries. Int J Ment Health Syst, 5(1):3.

30 Araya R, Pedro Z (2014) The impact of universal health programmes in improving access to health care for depression and other chronic diseases in Chile. Under review.

31 Araya R, Rojas G, Fritsch R, Gaete J, Rojas M, Simon G, et al. (2003) Treating depression in primary care in low-income women in Santiago, Chile: a randomised controlled trial. Lancet, 61(9363):995–1000.

32 Fritsch R, Araya R, Solis J, Montt E, Pilowsky D, Rojas G (2007) A randomized trial of pharmacotherapy with telephone monitoring to improve treatment of depression in primary care in Santiago, Chile (in Spanish). Rev Med Chile, 135(5):587–95.

33 Rojas G, Fritsch R, Solis J, Jadresic E, Castillo C, Gonzalez M, et al. (2007) Treatment of postnatal depression in low-income mothers in primary-care clinics in Santiago, Chile: a randomised controlled trial. Lancet, 370(9599):1629–37.

34 Araya R, Flynn T, Rojas G, Fritsch R, Simon G (2006) Cost-effectiveness of a primary care treatment program for depression in low-income women in Santiago, Chile. Am J Psychiatry, 163(8):1379–87.

35 Araya R, Alvarado R, Sepúlveda R, Rojas G (2012) Lessons from scaling up a depression treatment program in primary care in Chile. Rev Panam Salud Publica, 32(3):234–40.

36 Chatterjee S, Pillai A, Jain S, Cohen A, Patel V (2009) Outcomes of people with psychotic disorders in a community-based rehabilitation programme in rural India. British J Psychiatry, 195(5): 433–9.

37 World Health Organization (2008) mhGAP: Mental Health Gap Action Programme: scaling up care for mental, neurological and substance use disorders. Geneva: WHO.

38 Lund C, Tomlinson M, De Silva MJ, Fekadu A, Shidhaye R, Jordans M (2012) PRIME: a programme to reduce the treatment gap for mental disorders in five low- and middle-income countries. PLoS Med, 9(12).

39 Craig P, Dieppe P, Macintyre S, Nazareth I, Petticrew I (2008) Developing and evaluating complex interventions: the new Medical Research Council guidance. BMJ, 337:a1655.

40 McCrone P, Craig T, Power P, Garety P (2010) Cost-effectiveness of an early intervention service for people with psychosis. Br J Psychiatry, 196(5):377–82.

41 Bonell C, Hargreaves J, Cousens S, Ross D, Hayes R, Petticrew M, et al. (2011) Alternatives to randomisation in the evaluation of public health interventions: design challenges and solutions. J Epidemiol Community Health, 65(7):582–7.

Index